Mosquito Trails

Mosquito Trails

ECOLOGY, HEALTH, AND THE POLITICS
OF ENTANGLEMENT

Alex M. Nading

UNIVERSITY OF CALIFORNIA PRESS

University of California Press, one of the most distinguished university presses in the United States, enriches lives around the world by advancing scholarship in the humanities, social sciences, and natural sciences. Its activities are supported by the UC Press Foundation and by philanthropic contributions from individuals and institutions. For more information, visit www.ucpress.edu.

University of California Press
Oakland, California

Library of Congress Cataloging-in-Publication Data

Nading, Alexander M., III, 1979– author.
    Mosquito trails : ecology, health, and the politics of entanglement / Alex M. Nading.
        p. ; cm.
    Includes bibliographical references and index.
    ISBN 978-0-520-28261-2 (cloth : alk. paper)
    ISBN 978-0-520-28262-9 (pbk. : alk. paper)
    I. Title.
    [DNLM: 1. Dengue—Nicaragua—Personal Narratives.   2. Environmental Health—Nicaragua—Personal Narratives.   3. Health Knowledge, Attitudes, Practice—Nicaragua—Personal Narratives.   4. Politics—Nicaragua— Personal Narratives. WC 528]
    RA644.D4
    614.5′8852097285—dc23   2014008933

Manufactured in the United States of America

23 22 21 20 19 18 17 16 15 14
10 9 8 7 6 5 4 3 2 1

The paper used in this publication meets the minimum requirements of ANSI/ NISO Z39.48-1992 (R 2002) (Permanence of Paper).

CONTENTS

ILLUSTRATIONS

ACKNOWLEDGMENTS

I want to begin with a quick note about anonymity and its absence. I have obscured the names and in some cases the identities of most of the Nicaraguans who consented to let me walk, ride, talk, and learn alongside them. There are a few people, however, whose help was too valuable not to receive mention. I am forever grateful to Gertrudis Zepeda, Maria de Jesus Zepeda, and Rene Gutierrez. *Gracias* does not begin to cut it when it comes to Haydée Abarca and Marvin José Angulo Sosa (QEPD)—you were so much more than research assistants; you were close friends, sounding boards, and inspirations. Kamila Arias and Aura Lila Vargas taught me the value of humor in the face of absurdity. I am also indebted to the staff and directors (too many to mention) of the Hospital Nilda Patricia Velasco de Zedillo and the Alcaldía de Ciudad Sandino who supported this project. Finally, to Rafael Morales and the extended Morales/Vargas family, thanks for welcoming me to Nicaragua both during my fieldwork and, in a way, many years before. I should note that I have *not* chosen to create a pseudonym for one of the main subjects of this book, Ciudad Sandino. Trying to obscure the identity of so large a place seems counterproductive.

Like any worthwhile exercise, the making of this book has been a transformational experience. I did not intend to write a book that focused so intently on interspecies relations and their implications for health, even if I did think (vaguely) that I would study how people in urban Nicaragua came to understand dengue through their engagement with the urban environment. It was not until midway through my fieldwork that I came to realize how profoundly human social relations in Nicaragua and elsewhere are mediated by nonhuman beings. (Bad anthropologist! This should have been obvious.)

This brings me to my next, rather awkward, thank-you. It goes to Floyd, the cat that ended up being my field companion, messmate, antagonist, and friend over sixteen months in the field and for many years after. I adopted Floyd (who is female—long story) in a moment of fieldwork-induced loneliness and vulnerability. To say that she is difficult to love is putting it mildly. Floyd has a cerebral dysfunction that makes her behavior erratic and quite violent—I have the scars to prove it. Her head persistently tilts to one side, and one eye constantly drips dark-colored cat tears. She is also perhaps the least intelligent and coordinated cat alive today. She routinely falls off of countertops and chairs. Floyd has, in the six years of her life, been mauled by a dog (and saved by a Nicaraguan veterinarian's medicine—or by a charismatic preacher's laying on of hands, depending on who you ask), ingested bleach, taken Prozac, and been hit by a car. Her behavior and life have been steeped in violence, negativity, and quite a bit of misery. In this, she is not unlike a mosquito.

But trying desperately to keep Floyd alive amid her travails, and what seemed at times like fate itself, ended up bringing me into the lives of Nicaraguan neighbors and health care workers, and into Ciudad Sandino's wider landscape. In retrospect, I do not think I would have been a successful fieldworker had I not become attached to this shrieking, antagonistic, partially blind, five-pound monster. She brought out my emotions. She forced me to shed my know-it-all defenses. She improved my Spanish. She helped me test anthropological theories about human-animal relations. Floyd, my animal companion and mascot, though you cannot ever understand me, I thank you.

Back to human and institutional acknowledgments. At various stages between 2006 and 2013, research and writing for this book were supported by a Fulbright-Hays Doctoral Dissertation Research Abroad Award; an International Dissertation Research Fellowship from the Social Science Research Council, funded by the Andrew W. Mellon Foundation; National Science Foundation Doctoral Dissertation Improvement Grant 0849650; and several centers within the University of Wisconsin–Madison, including the Graduate Student Collaborative; Transdisciplinary Studies in Health and Society Working Group; Latin American, Caribbean, and Iberian Studies Center; Global Studies Center; Center for World Affairs and Global Economy; and Center for Culture, History, and Environment. Franklin and Marshall College provided funds for research, writing, and travel in the latter stages of research. The final months of writing were supported by a Hunt Postdoctoral Fellowship from the Wenner-Gren Foundation for Anthropological Research and a Fernand Braudel fellowship from the Fondation des Sciences de L'Homme and the European Commission. During brief research trips to the Centers for Disease Control and Prevention (CDC) Dengue Branch in Puerto Rico, I was generously hosted by Dr. Kay Tomashek and Dr. Carmen Perez. At the CDC in Atlanta, Mary Hilfertshauser, Randall Neilson, and Dan Rutz made my weeks of archival research pleasant and productive.

I began research for this book as a doctoral student in the Department of Anthropology at the University of Wisconsin–Madison. My adviser, Sharon Hutchinson, was everything a student like me needed: no-nonsense, sensitive, and unwavering in her ethical and scholarly standards. At every stage of my academic career, I have been confident that if I could convince Sharon about something, I was probably on the right track. Special thanks are due also to Claire Wendland, who arrived at the University of Wisconsin–Madison during my second year and was a de facto "second adviser" from the moment she moved into her first office in the human osteology lab. Claire introduced me to medical anthropology, held nearly weekly advising-cum-therapy sessions during the writing up of my research, and remains a go-to source for advice and counsel. I am honored to call her a mentor and friend. I met Paul Nadasdy as a prospective graduate student, and I am grateful for his continued support and mentorship. Linda Hogle's kind interest and support have been extremely valuable over the years. Special thanks are also due to Maria Lepowsky and Christina Ewig, as well as to anthropology department members past and present, including Katherine Bowie, Kenneth George, Anatoly Khazanov, Kirin Narayan, Larry Nesper, and the late Neil Whitehead. Thanks also to Peg Erdman, Maggie Brandenburg, and Jan Holmes. My former University of Wisconsin graduate student colleagues continue to be among my closest friends and intellectual interlocutors. Thanks to Chris Butler, Tony Chapa, Jim Hoesterey, Aaron Perkins, Natalie Porter, Erika Robb-Larkins, Susan Rottmann, and Noah Theriault.

Outside the University of Wisconsin anthropology world, I was fortunate to find a vibrant community of scholars interested in health, the environment, and science, particularly in the university's Center for Culture, History, and Environment and the Department of Geography. A humble thanks, for her years of support and friendship, goes to Abigail Neely, who has been a reader, critic, and now coauthor. Thanks also to Mitch Aso and Andrew Case, whose comments and support were crucial on the homestretch of dissertation writing. I would be remiss if I did not make special mention of Denise Wiyaka, or of Jamie Saul and Alex Delucenay, without whom I would never have made it through many things—graduate school is just one.

As a faculty member, I have benefited from the support and stimulation of the Department of Anthropology at Franklin and Marshall College. My thanks to the students in my courses who acted as sounding boards for many of the ideas herein. I am also grateful to my department colleagues, past and present, including Tania Ahmad, Misty Bastian, Michael Billig, Tate LeFevre, Mary Ann Levine, Sonja Schwake, James Slotta, Scott Smith, and Jim Taggart. At Franklin and Marshall, I have benefited from the support and advice of Doug Anthony, Dick Fluck, Jerome Hodos, Cynthia Krom, Stephanie McNulty, Gayatri Menon, Maria Mitchell, Judith Mueller, Nola Semczyszyn, Tim Sipe, Pam Snelson, Lisa Stilwell, and Jim Strick. Thanks also to Maribel Perez, Roberta Strickler, and—last but certainly not least—the indefatigable Kathy Clark.

In 2013–14, I was honored with an invitation to write and research at the Maison des Sciences de L'Homme in Paris, France. Nathanaël Cretin, Gilles Desfeux, Dana Dimenescu, Benedicte Rastier, and Nathalie Schnur gave me a warm welcome and technical, practical, and linguistic support. It has been a pleasure to work and think with Chun-Yi Chang, Sara Guindani-Riquier, Brian Milstein, Ben Nienass, Ingrid Noguera, and Sabine Selchow. There is no way of expressing my full appreciation to Frédéric Keck and Vinh-Kim Nguyen, who offered me the chance to come to Paris. Their intellectual and personal generosity is a major reason that this book found its way to completion.

Over the years, a number of other people have contributed to this work with advice, comments, or personal and emotional support. I presented versions of this book as papers at several conferences and workshops, and a version of chapter 4 is reprinted with the permission of *Cultural Anthropology*, where it appeared under the title "Dengue Mosquitoes Are Single Mothers: Biopolitics Meets Ecological Aesthetics in Nicaraguan Community Health Work."

For more provocations, conversations, contributions, and general encouragement, I want to thank Nikhil Anand, Hannah Appel, Ira Bashkow, Crystal Biruk, Dominic Boyer, Ashley Carse, Eric Carter, Mike Cepek, Fred Damon, Eve Danziger, Geert de Neve, Joe Dumit, James Faubion, Josh Fisher, Jill Fleuriet, Gertrude Fraser, Chris Garces, Katy Gardner, Jeremy Greene, Sherrine Hamdy, Tracey Heatherington, Chris Hewlett, Linda Hogle, Cymene Howe, Ali Kenner, Alan Klima, Andrew Lakoff, Julie Livingston, Rob Lorway, Theresa MacPhail, Ramah McKay, Susan McKinnon, George Mentore, Colin Milburn, Don Mitchell, Gregg Mitman, Sarah Moore, Eileen Moyer, Viranjani Munasinghe, Lisa Onaga, Jonathan Patz, Eric Plemons, Peter Redfield, Dan Reichman, Paul Robbins, Elizabeth Roberts, Elsa Rodeck, Dennis Rodgers, Robert Samet, Harris Solomon, Noelle Sullivan, Catherine Trundle, Sjaak Van der Geest, Marina Welker, Kath Weston, Matt Whiffen, and Austin Zeiderman.

At the University of California Press, I have been bowled over by the careful editorial attention that Stacy Eisenstark has given to this project. I am also grateful for the work of Reed Malcolm, Kate Warne, and the editorial staff at the press, as well as Debbie Masi and Trish Watson. Eric Carter, Sean Brotherton, and the anonymous reviewers have made this work stronger and provided me with a wealth of thoughtful, critical commentary. All errors, of course, remain my own.

There is no substitute for a family that believes in what you do, even when they may not fully understand it. Thanks to my parents and to the extended Beskys, Bonkowskis, Bromstads, and Nadings, as well as to Kitty and Sidney. Above all, my love and gratitude go to Sarah, whose sacrifice, support, and affection—even for Floyd, though she may deny it—are infused in these pages.

ASORENIC	Asociación de Recicladores de Nicaragua (Association of Recyclers of Nicaragua)
CDC	Centers for Disease Control and Prevention, formerly Communicable Disease Center, U.S. Department of Health and Human Services
CDS	Committees for the Defense of Sandinismo
CIA	Central Intelligence Agency (U.S.)
CIET	Community Information and Epidemiological Technologies International
CNDR	Centro Nacional de Diagnóstico y Referencia (National Diagnostic and Reference Center [Nicaragua])
COMBI	Communication for Behavioral Impact, a community-based health strategy devised by the WHO
CPC	Consejos del Poder Ciudadano (Councils of Citizen Power), FSLN-affiliated community action groups
FSLN	Frente Sandinista de Liberación Nacional (Sandinista National Liberation Front)
MCN	Movimientos Comunales de Nicaragua (Nicaraguan Community Movements),

	the nongovernmental community action organization formed after the 1990 electoral defeat of Nicaragua's Sandinista government
MINSA	Ministerio de Salud (Ministry of Health), Nicaragua
OPEN	Organismo Permanente de Emergencia Nacional (Permanent National Emergency Agency)
PAHO	Pan American Health Organization
PROMAPER	Proyecto Integrado Managua Periferia (Integrated Project for Peripheral Managua)
SEPA	Socializing Evidence for Participatory Action, a community-based method for dengue surveillance, elaborated by CIET
SILAIS	Sistema Integral de Atención en Salud (Local Health System)
WHO	World Health Organization

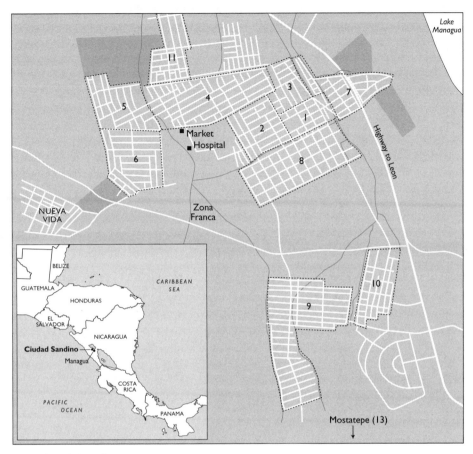

Map of Ciudad Sandino

Introduction

DENGUE IN THE LANDSCAPE

FATIMA'S SYMPTOMS—soreness and coughing—appeared on a Monday. Her parents initially thought she had a throat infection, but by Wednesday, her fever and joint and muscle aches had gotten worse, and she had developed a faint skin rash. On Saturday, she was bleeding through her nose. Fatima was admitted to a private hospital, where she remained for three days and nights. On Tuesday, she was back at home, in her family's small house in Ciudad Sandino, Nicaragua. Her fever was finally abating, but her body aches, rash, and nosebleeds indicated that she had contracted dengue fever. The Nicaraguan Ministry of Health (Ministerio de Salud, henceforth MINSA) received word of Fatima's case indirectly. Her family's neighbors informed a team of community health workers, who were carrying out a house-to-house antidengue campaign in the area. As part of the response, I accompanied a MINSA nurse to Fatima's home, where we asked her mother and grandmother to help speculate on how she might have contracted dengue.

Fatima's house was typical of Ciudad Sandino. Almost all the homes in the city occupy ten- by thirty-meter lots. Ciudad Sandino is located just north of Managua, Nicaragua's capital, on the flat plain between Lake Managua and the ridge that divides the rest of the country from the Pacific Ocean. It is home to more than 100,000 people, but, to the untrained eye looking down from the ridge, it does not look particularly "urban." There are no large buildings. Automobile and bus traffic is steady but not overwhelming. Trees are everywhere. They look green and healthy, especially at this time of year, December, when moisture from the rainy season remains heavy in the soil and air. December is a time of relative comfort. Temperatures remain low—peaking above eighty degrees Fahrenheit—until the end of January. Then the winds die and the sun heats up, leading to the *temporada polvada,* the hot, dusty dry season in February, March, and April, when thermometers routinely break 100.

At the bottom of the ridge in Fatima's neighborhood, many of the trees bear fruits, including mangoes, avocadoes, oranges, and limes. Cattle and horses walk up and down the streets, sometimes tethered to human minders, sometimes alone. Amid the swirls of dust that rise from the alleys, dogs hungry for scraps of food forage in gutters and tear open forgotten garbage bags. The claws of cats tingle over the galvanized roofs, which, even in the cooler months, visibly radiate heat conducted by the persistent sunlight. Snakes, mice, rats, and insects—including several species of mosquito—are all in abundance. As a thickly inhabited space, Ciudad Sandino is far from unique. Like all urban spaces, this one is thoroughly natural.

It is also thoroughly social.[1] City planners have parceled Ciudad Sandino's uniform, three-hundred-square-meter house lots into fourteen neighborhoods, known as *zonas*. The zonas all have names, usually those of heroes from Nicaraguan history or the 1979 Sandinista Revolution, in which a coalition of leftist groups toppled a dictatorship that had ruled the country for half a century. Officially, Fatima's zona was called Maura Clarke, after a Catholic nun of the Maryknoll order who came to the city in the 1970s to work as a teacher and community organizer in solidarity with the Sandinistas. In 1980, Clarke was brutally murdered along with three other missionaries with whom she had traveled to provide aid to victims of violence stemming from the civil war in neighboring El Salvador. Many knew the stories of Maura Clarke and other Sandinista "martyrs," but the MINSA nurse, Fatima's family, and nearly everyone else avoided using honorific titles for Ciudad Sandino's zonas. For them, Fatima's house was simply in *zona cinco* (zone 5).

A concrete wall, about eight feet high, surrounded the house. On the street side, Fatima's grandfather had installed a metal gate, painted in a fading green and wide enough to accommodate a car or light truck. The house, too, was constructed of concrete and was painted yellow. It sat back twenty or thirty feet from the gate. Between the house and gate was a patio, paved or tiled in most places, where Fatima's mother and grandmother potted tropical plants and flowers, and where a few faded pink and blue plastic toys lay strewn around. From this patio, I could see through the dimly lit, one-story house, and I could make out the family washbasin and toilet in the smaller open patio to the rear. The doors, ajar, were of heavy wood. The house's only two windows, glassless and screenless, were covered by thick steel bars, painted black.

So who might have brought dengue into Fatima's home? Her father worked as a laborer in a hospital in Managua that had also handled several dengue cases, but he had never had dengue. The adults of the house claimed that no one else in the family had either. As the MINSA nurse, doña Feliciana, discussed the case with the family, she raised the issue of mosquitoes, reminding Fatima's mother and grandmother that they must keep their patio free of standing water. *Aedes aegypti,* the mosquito that transmits the dengue virus to humans, lays its eggs in pools of stagnant water. The potted plants, the washbasin, the toilet, and the garbage were all places where a female mosquito might nest. After all, no matter which *human* had carried the virus into the house, a *mosquito* had delivered it into Fatima's body. The question of *who* brought the disease into the house was tangled up, ecologically speaking, with the question of *what* brought it there.

When the subject of the offending mosquito came up, the family pointed over the fading green wall to a neighbor's house, making clear that the most likely home of the offending insect was in *that* house. *That* house, they said, was minded by less conscientious people: drinkers, players of loud music, and, most offensive of all, people who hoarded and sold recyclable plastic, metal, paper, and other items. Fatima's mother described her neighbors as lacking *educación* and *cultura,* terms best translated as "courtesy" or "manners." If doña Feliciana wanted to admonish someone about cleanliness and insect control, it should be the garbage scavengers next door.

After finishing up with Fatima's family, doña Feliciana and I visited these neighbors. Their house was built mostly of wood, surrounded by a ramshackle fence of barbed wire and sheet metal. Splatters of white paint dotted its gray, cracking walls. An old man sat out front repairing a wicker rocking chair. I recognized the owner of the house—a younger man with long hair braided into a ponytail—not as a garbage scavenger but as a cheesemonger from the local market. He was tall, with a pronounced underbite that turned his face into a permanent grimace. His countenance and his decision to block the front door with his lanky body signaled clear hostility to doña Feliciana's request that she be allowed to inspect his patio. But doña Feliciana, like most MINSA nurses, was used to such initial resistance. She introduced herself curtly but politely, flashing her MINSA credentials. She glanced at me with a knowing and slightly impatient smirk as the man retreated into the house, returning with a bottle containing an oily white substance he said would kill all mosquitoes. He explained that he sprayed the house daily. He was "responsible." Doña Feliciana was prepared for this. She knew how to talk her way inside.

"If there are no mosquitoes, there is no problem, right?" she asked with a smile. She was less than five feet tall and spoke with a plaintive lilt. "Just let me take a quick look, *amor,* then I'll be able to complete my report." She waved her clipboard underneath his chin, choosing to adopt the persona of an overworked bureaucrat rather than that of a hygienic scold.

In the back of the three-room structure, we found an all-dirt patio. A latrine, located on the side of the patio closest to Fatima's house, was its most prominent feature. Water from a washbasin was overflowing onto the ground, under the sheet-metal fence, and out to the sidewalk. Next to the latrine was a rather large pile of plastic soda bottles, which would sell for about ten cents per pound at the local scrap dealer. Doña Feliciana, now confident that she could dismiss the white spray bottle still dangling from the man's hand, lectured the owner about mosquitoes and their breeding habits.

When she informed the man of Fatima's dengue case, his reaction was not sympathetic: "So they found out their kid has dengue and they complain about *us?*" There wasn't any way doña Feliciana could be sure, he protested, that his house or "his" mosquitoes had anything to do with it. "What about all the puddles in the streets?" the man asked. "There are clouds— *clouds* of mosquitoes that come from out there!"

The neighbor was hostile, but he was correct—at least in part. He pointed out a problem that confronted many health workers in Nicaragua who attempted to trace the origins of dengue cases. Thanks to the dedication of a few well-connected Nicaraguan doctors and a handful of scientists working with funding from a global dengue vaccine-development consortium, it was possible at that time—late 2007—to perform immunoglobulin assays— tests that detected dengue antibodies—on Fatima's blood. These assays would indicate whether or not dengue was indeed what had made her sick. But the results of such tests could take weeks to come back from Managua, even though MINSA's national diagnostic laboratory was less than an hour's drive away. Moreover, finding out how that particular dengue virus made it into Fatima's body, of all bodies, was almost impossible. If Fatima's brothers, sisters, or any of the other human inhabitants of her house had been known carriers of dengue, the case would have been simpler to solve. But they weren't. Or at least they said they weren't. And, as the neighbor said, it seemed like mosquitoes were everywhere. Pinning the case on an individual insect was futile, but finding an individual human carrier was also difficult.

In the majority of dengue cases, as I later learned, the human carriers present no symptoms. Given that Fatima and her family moved around the zona and across the city from home to school to work to church to market, singling out the neighbors made little sense either. The linked questions of *who* and *what* caused Fatima's illness produced a third question: *Where* did Fatima become ill? This book is an examination of the entangled whos, whats, and wheres of dengue. It is a story about people, insects, viruses, and the trails—the lines of bodily, ecological, and epistemological connection—that constitute their world.

DENGUE IN PLACE

Ciudad Sandino, like other dengue-endemic communities, is home to plenty of mosquitoes, and it contains plenty of places for them to hide and breed. Estimates of formal unemployment in the city range from 50 to 75 percent, and scavenging and selling recyclable materials is a common livelihood strategy. The houses of Fatima and her neighbors were typical. While Fatima's family home had walls of concrete, and its patio had a few more adornments, their house, like that of their next-door neighbors, was an open-air structure. Neither family had screens to protect the indoors from mosquitoes, and each ten- by thirty-meter lot directly abutted the next. *Ae. aegypti* mosquitoes prefer such close-knit spaces. Houses in urban Nicaragua contain a reliably high number of small, relatively clean water containers, like the pots for Fatima's mother's and grandmother's plants and the washbasin of her neighbors. Female *Ae. aegypti* tend to lay their eggs in such containers, and they feed almost exclusively on human blood. Blood is essential to the mosquito's reproductive process. The metamorphic cycle of the mosquito, from egg to larva to pupa to adult, can be as short as eight to ten days. Newborn mosquitoes can take refuge in garbage piles or weed patches while they dry their wings and mature into adults. The adult female of the species is capable of carrying the dengue virus, which has become a growing public health threat across urban Latin America. Indeed, dengue is so common in urban Nicaragua that most adults—whether or not they know it—have likely been exposed to the virus by the time they reach twenty years of age.[2]

As soon as doña Feliciana raised the issue of insect habits, Fatima's family inserted them into their complaints about human ones. The neighbors countered with the insight that, given the sheer number of mosquitoes and their unpredictability, none of us really knew, *for certain,* how housekeeping habits played into Fatima's illness. The neighbors also knew that not everyone looked at the garbage scavenging business as negative. Some in Ciudad Sandino told me that garbage traders' willingness to cart away unwanted material was helping keep their patios and houses clean and safe.

In his refusal to take responsibility for "his" mosquitoes, Fatima's maligned neighbor questioned MINSA's focus on household hygiene. After all, as he and other neighborhood residents—and even MINSA workers—pointed out, there was a constant glut of garbage in the streets and open sewers of the barrio. Didn't mosquitoes breed there? Who was responsible for them if they did? If someone wanted to clean up that garbage and sell it, wouldn't the city be healthier and more prosperous? People frequently described the street as a gathering point *(foco)* not only for undesirable people given to antisocial behavior but also for undesirable creatures. A woman on Fatima's block told me that she was fed up with people using the street and the sewer as dumps. Garbage harbored *animales* (insects) and *microbios* (a general term for *germ*). The sad state of the sewer also made it attractive for small-time gang *(pandilla)* youth, who lacked *educación* and *cultura*.[3] To add to the apprehension of people like Fatima's neighbor, the identities of these antagonists were constantly shifting. Should she worry about *Ae. aegypti*, the dengue vector? An *Anopheles* mosquito, the malaria vector? Influenza? Rabies? Or potential robbery or gun violence? As another woman told me, referring to a dump near her home, "You can find all the sicknesses there."

These women's complaints were about the seeming failure of some neighbors to live responsibly in a thickly settled urban environment. They were also about a sense of simultaneous loss: of safe public space, on the one hand, and of genuinely private space, on the other. Dengue epidemics have made it commonplace for operatives of the Nicaraguan state (at the height of the 2007 dengue epidemic, these included not only MINSA nurses but also army officers and the national police) to enter homes, document the presence of potential mosquito habitats, and report their findings to medical authorities. In Ciudad Sandino, the presence of a virus transmitted by a pesky insect that lived in piles of refuse stoked intraneighborhood suspicion. MINSA had no institutional mechanism for monitoring food quality, waste disposal, or hygiene. Instead, the vast majority of environmental and health problems came to the ministry's attention through citizen reports.

It was such a report that brought us to Fatima's house on that December day. To manifest the public health system in their lives, people like Fatima's neighbors felt they had to report one another to the authorities. A report about the goings-on in Fatima's house, however, ended up drawing attention to the goings-on next door. The seeming ubiquity of street waste and mosquitoes made it easy to presume that neighbors had either chosen to dwell with them in their midst (the lack of *cultura* explanation common on the streets and in neighborhood homes) or failed to control them due to ignorance (MINSA's explanation).

Either way, the onus for engaging either the government or one's neighbors in solving health problems had fallen almost completely onto individual residents. The problem was that engaging the former could make it difficult or impossible to engage the latter. From the point of view of people like Fatima's neighbors, garbage and insects—resilient, persistent, and prolific—were exacerbating the worst aspects of living in a place where labor migration, divergent social histories, and abiding fears of violence meant that people just didn't know each other very well. Many thought of Ciudad Sandino as a *dormitorio público,* a "bedroom community" where most people lived and slept, only to rise each morning and head for work in the markets of nearby Managua or the apparel factories, also called *zonas francas* or *maquiladoras,* that dotted the outskirts of the city. Lives in Ciudad Sandino seemed physically and biologically connected but, at the same time, socially and economically fractured.

DENGUE AS ENTANGLEMENT

Dengue has been known to medicine for some time. It was first described over two hundred years ago, but it has become recognized as a grave health problem in Latin America only in the past twenty-five years.[4] Dengue is a flavivirus with four known subtypes, or serotypes.[5] The four serotypes share about 65 percent of the same genetic material, which means they are about as closely related to one another as the West Nile virus is to the Japanese encephalitis virus. Unlike West Nile and Japanese encephalitis, however, the four dengue serotypes lead to remarkably similar symptoms, the most common of which are fever and joint and muscle pain. All four serotypes are spread by *Ae. aegypti.*[6] First exposure to any one of the serotypes usually results in a mild to severe fever, while later exposures can lead to dengue hemorrhagic fever (DHF), the more severe form of dengue, marked by internal and sometimes external bleeding. The name "hemorrhagic fever" is a bit misleading. Fatima had nosebleeds, but these may have been epiphenomenal. Insidiously, the symptoms of dengue-related hemorrhage often do not present themselves until *after* high fevers subside. Unchecked, internal plasma leakage can lead to death. Fatima was recovering, then, but her fever was recent enough that the most dangerous stages of the disease might still lie ahead.[7] As it happened, her recovery was smooth, and the disease that struck her did not fit the clinical definition of DHF.

From 2006 to 2011, years in which I made four separate field visits to Nicaragua, the dengue caseload, both in Ciudad Sandino and across Nicaragua, continued to rise. In 2006, Ciudad Sandino's health center reported 124 suspected cases of dengue, with 3 confirmed, and one case of DHF. The next year, the number of suspected cases rose to 212, with 20 confirmed, and four DHF cases. In 2008, the numbers went up again: 239 suspected cases, 29 confirmed, four DHF cases, and one fatality. This amounts to a 93 percent increase in suspected cases over two years. Counting suspected cases in Nicaragua was important. Because of constraints in time and materials, most cases would not undergo full laboratory testing. If the number of cases still seems low, it is important to remember that most dengue fever still goes both unsuspected and undiagnosed. A long-term study published in 2010 estimated that Nicaragua's health system may have underestimated the national caseload by as much as twenty times, due to failure to report mild or latent cases and a lack of capacity for thorough testing.[8] Even according to MINSA's official numbers for 2007–2009, the confirmed case rate in 2008 was 3.25 per 10,000 residents. Dengue became even more serious in 2009, when a dengue epidemic coincided with the outbreak of H1N1, or "swine flu," stressing the fragile Nicaraguan health system even further. What is clear is that in Nicaragua, as in most every other part of the tropical world, dengue fever is becoming more common and more deadly with each passing year.

This book uses stories from a series of dengue fever epidemics in Ciudad Sandino to track the changing relationship between health and the urban environment. In Ciudad Sandino, the search for health entailed political struggles over how to confront the connections not only between citizens and institutions but also among people, mosquitoes, viruses, and their shared habitats. Much of this book is based on fieldwork I conducted with a group of twenty-four low-level community health workers, known as *brigadistas*. The brigadistas, all poor and predominantly female, carried out house-to-house dengue prevention campaigns for MINSA. Modeled on best practices for dengue prevention promoted by the World Health Organization (WHO) and Pan American Health Organization (PAHO), these campaigns sought to use a combination of technology and community education to suppress the population of *Ae. aegypti* and thus limit the spread of the virus. Importantly, these campaigns put the onus for mosquito control onto householders. In practice, if not by design, women in Nicaragua and elsewhere ended up being the primary deliverers and targets of dengue control strategy. The strategy was designed not only to discipline the population by instilling hygienic habits but also to protect it from what most experts agree is among the fastest-growing disease pandemics on Earth. For the predominantly female brigadistas, however, dengue control was not always a matter of disciplining or protecting bodies. Instead, their experiences led them to conceive of disease control as a search for ways to *open* bodies to new forms of attachment.

This search for openness runs counter to standard public health narratives about infectious disease in general and animal-borne disease in particular. Recent accounts, including several from anthropology, have analyzed how governments and communities react to the emergence of epidemics like dengue, malaria, and avian influenza. These diseases all have something in common; namely, they involve the transmission of a pathogen through the bodies of both animals and people. Critical analyses show how national health policies, underwritten by global health organizations, work to *insulate* people from viruses and parasites, the animal vectors that transmit them, and even one another.[9] It is certainly true that disease control protocols conceived by global health institutions, including the Bill and Melinda Gates Foundation, WHO, and PAHO, have resonance in Ciudad Sandino. But the city's physical landscape and Nicaragua's volatile political and environmental history continue to color local people's conceptions of what health should mean and how they should participate in it. Thus, it is too simple to say that people in Ciudad Sandino are simply responding to dengue control programs devised in distant centers of national or global policy. Instead, they have become engaged as medical and environmental subjects, taking it upon themselves to put disease governance into action, even if that means adjusting policies to the contingencies of local life.[10] While global "best practices" for dengue control imagine discrete spaces, institutions, and spheres of ecological and social action, the reality in contemporary Nicaragua is more fluid than policy makers seem willing to imagine. Brigadistas are also householders. Epidemiologists are also political actors. Garbage scavengers are sometimes brigadistas. And their lives are all entangled with those of viruses and mosquitoes.

This book brings theories from the interdisciplinary field of political ecology into dialogue with those of critical medical anthropology. One important strain of critical medical anthropology focuses on what Margaret Lock calls "local biologies," the ways in which material and social conditions are dialectically reproduced in the space of the body. Political ecology is about how the material and the social, mediated by political economic structures, are dialectically produced in something we call nature.[11] Sicknesses like Fatima's thus seem to be explainable in two ways: as a result of shortcomings in intimate, *local* forms of attachment, such as urban planning or neighborhood social cohesion, and as the outcome of painful partialities in people's ability to participate in seemingly more *global* forms of attachment. These global forms include those of the market: the trade in garbage and used car tires that transmits dengue mosquitoes, and the mix of industrial agriculture, tourism, and labor migration that contribute to the spread of viruses. The scientific techniques of global health, namely, pandemic planning and viral tracking, also work to form local and global attachments. Combining ideas about local biologies with political ecology helps reveal how bodies and environments are not just *related,* such that environmental conditions affect health or that human actions affect landscapes, but *entangled,* such that changes in bodies reverberate through landscapes, and vice versa.

My argument is that dengue renders the scalar distinction between local and global infrastructures, bodies, and forms of knowledge increasingly difficult to maintain. Dengue makes the ostensibly intimate operations of home life a public concern, and it drives public concerns into the center of intimate life.[12] Places like Ciudad Sandino and bodies like Fatima's are not simply sites where dengue epidemics occur. They are themselves entanglements of relationships.[13] Thus, I argue that dengue is best understood not as the outcome of a pathological clash between independent antagonists (mosquitoes, viruses, and people) but as a set of *attachments*—some positive, some negative, and some ambiguous—among them.[14] In philosopher and historian of science Donna Haraway's understanding, a focus on presumably stable objects or entities can produce a misleading picture of how the world works. Instead, she encourages scholars to think of "relationships" as "the smallest patterns for analysis."[15] Too often, dengue and other emerging infectious diseases (EIDs) are studied in a bifurcated manner. Certain scholars focus on their human dimensions, and others interrogate their ecological dimensions. While research agendas and public health interventions have long attempted to bridge the two by emphasizing the social aspects of ecology and the ecological aspects of sociality, I choose the analytical framework of entanglement to disrupt this tendency.[16] A disease like dengue constitutes not simply a socioecological system, in which human activity has bearing on nonhuman behavior and vice versa, but a heterogeneous knot of connections that undermines simple spatial, social, and species barriers. Dengue provides a lens for rethinking health as the set of practices by which bodies and environments become attached to one another. In the context of dengue, questions about mosquito habitats are bound up with the regulation of human well-being. People negotiate and redefine health as they—in cooperation with or resistance to various kinds of authorities—develop and deploy knowledge about what kind of life (mosquito, viral, human) is worth monitoring, preserving, and reproducing.[17]

I define entanglement as the unfolding, often incidental attachments and affinities, antagonisms and animosities that bring people, nonhuman animals, and things into each other's worlds.[18] Entanglement is at once a material, temporal, and spatial condition. The material connotation of entanglement comes from quantum physics. Physicists use the term to explain how, in the words of anthropologist Kath Weston, "a change in one particle is accompanied by a parallel change in the state of the other, even when the two particles are nowhere near each other in any sense that could be explained by the principles of classical mechanics."[19] I find this understanding useful for understanding dengue at an ontological level—as a phenomenon of study and of experience. In dengue, human and mosquito bodies, like mosquito and viral bodies, are both two and one at the same time.

Entanglement also has a temporal dimension. Dengue epidemics in the present are the results of contemporary material attachments, but people caught up in dengue epidemics inevitably understand those contemporary attachments by recalling past ones.[20] Nicaragua's revolutionary and post-revolutionary periods directly parallel the history of Ciudad Sandino, and people's senses of the meanings of health continue to be driven by engagements with the country's volatile past. Indeed, that past is written into the landscape that people and mosquitoes inhabit. As a disease, however, dengue is dangerous to people and confounding to scientists because of another, more direct temporal feature. People who have been exposed to one of the four serotypes of the disease have long been thought to run a high risk for severe infection on exposure to a second.[21] In a phenomenon called "antibody-dependent enhancement," the immune system fails to recognize the new serotype as distinct, and its response facilitates, rather than mitigates, the propagation of the virus in human cells. Thus, even years after recovery, the immunological memory of past infections shapes future ones. In Nicaragua, brigadistas and doctors drew on this understanding of dengue's trajectory, and they often told their neighbors, "Dengue makes you sick the first time, but it kills you the second."

At a spatial level, dengue epidemics, to paraphrase geographer Paul Robbins, seem to strike everywhere and nowhere at once.[22] They are "rhizomatic" phenomena—without clear beginnings, middles, and ends. Fatima's case, then, offers as convenient a trailhead as any for an ethnographic exploration of dengue. The story of Ciudad Sandino is both the story of a community's struggle with a "global" pandemic and that of a highly local set of problems, from earthquakes and floods to gang violence and municipal politics. The story of Fatima's case leads us in multiple directions, and into the stories not only of other humans but also of swarms of mosquitoes, viral assemblages, piles of garbage, and networks of power.[23]

A POLITICS OF ENTANGLEMENT: INFRASTRUCTURES, BODIES, AND KNOWLEDGE

Transmitted by house-dwelling mosquitoes, the dengue virus infects over 250 million people per year, from Singapore to South Florida. As with other EIDs, funding for research on new ways to insulate people from dengue viruses and *Ae. aegypti* has soared over the past two decades, particularly in the areas of vaccine and rapid diagnostic technology. Much of this research, in one way or another, has involved Nicaraguans like Fatima and her neighbors. Since the 1990s, Nicaragua has been a site of field and laboratory research on the virus, on people's immunological reactions to it and their hygienic responses to mosquitoes, and on new forms of epidemic management. A variety of prevention strategies, from the pesticide DDT to participatory mosquito control to vaccines, have all either been tested or implemented there. The latest efforts have tended to be labeled as "global health" projects.

The ascendance of the contemporary global health complex, a humanitarian, intergovernmental effort to eradicate dengue and other EIDs, has been well documented. In brief, it involves attempts by academic and state scientists to bring the biomedical technology normally directed toward diseases of wealthy countries to bear on diseases such as HIV/AIDS, malaria, tuberculosis, and influenza: diseases associated with the Global South but whose continued spread makes them of worldwide concern.[24] Global health hinges on the formation of "partnerships" between local communities and research groups, among governments, and between northern and southern academic institutions. These partnerships are intended to go beyond conventional donor-recipient relationships.[25] The partnership between MINSA and a series of nongovernmental and corporate organizations that produced the possibility of a dengue diagnosis for Fatima is one such example. Making health "global" thus entails forging both an encompassing geographical reach for biomedical technology and a universal epistemology, a "global" way of understanding what health means. Even as global health complexes attempt to improve infrastructures and thereby insulate bodies from infectious diseases, diseases themselves create new entanglements.[26] Fatima's illness prompted her family to contemplate their relationships not just with their neighbors and with their government but also with mosquitoes, garbage, streets, viruses, and water.

Put another way, the processes by which bodies and environments come into being are always interconnected.[27] Such a perspective has important implications for critical medical anthropology, which has been particularly attentive to the ways in which biomedical and other forms of healing intersect. Much of the field uses ethnographic accounts of this intersection to push back against the kinds of universalizing conceptions of illness and wellness that drive global health.[28] Critical studies highlight the broader forces, notably colonialism and capitalism, that produce unequal relationships between different kinds of (gendered, raced, cultured) bodies. In a way, then, much critical medical anthropology is about a politics of entanglement—the persistent inequalities that attend attachments between people, places, and ways of knowing.[29] The field has been slow, however, to examine the more-than-human aspects of entanglement. The three parts of this book explore three important more-than-human elements: infrastructure, bodies, and knowledge.

Infrastructure

Water pipes, roads, sewers, and waste streams connect city dwellers with their human and nonhuman neighbors. In places like Ciudad Sandino, dengue thrives because of partialities in these infrastructures. There, as in other dengue-endemic places, water, garbage, and sewage routinely fail to circulate. The area now known as Ciudad Sandino was once a cotton and wheat plantation. It became an urban settlement when a 1972 earthquake destroyed most of nearby Managua. Its population swelled after a series of environmental disasters in the 1980s and 1990s, most notably Hurricane Mitch in 1998. The story of its people's struggle with dengue is instructive for understanding other similar sites and sociopolitical responses to vector-borne diseases in general, but this particular landscape and its history also give dengue a place-specific significance that confounds globally standardized visions of disease control.

Part 1 of the book traces how the meanings of public health in Ciudad Sandino have changed, from the coming of the 1979 Sandinista Revolution, through the U.S.-backed counterrevolution of the 1980s (known as the *contra* war), and into the 1990s and early 2000s, a period of structural adjustment and state austerity. These changes created new material, social, and political economic attachments among the city's human and nonhuman residents. Since the 1990s, Ciudad Sandino has become a hub in the formal and informal circulation of goods and people in and out of Nicaragua. Today, zonas francas, or free trade zones, mostly occupied by international apparel factories, dot the city's outskirts. Ciudad Sandino is also the site of a sizable trade in recyclable garbage, and it is home to many migrant laborers. "People come here to *sleep*," one woman explained to me in an interview. "They go to *work* in Managua, Costa Rica, Panama, North America." In Ciudad Sandino, dengue emerged thanks to migrations of several kinds into and out of the city, a place tenuously implicated in the process scholars often call globalization.

Dengue was a predictable part of life in Ciudad Sandino, even if no one could say who would become sick next. In many ways, the disease united the community. After all, the virus moved through blood and across property lines, borne by a mosquito that traveled along with people as they circulated. The things they bought and sold—including garbage—crossed not only municipal borders but also mountains and oceans on worldwide trade routes. Dengue's ecology, then, was the product of an age in which trade was rapid, urbanization was uneven, and social and economic inequality was on the rise. Dengue united patients, state authorities, formal and informal economic actors, medical entomologists, and urban planners, but as Fatima's story illustrates, it also raised ethical questions about the relationships among them. Ciudad Sandino was a low-income city, but it was not what most outside observers would call a slum. In fact, during the course of my fieldwork, the city's infrastructure was improving. Pipes, electrical wires, and the garbage system were producing new connections among households. These supposedly modern trappings of urban infrastructure sparked new debates about the relationship between people and mosquitoes.

Bodies

The bodily element of entanglement involves less visible pathways. House-to-house mosquito control measures such as the ones taken in Fatima's case are humanitarian endeavors, but they also are political ones.[30] They seek to impose rationality on the landscape and, in so doing, to control cities and their inhabitants. Crucially, this controlling work is aimed not just at the bodies of human beings but at a "multispecies" environment.[31] The vitality of human beings is routed through the vitality of mosquitoes and microbes.[32]

The politics of bodily entanglement has a distinctly gendered dimension. In Fatima's case, as in many of those I describe in this book, women found themselves taking primary responsibility for controlling mosquitoes and for regulating urban space. Dengue was never explicitly couched in Nicaraguan or global health policy as a "women's issue," yet community health workers and citizens saw it through a gendered lens. Ninety percent of the brigadistas in Ciudad Sandino were female, and all lived in the marginalized barrios of Ciudad Sandino. Those most directly responsible for dengue prevention in the city were also very often single mothers and/or the de facto heads of their households. Their experience of urban space, like their work in dengue prevention, amounted to a series of house-to-house tasks: trading piece labor like washing and ironing for money, selling food or caring for children on behalf of neighbors, and distributing medical care and advice.

MINSA protocols for the control of *Ae. aegypti* hinged on an aesthetic ordering of the urban household: one in which mosquitoes, like garbage and dirt, did not belong. Management regimes such as this, which are common around the dengue-endemic world, seem to rely on an alienation of people— in the case of dengue, women in particular—from the urban natures in which they live. For brigadistas, however, mosquito abatement involved an opening up, rather than a closing, of the landscape. As I argue in part 2, female brigadistas took deep pleasure in learning about mosquito-human lifeworlds and in forming new relations through mosquito control work, a pleasure I call "ecological aesthetic." Ecological aesthetics—patterns of connection that are visible only through action—contrasted to the more rigid aesthetics identifiable in MINSA's ordering of the household. While the latter aesthetics has human control *over* life at its core, the former emphasizes a relational knowledge *of* life.

Knowledge

Entanglement calls attention to competing ways of knowing about bodies and the environment, particularly ecological models of mosquito development, epidemiological models of risk, and political calculations about the value of prevention. It brings Nicaraguan ideas about *educación* and *cultura* together with epidemiological and biomedical ideas about prevention and infection. In part 3 of this book, I use accounts of a series of dengue epidemics and prevention projects in Ciudad Sandino to show how the techniques of epidemiology and public health were entangled with those of Nicaraguan street politics. I explore how brigadistas and others operationalized three technical/political concepts in the course of routine dengue control. First, I examine the preventive work of brigadistas in further detail, showing how the logics of public health "surveillance" dovetailed with those of political surveillance. I describe the ways in which brigadistas and other health workers deployed ideas about political identity in their day-to-day interactions with neighbors. Second, I trace the changing meaning of "participation" in the context of the return of the Sandinistas to political power in 2007, showing again how the seemingly neutral concept of community engagement, perennially popular in global dengue policy, took on particular political meanings in Ciudad Sandino. Finally, I show how people reacted to seasonal dengue epidemics. Dengue is a "seasonal emergency" in Nicaragua. Epidemics occur yearly, during the rainy season between September and December, a time when mosquito populations expand in predictable cycles. Amid seasonal emergencies, people in Ciudad Sandino found themselves confronting the uneven and often unequal roles of national health policy, global health technology, and economics, not just in responding to climatic and ecological cycles but in reproducing them.

FINDING TRAILS: ENTANGLEMENT, LANDSCAPE, AND METHOD

The gridded nature of Ciudad Sandino's streets, as shown in the map in the front of this book, make it stand out from other parts of Managua, where streets begin and end in a much more haphazard fashion. Still, like the streets of Managua, the streets of Ciudad Sandino have no names. Residents navigate their daily comings and goings with a "popular geography," giving directions using highly specific landmarks and idiosyncratic cardinal points.[33] In central Managua, a set of alternative cardinal directions pertains, whereby north becomes *al lago,* or toward Lake Managua; east is *arriba,* or "up" in the direction of the central mountains; and west is *abajo,* "down" toward the Pacific. South normally remains *al sur.* Ciudad Sandino's residents continue to use these terms in alternation with the normal cardinal directions, even though, as I would point out to friends, "al lago" and "arriba" were actually in the same direction, given Ciudad Sandino's location on the western shore of Lake Managua. Most addresses in Managua include no official postal or bureaucratic references. In Ciudad Sandino, as the map shows, barrios are known by numbers (zona 1, zona 7, etc.).[34] A typical address in Ciudad Sandino was something like, "De donde fue el Mini Cine. Dos cuadras abajo. Una cuadra al sur. Tercera Casa. Mano derecha," or "From where the Mini Cinema was, two blocks down, one block south, third house on the right."

In Fatima's case, the complexity of local geography became a tool in a preexisting dispute between neighbors. Fatima's family's circumstances (i.e., father with a hospital job in Managua, paved patio) were slightly more comfortable than those of her neighbors, whom Fatima's mother and grandmother described as lacking *cultura.* It seems more than convenient or coincidental that the complaints about the bad neighbors flew at about the same range as *Ae. aegypti* (ten to thirty meters). In an urban area with a history of disease and insect problems, the mosquito had made itself a player in a human conflict. As soon as the issue of insect habits came up, members of Fatima's family inserted it into their complaints about human habits. The neighbors countered with the insight that, given the number of mosquitoes and their unpredictability, none of us really knew how they played into Fatima's illness. They both used talk about mosquitoes and viruses to call attention to the dilapidation of streets and the failure of the garbage service, making claims about the insufficiency of infrastructure. The conflict between the neighbors was certainly political, and in hundreds of subsequent home visits with MINSA officials, I saw similar scenarios repeated. Blame circulated along with illness, yet those circulations were never straightforward.

For this reason, I place a methodological emphasis on the trails—material as well as symbolic—by which dengue and knowledge about it flowed through Ciudad Sandino. My method of learning about garbage scavengers, brigadistas, city garbage collectors, and MINSA doctors and hygienists was "house-to-house" ethnography, just as the work they undertook was of a "house-to-house" nature. (This methodological choice draws directly from the theoretical ideas about entanglement that I outline above, but readers looking for deeper theoretical insights should consult the endnotes to each chapter.) This does not mean that I carried out surveys or interviews in each house. Rather, it calls attention to the fact that houses were the dominant physical form of Ciudad Sandino. They were the site and direct object of antidengue and antigarbage campaigns. My work took place in houses, but it also took place on rides in garbage trucks, on walks through streets, and in examinations of epidemiological charts and maps. The story of dengue takes place not just at particular sites but along the well-worn paths that link them.[35] More than its health centers or its dump and junk brokerages, Ciudad Sandino's houses and the trails that connected them were, collectively, my field site.

I spent four months in the company of Ciudad Sandino's corps of approximately twenty-five garbage collectors, riding along on garbage collecting routes, attending union and planning meetings, and occasionally assisting in the collection and redistribution of waste. I dedicated another eight months of my study to dengue prevention campaigns, working mainly with the group of twenty-four brigadistas hired by the local MINSA health center. Like the garbage work, the dengue prevention work involved house-to-house visits throughout Ciudad Sandino's fourteen zonas. Finally, I worked over several months with garbage scavengers and brokers, on the streets of Ciudad Sandino, in household junk brokerages, and in the city's dump. The number of scavengers in the city fluctuated, since participants often drifted in and out of the economic sphere depending on personal circumstances. Normally, however, the city counted about seventy to eighty scavengers working in the main municipal dump, and another fifty to eighty plying the streets, parks, storm sewers, market, and informal dumps.

All of this work was circulatory. I moved in and out of neighborhoods, houses, junk brokerages, and public and private spaces with my interlocutors, carrying on conversations, sometimes taking photographs and making recordings, and maintaining notes of the activities. The notes were often of a highly descriptive nature, a kind of "nondirective" research, pursuing "questions about events and practices that people were already discussing or actively engaged in at the time."[36] This method allowed me not only to identify those with a willingness to talk but also to make the interviews rather unstructured and free-flowing. Some of the conversations in this book are reconstructed from notes taken in situ, but many of the interviews represent seated reflection on what my interlocutors and I had done together. The work I observed and in which I sometimes participated was repetitive and cellular. The people I joined circulated objects, ideas, and values from point to point and from house to house.

With that circulation in mind, I want to use the trope of the trail—a mark on the landscape that may be anthropogenic but may also be created by a plant or animal—to call attention to the role of people and other living creatures as place makers. "Minimally," the philosopher Edward Casey argues, "places gather things in their midst—where 'things' connote various animate and inanimate entities. Places also gather experiences and history, even languages and thoughts."[37] In this sense, a place can be a political locality, like Ciudad Sandino, but it can also be a house within such a locality. My choice of methods allowed me to see how people, blood, resources, waste, money, and mosquitoes did more than simply appear in houses. These things all left important social and physical marks between houses. They thus actively entangled one another. But houses were the spaces in which a tension between individualistic self-preservation and collective cooperation became most apparent. As agents of MINSA, the brigadistas whose stories comprise much of this book had to hunt out mosquito colonies and document their presence in the intimate spaces of their neighbors' houses. They had to reconcile the systematic languages of epidemiology, public health, entomology, and urban planning with the gendered realities of everyday life in urban poverty. An anthropology of entanglement can help us understand the limits of this reconciliation.

The landscapes of disease are cocreated by active human and nonhuman elements. Analytically separating the human aspects of such landscapes from their nonhuman ones requires adopting rigid categorical views of the relations between humans, nonhumans, and the material world.[38] Inhabited landscapes do not fit these categories. Inhabited landscapes are fluid and "weedy," neither wholly natural nor wholly cultural, neither productive nor reproductive.[39] They are inherently unstable. A focus on entanglement calls attention to the "gaps" between the categories we traditionally use to think about landscapes, gaps between domestic and wild, nature and culture, *polis* and *oikos,* waste and resource. These are the gaps occupied by dengue mosquitoes, to be sure, but they are also occupied by people. These gaps, I suggest, are the norm. It might be easier to study inhabited landscapes if we focus on the marks—invisible and visible—left behind by the intertwined movements of people, things, nonhuman animals like *Ae. aegypti,* and quasi life forms like viruses. My contention is that it is possible and worthwhile to attend to such marks—the "trails" I have in mind in this book's title—because they tell a story about disease that belies easy separations like local/global or body/environment. The marks on Fatima's body provide a perfect example. How could doña Feliciana begin to understand the rash on her skin without seeing it as connected to a mosquito's feeding and breeding habits, her father's job in a hospital, and the national and international dengue diagnostic network? That trace of skin inflammation contained, to use Tim Ingold's term, a "meshwork" of material, symbolic, and political threads.[40]

In Ciudad Sandino, the house itself—another key ecological gap filled by the dangerous mosquito vector—was also full of such traces. The visible traces of the circulation of garbage from dump to household to global marketplace were not included in the brigadistas' script for teaching people about dengue and mosquitoes. In that script, the house was a static site of leisure, rest, and reproduction. The house contained contradictory impulses, toward cleanliness, on one hand, and toward economic production, on the other. Through attention to the daily comings and goings of insects, people, and things, I began to see dwellings as "houses in motion."[41] In addition to houses, I worked to trace the roadways, garbage collection routes, and health care visits.[42]

Even when I made maps available to people in Ciudad Sandino, maps didn't seem to help them understand where they were. Rather, the brigadistas and scavengers understood the city through specific kinds of movement. Going house-to-house teaching about and looking for mosquitoes was a task that Morena Sanchez, one of the brigadistas with whom I interacted most closely, described as "negotiation." Knowing that her neighbors wouldn't always be happy to see her (Morena did represent the state, after all), she would walk through their houses, complimenting them on elements she liked: an adornment or a fruit tree. This paid off in cooperation, but also in material exchange. Morena and other brigadistas would frequently finish a day on the trail of Ciudad Sandino's mosquitoes with sacks of mangoes, limes, or even aluminum cans, in addition to a neat bureaucratic record of insect habitats and their locations. If some of the piles of garbage were left off the record, this only seemed fair. The ability to navigate neighborhood streets in multiple ways—the ability to make community health work productive both of knowledge and of economic value—was essential to being an effective brigadista. Knowledge of what was in the landscape was more than a matter of fitting observations to categories. Deftness at walking the trails that connected the health center to the household, the household to the dump, the dump to the junk buyer, and so forth, was crucial for Morena to making a living, and for me as the anthropologist to understanding how health and environmental politics converged.

WAYFARING AND CONNECTING:
LIFE IN THE FIELD AND ON THE TRAIL

Nicaragua has long been known as a welcoming place for *internacionalistas,* or foreign solidarity workers. Attempts to remake foreign aid as social work, from participatory action in public health to the formation of fair-trade coffee cooperatives, can be traced back to the earliest days of the Nicaraguan revolution.[43] In 1979, the Sandinistas succeeded in toppling the Somoza dynasty, which ruled Nicaragua from the 1930s to the 1970s. They did this despite the fact that the Somozas enjoyed the material and financial backing of the United States for most of that period. Still, leftist and centrist activists from poor and middle-class Nicaraguan families were united under the banner of the Frente Sandinista de Liberación Nacional (FSLN). After the successful overthrow, the Sandinistas became a cause célèbre of the American and European left, even winning the tacit support of the administration of U.S. president Jimmy Carter. But the administration of Ronald Reagan, who took office in 1981, openly supported (and covertly supplied) an army of counterrevolutionaries known as *contras.* During the 1980s, nearly fifty thousand people (including a handful of internacionalistas) died in the war between the revolutionary government and the CIA's proxy army of contras. The draining war, combined with crippling economic sanctions and political maneuvering on the part of the United States and paranoia and vanguardism among the FSLN political elite, led to an electoral defeat of the FSLN in 1990 and the end of the revolution.

As a foreign researcher, I benefited from the goodwill of the hundreds of internacionalistas who preceded me. Still, as I found out, global health projects in Nicaragua have had difficulty dealing with the politically and morally charged relationship between Nicaraguans and people from more powerful nation-states, particularly the United States. Both global health and *internacionalismo* have two sides. On one hand is *solidarity,* a humanitarian impulse to do good in partnership with those in need. On the other hand lies a set of calculated efforts at *control*.[44] In the case of American relations with Nicaragua, the work of internacionalistas was tempered by covert and overt attempts to steer politics away from the socialist left through the contras. By contrast, global health tends to present itself as apolitical, or antipolitical.[45] In the case of global health, control means doing research in places like Nicaragua not only to cure diseases that affect poor Latin Americans and others in the Global South but also to manage the spread of emerging pathogens north to the United States. It does not mean getting involved in revolutionary politics (at least not directly).

Like many of my colleagues in medical anthropology, I have good reason to be suspicious of the facile use of "global health" and "emerging infectious disease" as pedagogical rubrics, as research programs, and as bases for new policy initiatives. After all, dengue epidemics are nothing new in places like Ciudad Sandino. As Paul Farmer has pointed out, the adjective *emergent*, when used to describe diseases, often masks the unsettling reality that people like Fatima and her family have been dealing for some time with diseases we couch as novel or "outbreaking."[46] The rise of market-driven globalization and uneven urban development has made them more common and more deadly in places like Nicaragua, but more importantly, this rise has forced the governments of wealthy northern countries (especially the United States) to reckon with the possibility that "tropical" diseases may threaten their residents, their economies, and their households. The unchecked spread of dengue, including recent outbreaks in middle-income and wealthier countries, has undeniably been a driver of the recent explosion in international research on it. The growing interest on the part of scientists, donors, and corporations in finding a cure thus seems to be at least partly self-serving.[47]

During my fieldwork, I spent hours among residents of Ciudad Sandino, doctors, nurses, epidemiologists, city planners, garbage scavengers, and, most of all, with a group of brigadistas. I lived in one of the zonas of Ciudad Sandino, renting rooms from a social activist and former brigadista, whom I call doña Eugenia. Doña Eugenia was a psychologist working within MINSA's local health center, but she was also deeply involved, through a few different nongovernmental organizations (NGOs), in the recruitment and organization of modern-day internacionalistas, mostly American missionaries and students. I first came to Nicaragua as such an internacionalista, wondering whether I was better suited to long-term anthropological fieldwork or to development work. I had heard stories from professors and activists just a few years older than myself of the heady days of the "solidarity movement," the loose affiliation of left-leaning (and even radical) Americans and Europeans who came to Nicaragua to support the Sandinistas. As a child in the 1980s, I vaguely remember nightly news reports about the Sandinistas and the contras, but not surprisingly, internacionalistas were not regular features.

Doña Eugenia was a political agnostic. She was a devout evangelical Christian, weary and suspect of the "immorality" she saw in Nicaraguan politics. Politicians were conspicuous consumers and drinkers, and even in the days of the revolution, the relationship between *militantes* from the Sandinista party and internacionalistas was predicated on alcohol, womanizing, and carousing. In the 2000s, this romance had been repackaged by ex-revolutionaries like the folk singer Carlos Mejía Godoy, who ran a popular, *gringo*-friendly nightclub in Managua. Many students I met in the 2000s willingly partook in this partial legacy of internacionalista life, but talk of politics and social justice was largely absent from their discourse. Much like the missionaries I met, the modern-day internacionalistas wanted to "do some good," "fulfill a need," "teach," or "help a family," without thinking much about the social, political, or economic context of those actions, or of that need.

A sizable portion of this new generation of internacionalistas was composed of undergraduates or recent graduates with aspirations to attend medical schools. What they sometimes called the "primitivism" of Nicaragua's health system disturbed them, but it did not always shock them. As I found out, an appreciable number had been inspired to visit Nicaragua by medical anthropology classes in which they encountered writing by or about anthropologists like Paul Farmer and Jim Yong Kim. These young volunteers aspired to, as one student told me, "do a Partners in Health kind of thing." I wanted life for my acquaintances and friends in Ciudad Sandino to get better, too, but I became quickly disillusioned by the absence in my conversations with other internacionalistas of what I considered to be the most pressing issues: how harsh international debt restructuring terms had undermined the gains that the FSLN had made in health care by imposing privatization, fees, and wholesale cutbacks; or how the proliferation of zonas francas allowed international commercial concerns to poach (tax-free) a needy and oversized labor force of young people (mostly women); or how those same laborers were consistently punished for attempting to organize unions.

At the time of this writing, the places of these young internacionalistas in internships and service-learning organizations have now been taken by women and men like my own students. I find the new generation of internacionalistas instinctively generous and infectiously curious. Like me, they have little to no firsthand memory of *La Revolución,* but sitting somewhat between them and the generation of internacionalistas that preceded me (the ones who worked on coffee harvests and Sandinista literacy campaigns), I hope that with this book I can alert my students and other potential internacionalistas to some of the deeper dynamics of urban life and health in Nicaragua. The internacionalistas I met during my fieldwork saw themselves as part of a network of potential professionals (mostly doctors, but also economists, teachers, and engineers) with sights set on making work not just *for* the poor but *with* the poor a central phase of their careers. I greatly admire this aspiration, even if I remain cynical about the possibility that short stints of service learning in places like Ciudad Sandino will lead to meaningful structural change of the kind that Farmer and others advocate.[48] I felt—and still feel—that understanding how health and illness are experienced within a supposedly needy population like that of Ciudad Sandino is of profound value, especially if those populations are to become something more than targets for North-to-South interventions.

On the other hand, I sympathized with doña Eugenia's feelings about Nicaraguan politics. Local narratives about life in Nicaragua remain colored by tension between nostalgia for a past marked by social solidarity—often framed in the religious idioms of liberation theology that drove much of the Sandinista rank and file—and laments for a present marked by selfishness and greed.[49] Politics was marked by entanglements between these memories and experiences. Nicaragua's political culture in the middle to late 2000s was shaped in large part by what Nicaraguans refer to as "the pact" *(el pacto)* between its two main political bosses *(caudillos).* In brief, Arnoldo Alemán, leader of the Constitutional Liberal Party and president of Nicaragua from 1996 to 2001, struck a fairly blatant political deal with Daniel Ortega, Sandinista president from 1984 to 1990. By the terms of the pact, Ortega promised not to use the considerable power of the Sandinistas in the National Assembly and judiciary to prosecute Alemán for a series of well-documented crimes, including embezzlement of state funds and criminal mismanagement of the bureaucracy. In exchange, Alemán assented to a constitutional change that would allow Nicaraguan presidents to be elected with a plurality of the popular vote, rather than a simple majority. Both sides wagered that, given their considerable party apparatuses, they could muster such a plurality. The pact thus ensured the dominance of the liberals and the FSLN over more progressive elements, particularly the sizable dissident center-left Sandinista movement known as the Movement for the Renovation of Sandinismo.

Ortega ended up getting the better of the deal, winning election to a second presidential term in 2006 (with just 38 percent of the popular vote) and manipulating the national constitution (again, with Alemán's cooperation) to permit his reelection in 2011. Ortega's return to the presidency after sixteen years of center-right rule provides the political backdrop for much of this book. I say more about it in subsequent chapters, but it is sufficient to note here that, as a researcher and as someone concerned with the conditions of life in urban Nicaragua, I was reluctant to throw my lot in with Ortega, as a previous generation of internacionalistas had done.

I was continually drawn out of my disillusion and cynicism by a peculiar Nicaraguan penchant for making personal, material, and emotional connections. Nicaraguans have a saying that goes, *Mejor solo que mal acompañado,* or, "It's better be alone than in bad company." When I first heard this expression, I dutifully jotted it down in my field notes and interpreted it as an argument for self-reliance—the kind of do-it-yourself attitude that would make one suspicious of politicians who promised, as Ortega did, solidarity with *los pobres* while they flaunted the material wealth that political power had brought them. Such individualism seemed like a rational reaction to the revival of patron-client politics that has defined postrevolutionary Nicaragua. My experiences in the field, however, militated against such an interpretation. If there was a good life to be lived in Ciudad Sandino, it came from being in good company. When I told people that I lived alone (as I did for most of my time in the field, sharing an apartment with an ill-tempered cat and a Nicaraguan roommate who was nearly always with family, a girlfriend, or his church group), they would show pity both verbally and visually. Kin and social attachments were essential not just to a satisfying social life but to survival. These attachments often spanned across geographical space. Thus, while houses on my street were almost always bolted shut, and my neighbors would constantly express fear of the "violence" and "danger" that lay outside, especially at night, they also pitied and suspected anyone (like myself) who lived alone.

A *lack* of entanglement, as I found out, was perhaps the most unhealthy thing that could befall an urban Nicaraguan. One of the two brigadistas I knew best explained it this way: "The thing that kills more people than anything here in Nicaragua is depression. Depression is what makes you sick; loneliness makes you sicker." In this book, I expand on this idea, though I depart from the psychological idiom that this brigadista invoked, to resolve the reservations my Nicaraguan friends and I have (and which other anthropologists also have) about the state of international development work—and global health in particular. For people in Ciudad Sandino, the search for improvement in health, in education, and in environmental conditions was not always a matter of severing connections between human bodies, mosquitoes, and viruses. Rather, it was about building quality attachments.

PART ONE

Infrastructure

Nothing was donated. It was all a struggle.

DON MIGUEL RAMOS, *2009*

How would it be if we didn't live this way? We'd really be the worst city in Nicaragua.

GARBAGE SCAVENGER, *Ciudad Sandino, 2008*

———

ONE

City of Emergencies

THE TOYOTA TRUCK came to a stop at the end of a rutted, narrow dirt lane, where the section of Ciudad Sandino called Mostatepe, or zona 13, met a long, paved stretch of highway. The truck's driver, don Gilberto, checked his rearview mirrors and whistled out the window, partly in the direction of the group of women awaiting a bicycle taxi to carry them to the nearby bus stop, and partly in that of the two *recolectores* (collectors) who were trailing the truck on foot, picking up refuse stuffed into old fifty-pound rice sacks from the houses we passed. The *recolectores,* clad in oversized yellow jump-suits and frayed cloth gloves, hurled the last pair of rice sacks up to a third man, who was perched in the truck's bed. The third man dumped the leaves, food waste, and other garbage into the brimming hold and tossed the rice sacks down to the ground. At the sound of don Gilberto's whistle, the two *recolectores* latched themselves onto the handles on each side of the already-moving truck.

As we sped down the smooth highway toward the dump, don Gilberto began telling me about local history. It had just been a few days since I began riding along with the garbage team, hoping to learn something about the connection between dengue, mosquitoes, waste, and the city's geography. Don Gilberto, like most of the drivers I would meet, seemed to like having someone to talk with in the cab of the truck, and he took it upon himself in those early days to teach me something about the city. On that day, as we bounced along, with leaves and mango skins flying into the wind, he told me that to understand Ciudad Sandino was to understand that it was a "city of emergencies."

Like most residents, don Gilberto could recall two key moments in Ciudad Sandino's history. The first was November 5, 1970, the day a flood destroyed homes in the slums *(asentamientos)* of La Tejera, Miralagos, Quinta Niña, and Acagualinca in north and east Managua.[1] For most Nicaraguans, that flood was probably unremarkable. Floods are yearly occurrences in the capital, and its *asentamientos* are always the most vulnerable areas. But that particular flood, which left several families homeless, prompted the Nicaraguan Organismo Permanente de Emergencia Nacional (Permanent National Emergency Agency) to create a new settlement just north of town, near a small village called Bello Amanecer. The Organismo Permanente de Emergencia Nacional settlement, known by the acronym OPEN, formed the seed of what would eventually become Ciudad Sandino.

While the 1970 flood is alive in the memory of just a handful of families in present-day Ciudad Sandino, the second key moment remains a historical touchstone for all Nicaraguans. On December 23, 1972, a massive earthquake destroyed 90 percent of Managua. After the earthquake, which left tens of thousands of people without shelter or livelihoods, the OPEN became home to a new influx of migrants.

Catastrophe is at the center of Nicaragua's national narrative. In 2008, my friend doña Eugenia helped host a group of American college students who had come to Ciudad Sandino to volunteer on an "alternative spring break" trip. As part of their orientation, she asked a professor from the Universidad Centroamericana to teach them a bit about Nicaragua's history. He began his lesson on what Nicaraguans call the "land of lakes and volcanoes" *(la tierra de lagos y volcanes)* with the story of another tropical storm. In 1502, after they had spent several days battling a hurricane, Christopher Columbus and a crew of sailors landed in the area that is now Nicaragua's North Atlantic Autonomous Region. The storm must have been abnormally strong, given that they named the spot at which they finally found refuge Cabo Gracias a Dios (literally, Cape Thank God).

The 1502 hurricane might be written off as force majeure. The inclusion of Nicaragua in a colonial system, though socially catastrophic, was of course intentional. Over the five centuries since that landing, Nicaragua has remained a target for international interlopers. The professor went on to tell the students the story of William Walker, the American white supremacist and filibuster who briefly ruled the country in the mid-1800s. In 1856 Walker overran Nicaragua with a private army and installed himself as dictator, legalizing slavery, among other things. He was ousted after less than two years, but violent foreign incursions did not cease. The professor told the students about the U.S. and British fruit companies that transformed much of the

Atlantic region into plantations in the twentieth century, the U.S. Marines that supported agricultural elites in the 1930s, the CIA-backed contra army that fought the Sandinistas in the 1980s, and the transnational corporations, including Unilever, Cargill, Wal-Mart, and Texaco, which now have warehouses, plantations, and refineries in the country.[2] The professor's history was peppered with references to hydrological and geological instability, as well as human-induced land degradation and pollution.[3]

Ciudad Sandino is a young city, just forty-five years old at the time of this writing. Its evolution from a loose collection of refugee houses to a city of nearly 150,000 people happened within the living memory of many of its residents.[4] The history of Ciudad Sandino is, quite literally, a history of the building of streets, as well as of pipes, water pumps, and power lines.[5] It is the story of how its inhabitants forged attachments to one another, linking public spaces and activities to intimate ones. Infrastructures are "demanding environments." As technologies and techniques of entanglement, infrastructures, like public health systems, steer people into certain ways of behaving and knowing the world.[6] They have the potential to create social solidarity by establishing formal lines of affiliation between otherwise isolated houses, families, and social groups.[7] But in Nicaragua, as elsewhere, neither infrastructures nor public health systems come into being in a vacuum. Rather, people build them on top of already-existing technologies and techniques of entanglement. Historian Julie Livingston, examining how new medical technologies changed social life in periurban Gaborone, Botswana, found that urban Botswana had a long-standing sense of the moral tension between concern for individual survival and concern for collective well-being. What it meant for people in Gaborone to *care* at once for themselves and for one another—their sense of public health—emerged amid that moral tension. The meaning of care changed with the adoption of new technologies of attachment.[8]

The story of Ciudad Sandino's public health, its infrastructure, and of the changing role of community members in it—particularly that of community health workers called brigadistas—is similar. It is the story of a landscape-as-palimpsest: of the (partial) erasure of old technologies of entanglement by political and ecological catastrophe, followed by the (partial) installation of new ones. Attention to the lived experience of urban construction *and* destruction shows how public health and infrastructure, for all their potential to create solidarity, have an equal potential to promote isolation and fracture.[9] The building and replacement of streets, sewers, pipes, and electrical grids has frequently been disrupted by nonhuman forces of geology, weather, and—most relevant for Ciudad Sandino's recent history and for this book—circulating pathogens. As Ciudad Sandino's physical infrastructure changed—from its founding, to the earthquake, to the Sandinista revolution, and into the era of dengue epidemics—so too did residents' ways of thinking about health. New systems of public health were built alongside—and sometimes within—the relics of old ones, and in the process, new forms of care and concern became entangled with old ones.[10] The story of Ciudad Sandino is the story of people's struggles to maintain a sense of collective concern in the face of forces that pushed them toward self-preservation. Understanding those struggles is essential for understanding Nicaraguan experiences with dengue.

SOMOZA STONES

As don Gilberto and I discussed the history of emergency and infrastructure, I let myself stretch a bit. After two hours plodding along the jarring, unpredictable roads of Mostatepe, a few minutes on a paved highway felt luxurious. Ciudad Sandino contains all kinds of streets. Most are made of dirt, occasionally graded but mostly taking shape in response to the less regimented tracings of footfalls and car tires. A few of the city's central arteries are paved in asphalt, which permits a rapid (and some say dangerous) flow of buses and taxicabs, decorated with vivid decals that range from graphic depictions of the Passion of the Christ to copies of the Rolling Stones' famous tongue-wagging logo. The houses that line the paved streets that run along the road between the plaza and the market echo with the sounds of revving engines and novelty car horns, interrupted by the whistles and shouts of the bus touts, slender young men in baggy jeans who swing out the doors of re-purposed American school buses. Leaping into the crowd of waiting passengers, they list the route's upcoming stops in staccato Spanish while they prod people, baggage, and the occasional animal into the child-size seats and aisles: "El dos-diez; Velez Pais; Siete Sur; Zumen; Julio Martinez, La UCA; Metrocentro! Managua, Managua, Managua!"

Most other streets are made of "Somoza stones." In 2007, when Daniel Ortega and the FSLN returned to power after a decade and a half in opposition, they sought to make good on promises to undo a period of austerity and inattention to urban planning. The FSLN initiated numerous infrastructure campaigns, and Ciudad Sandino received funding to improve some of its roadways. In an initiative Ortega called Calles Para el Pueblo (Streets for the People), dirt and gravel thoroughfares in the city began to be covered with stones. Anyone who has traveled in Nicaragua probably remembers these stones, hexagonal in shape, laid together in a patchwork down the street. Though preferable to mud and gravel, they are still hell on the shock absorbers of cars and buses. These stones are not generally sealed with cement. This makes them cheaper to install than asphalt or concrete pavement. As my neighbors explained to me, stone streets also require more labor to build, which means that such projects can employ more people.

The stones have symbolic importance for Nicaraguans as well. For many, they are signifiers of poverty. My neighbors knew that even the backstreets in wealthier parts of Managua had "real" pavement, made of concrete or asphalt. Hexagonal stones were an old technology, relegated to poor neighborhoods. But the stones were also reminders of a history of urban resistance to political repression. In the 1970s, the only company that made them was owned by the family of Anastasio Somoza Debayle, the dictator who ruled the country from 1967 to 1979. Stones were the primary material used in the reconstruction of Managua's streets after the 1972 earthquake, and the cement company profited significantly from the reconstruction.[11] Partly because of numerous such self-serving schemes on the part of Somoza, the earthquake and its aftermath became catalyzing events in the acceleration of the popular revolution that overthrew the dictator. During the 1970s, the Sandinistas consolidated their base in poor urban neighborhoods like the OPEN, where the government's laconic and corrupt disaster response became a common point of discontent.[12] Over these new streets, Somoza's personal army, the Nicaraguan National Guard, carried out house-to-house raids in search of Sandinista insurgents. During the peak of revolutionary violence, insurgents would pull the stones off of the streets to build barricades to prevent the Guard from entering their barrios. In the first years of the new century, people in Ciudad Sandino still pulled them off the streets, to repair the pipes below or to prop up broken-down cars.

In many ways, the Somoza stones turned the city into a recognizable political unit, in which the space of public, productive life—the *polis* of streets and plazas—was clearly distinguished from that of private, reproductive life—the *oikos* of households and patios. But floods and earthquakes—not to mention dengue epidemics—confused this neat dichotomy. People felt the impact of environmental disturbances in the *oikos* as much as in the *polis*.

For people in Ciudad Sandino, infrastructure meant attachment to systems of political and economic power, but, as the Somoza stones graphically reminded them, even a modern-looking street could be a symbol of marginalization.

COTTON

There were other such symbols embedded in the landscape. As a child, don Gilberto told me, he moved back and forth between the OPEN and a small family farm north of the city. Traces of Nicaragua's agrarian past remained in evidence throughout Ciudad Sandino, even though the city was now the most densely populated part of Nicaragua. Horse carts were a common sight, and artisan dairies selling fresh, raw milk—much cheaper and more versatile than the pasteurized kind available in the market—were never more than half an hour's walk away. I had been living in Ciudad Sandino for nearly six months, however, before I first noticed the cotton shrubs.

I had walked down one of the rutted dirt roads to visit my friend Felipe, who lived in zona 11, on the northern edge of the city. I arrived early. Felipe was not at home, but his father, a frequently inebriated but friendly man, invited me to sit and await him in his patio. He stopped me and pointed to a tall flowerless plant at the center of the patio, saying, "Ya es la mediodia [It's noon]." He was indicating that the plant's shadow was falling directly at its base. I assumed aloud that this meant that the sun was at its highest point in the sky. "Asi se marca la hora en el campo [That's how we tell time in the country]," he replied approvingly. Then he showed me where the shadow would fall, on the wall of the house next door, around 4:00 P.M.

The plant looked unusual, and in the awkward silence that followed the brief lesson, I inspected it more closely. Whiffs of white were poking out of the end of one of its branches. I peered closer and tugged at them. "Algodón?" I asked. Could this be cotton? He smiled. Of course it was cotton. He then recalled that in the 1970s, there had been a big hacienda just outside what would have been the original group of houses that made up the OPEN. He added that the village of Bello Amanecer (later to become zona 9) used to have a hacienda as well. Back then, he said, cotton grew as close to Managua as the Las Piedrecitas Park, on the northern edge of town. Now, Las Piedrecitas sat across a busy highway from the U.S. embassy. At its gates, commuters weary of the crowded buses could pick up taxicabs for the seven-kilometer ride over the ridge from Managua to Ciudad Sandino.

Talk of *el campo* and cotton led Felipe's father to reminisce about his days selling *sorbetes* (fruit-flavored ices) in and around Managua. He said that his boss at the *sorbetería* would load up a cart with tubs of *sorbetes* on the weekends and send him into the streets to sell. In March and April, the hottest months of the year, when the cotton came in, he would go to the houses on the haciendas after the workday ended and sell great quantities of *sorbete*. He remembered when trains ran through the countryside, not far from where we were now standing. The tracks took people and plants in and out of the grand estates owned by the wealthiest families in Nicaragua, most of them close cronies to the Somoza family. Laughing, he recalled the time he got a ride on a large boxcar, *sorbete* cart and all, to a farm near Chinandega, in the far northwest corner of the country, some three hours' journey. There, too, he did very well at his sales.

Then he pointed out a little cotton sapling sprouting up near the wash sink in the patio. The bush by which he had told the time, he said, was abnormal in its height. Perhaps that was why it took me a while to recognize it as cotton. Demonstrating on this smaller bush, he showed me how each year, at harvest time, the workers cut the plants down to stumps, after which a tractor would come through and plow the fields. The haciendas had another machine, he said, for planting the new seeds, but even then, a worker— someone with skill and a good eye—had to come through and identify the weak plants, pulling them up so that they would not sap the soil. He told me that all plants I would see today were weak. In Ciudad Sandino, cotton was a relic.

At the time of the 1972 earthquake, the countryside to the north of Managua was still thick with cash crops, including cotton, peanuts, and wheat. The capital, on the other hand, was a thriving and in many ways "modern" city, home to a vibrant middle class.[13] The city was also home to a large urban underclass, composed of people who had left the farms in the northwest and the coffee plantations in the mountains that ran through the country's center. After William Walker was ousted in 1857, conservative governments took over the country, and in 1877, as part of a wave of decommunalization, the conservatives banned all forms of property except individual, state-recognized title. As Thomas Walker explains, "Communal indigenous properties as well as plots held previously under common law by the illiterate mestizo peasantry instantly became 'unoccupied' national territory that could be purchased by the agrarian elite. To add insult to injury, the cultivation of plantain, the banana-like staple food of the peasantry, was outlawed and 'vagrancy' was made punishable by forced labor in productive enterprises (often the coffee plantations that quickly replaced . . . communal farms)."[14] This dramatic reorganization of land tenure prompted a major influx of migrants to Nicaragua's towns.[15] Fifty years later, those in the delanded peasantry who had not fled to the cities formed the core of the guerilla army of Augusto César Sandino, who staged successful uprisings against the coffee elite and the U.S. Marines, who underwrote their power. Sandino became the namesake of both the FSLN and of Ciudad Sandino.

Sandino's ragtag army, which would become a model for people's revolutions across the globe, was eventually suppressed by the U.S.-trained National Guard. In 1932, the guard's leader, Anastasio Somoza García, after having Sandino assassinated, installed himself as ruler of Nicaragua. With the blessing of the Roosevelt administration, Somoza maintained power through the middle of the twentieth century, passing it first to his son Luis, and then to Luis's brother, Anastasio Somoza Debayle, whose company made the paving stones. Over that period, the Somozas used their unilateral control of the National Guard to consolidate power and eliminate enemies. All three Somozas were eager to grow the agro-export economy, and they did in the Pacific coastal plain what their predecessors had done in the coffee-growing mountains to the east of Managua: they consolidated landholdings in the hands of loyalists, intensified agriculture, and forced peasants to move either into waged agricultural work or into the *asentamientos* of Managua.

Recent satellite photos show little unpopulated land between present-day central Managua and Ciudad Sandino, yet just fifty years ago the land that is now Ciudad Sandino was, as the old man had explained to me, a hacienda.[16] Nicaraguan plantation owners were successful during the Somoza era in part because of their zeal for suppressing populations of pest insects. They were keen adopters of harsh but extraordinarily effective pesticides, and their temporary mastery over pests made Nicaragua the agro-export leader of Central America for most of the 1950s and 1960s. Profits and outputs soared, even as per capita incomes remained among the lowest in Central America.[17] Then the pesticides stopped working. New pesticides temporarily helped farmers recover the cotton crop, but by 1970 much of the land had been hopelessly overplanted and oversprayed.

In the winter of 1970, as the agricultural decline began, the Somoza fortune had risen to nearly half a billion dollars.[18] When the November flood came, few programs existed to help people recover from disaster. Neverthe-less, Anastasio Somoza Debayle, never one to shy away from a business oppor-tunity, responded by initiating a series of OPEN projects, encouraging disaster-affected families to resettle on the outskirts of the capital.[19] One group of refugees from the flood, led by the charismatic Alberto "El Gato" Aguilar, a folk singer and *asentamiento* organizer, were invited to purchase land from the estate of Julio Blandón García. The Blandón land became the third OPEN set-tlement, known for the next nine years by the "emergency" moniker OPEN III. Aguilar and the other founders realized that by buying land from an oligarch, they were putting money into the regime's coffers, but they also intuited that by taking advantage of the OPEN system, they could bypass the lethargic state and build their own community, complete with streets, pipes, and sewers. In-deed, according to local historian Pablo Barreto, a common desire for these basic trappings of urban life united the fledgling community.[20]

Somoza knew that the urban poor formed one important constituency of the Sandinista dissident movement against him, which had been stirring both in the cities and in the countryside since the early 1960s. He believed that to corral the restless poor in a new settlement and to make them legally contracted landowners might be a good way to control them. For Somoza, it was more lucrative financially to turn the refugees into rent-paying citizens. Plots of three hundred square meters were sold to the refugees for three thousand córdobas, payable in thirty-córdoba monthly installments. As an-other local historian recalled, "If a person didn't pay the rent at the con-tracted time, without pity they duplicated the debt, or the land was repos-sessed and sold to another buyer. . . . These lots . . . were covered in rocks, with divots and weeds and with dried out areas left by poorly managed cotton. . . . Some people were disappointed by all this and returned to the same barrios from which they came once the water receded and they were habitable again."[21] Most families, however, stayed in OPEN III, but instead of becoming an area in which refugees struggled with only their "bare lives" as testament to their belonging in the Nicaraguan state, the settlement be-came a site where poor people sought to assert full citizenship.[22] Much of their work was practical. They needed to get around town, so they built roads. They wanted to avoid floods and waterborne diseases, so they dug storm sewers. Workers needed to get to jobs in nearby Managua, so entre-preneurs started bus lines. Slowly, they turned the fallow of the Blandón ha-cienda into a more livable and more governable space. Much of this conver-sion happened thanks to house-to-house mobilization.

"Ciudad Sandino is known for its *cauces*," the MINSA nurse doña Feliciana once told me. The city's landscape was lined with them: deep, open sewer ditches that divided zona from zona. These trenches were the first bits of infrastructure to be built on the land (indeed, many of them were built when the land was still a hacienda), and they were key to preventing the kinds of flooding that besieged the *asentamientos* back in Managua. The *cauces* were, like the Somoza Stones and the cotton plants, bittersweet historical markers. If the city was "known" for its large network of *cauces*, doña Feliciana was not pleased about it. *Cauces* may have controlled flooding, but they were also places where people carelessly dumped garbage, left unwanted or sick animals to die or fend for themselves, bought and sold drugs, and hunted for scraps of recyclable metal or plastic. *Cauces* were also where drainpipes and gutters spilled out into the open air. Those pipes, particularly in Ciudad Sandino's central zonas, formed an impressive underground network. Back in 1970, the city's earliest residents had insisted upon the installation of *tubos madres*, or "mother pipes," which would carry potable water down the ridge from the aquifer near Las Piedrecitas. They also installed a system for carrying dirty water away from their houses and into the *cauces*.

My neighbor doña Josefina was part of one of Ciudad Sandino's founding families, and she remembered the struggle to install those systems. She lived near the city's main plaza, and on most afternoons she could be found in the front patio of her house, surrounded by children and grandchildren. In the past, she was regarded as a neighborhood health activist and trainer of brigadistas, though by the time I knew her she was retired. Still, like many residents of her generation, doña Josefina relished the chance to talk about the city's early days. Like many older Nicaraguans I would meet, she used nostalgia for a past of collective commitment to comment on what she saw as a present of individualism and "vanity."[23] In one interview, doña Josefina recounted the story of Padre Miguel, a Jesuit priest from one of the lakeside barrios, who accompanied the families to OPEN III. Padre Miguel helped the settlers access bricks, sheet metal, and wood for construction, but the founding families remained disorganized and spread out.

Between 1970 and 1972, the houses became more numerous, but as doña Josefina put it, the people tired of having to pay twenty córdobas to fill up their metal water barrels at the pumping stations near the highway, which still belonged to the hacienda. She told me of a people's movement to install running water:

JOSEFINA: So when ... [Padre Miguel] saw that some of us had lost everything, that we didn't come with anything but our arms, then he ... looked for help for the families that needed it most ... and so he looked for financing, support to pay for water pipes, mother pipes that we put in. He got us together; the whole community was involved in this, because by that time there was a good amount of people. There were close to fifteen thousand. ... Those of us who didn't have work, we went out and started digging ditches for the pipes. And ... the majority of those of us who worked in the ditches, 80 percent, were women ...

ALEX: Building ...

JOSEFINA: Women, some of us already with children, others single, that were ... single mothers that didn't work, and so to survive they began to dig the ditches. The community itself made the ditches for the mother pipes to get water ...

ALEX: And the mothers were ...

JOSEFINA: Fighting. When the government finally saw that ... the mother tubes were laid and that we had water, then they began to put a price on it, so we'd pay monthly, so the government began to demand that we pay twenty [córdobas] monthly. Padre Miguel joined the fight against this because we—the majority of us here, a good percentage ... were single mothers that came to live in OPEN III like a "public dormitory" [dormitorio público]. A dormitorio público is when the person only comes to sleep in her house and at five in the morning goes to work, to sell in the market, to sell in the streets. Okay? So, when he saw this, when Padre Miguel saw that we were families with little means, we began the "Ten Yes, Twenty No!" struggle, until we won. And we managed to pay only ten córdobas for our water. And so it began. So it began.

Aside from being an inspiring tale of neighborhood cohesion, doña Josefina's story hints at some themes that would recur as I discussed Ciudad Sandino's history with long-term residents. The first was that of "natural" events—for example, the flood or the later earthquake and hurricanes and dengue epidemics—being flashpoints for dramatic social upheaval. The second was that of infrastructure—in Josefina's story, water pipes—being built not because of systems of repressive political power but despite them. The third was that of women, and single or young "mothers" in particular, playing a vital role in the construction and reconstruction of the city.

Doña Emilia Suarez, who lived just three blocks from doña Josefina, didn't like to talk about this period. Doña Emilia ran her own *pulpería* (a small shop) out of the front of her house, and she sold tortillas and *nacatamales* (oversized boiled dumplings made of corn masa, stuffed with meat and vegetables, and wrapped in banana leaves). With income from these businesses, she supported her out-of-work partner *(marido)*, a mentally disabled daughter, an adopted daughter, and three grandchildren. Like many other women, she came to OPEN III alone, with a young son and two daughters. Word around Ciudad Sandino was that she had run a safe house *(casa de seguridad)* for the early Sandinista *guerilleros* whose clandestine movements took them from barrio to barrio during the 1970s. When I knew her, her marido, Miguel Ramos, and her children talked about her political activism, but she was reluctant. During my return visits to her house, she did, however, discuss the building of the pipes, *cauces,* and streets, activities in which Sandinistas joined non-Sandinistas, including don Miguel's family. In those early days, as doña Emilia explained, party affiliation had little meaning. Don Miguel and his family came from the Acagualinca section of Managua, but they were loyal to the liberals, the party of Somoza. They, too, bought land from the Blandónes.

Doña Emilia told me that though most of the "single mothers" who helped lay the original foundations of the city were—or ended up being—Sandinistas, they also included a great number of political agnostics and, in one case, the wife of a Somoza National Guardsman. Doña Emilia participated in two forms of house-to-house mobilization. As a Sandinista safe house operator, she was a node in a household network of insurgents that spanned the length and breadth of the country. As a participant in local infrastructure building, she was another fighting mother building mother pipes.

When I brought up the rent question in our interview, don Miguel was defensive. He acknowledged that the Blandónes were exploiting their new tenants, but he wanted to be clear that all of the founders of the neighborhood were "owners." "Nothing was donated," he pointed out. "It was all a struggle." As I later learned, that distinction, between individual donation and collective struggle, would prove to be a salient one in contemporary local politics.

Just as Padre Miguel was leading the residents of OPEN III in a fight against water gouging, the earthquake struck, destroying Managua's city center and displacing tens of thousands of residents. Managua's location on a fault line constitutes yet another instance of the conjuncture of environmental and political events. Historically, Nicaragua's elites have been divided into a liberal party faction, centered in the colonial city of León in the northwest, and a conservative party faction, associated with Granada, on the shores of Lake Nicaragua to the south. Managua, which lies between León and Granada, owed its large population and status as capital city to a geographical compromise the two parties made over one hundred years before the earthquake.[24] In December 1972, the Somozas were celebrating thirty-six years of keeping both parties at bay, often with the help of the United States. (Nominally, the Somozas were liberals, but party politics was effectively neutralized during their reign.) Anastasio Somoza Debayle pocketed millions of dollars in earthquake relief, seizing control of nearly all industries related to rebuilding or demolition.

OPEN III received hundreds more families after the earthquake, and it evolved into an organized and incorporated sector of the municipality of Managua. Government planners divided the city into numbered neighborhoods, the original zonas. As a refuge for Managua's poor and unrepresented urban population, OPEN III became a center for clandestine revolutionary activity. Increasingly, even self-described liberals like don Miguel's family began supporting the Sandinistas' efforts to oust Somoza.

The landscape bears the traces of that political uprising. Doña Feliciana once led me to a small aluminum plaque that stood along the broken sidewalk on a block in zona 8. The plaque commemorates a former Sandinista *casa de seguridad*. On a single bloody night in the late 1970s, Somoza guardsmen infiltrated the *casa de seguridad* and abducted seventeen young men and boys, all of whom "disappeared." Such house-to-house purges were frequent. The careful and legible construction of settlements like OPEN III allowed the guard to move in and out of neighborhoods efficiently. From the top of the ridgeline that runs along the west coast of Lake Managua, marking a physical border between Managua and Ciudad Sandino, it is possible to see the skyline of Managua through the plumes of smoke rising up from the capital's open-air garbage dump. The ridge is known as the Cuesta del Plomo (Lead Ridge). That ridge, locals say, was where the National Guardsmen disposed of the bodies of dissidents.

In 1979, just after the July revolution that ended the Somoza regime, OPEN III was renamed Ciudad Sandino. The idea came from "El Gato" Aguilar. On July 16, 1979, the night before the FSLN army marched into Managua, just one day after Anastasio Somoza fled to Miami in recognition of his impending defeat, "don Alberto ... in the company of Roberto Zapata ... put up a sign with the words CIUDAD SANDINO in the principal entrance to the city, even as the people of the *barrio* faced down the National Guard."[25] Turning around atop the Cuesta del Plomo, looking away from Managua, you can make out that entrance. There, a footbridge crosses the León highway, marking the spot where Aguilar and Zapata posted their sign. A giant statue of Augusto César Sandino greets the taxis and buses that turn off the highway and into the city. The bronze Sandino, usually decorated with a bright red bandana around his neck, stares defiantly at the Cuesta del Plomo.

LOS CACHORROS

Buses tend to halt for longer than usual along the Somoza-stone street that leads past the Sandino statue and into town. This gives the touts time to sprint across the road to punch time cards and deposit cash in a *pulpería*. Food sellers hawking *sorbetes,* churros, and peanuts swarm the buses. Riders toss coins in exchange for food, or perhaps water or juice, which comes in small plastic bags. The scene is one of momentary relief, as the passengers suck in the sugar and water. The buses speed off as empty containers fly from their tiny windows.

Just up the road, not far from the next stop, sits one of the few public buildings in town. Ciudad Sandino has a few health centers, a plaza, and a market, but apart from the overgrown park and baseball diamond in zona 8, there are few places for communal gatherings. The concrete and tin shell of Los Cachorros, a modest meeting hall and playground, named for the organization founded by the young soldiers who fought in the revolutionary army against the contras during the 1980s, stands out among the small house lots. During my fieldwork, Los Cachorros was in poor repair, but it remained a meeting place for youth activists, women's and veterans' groups, and, during public health campaigns, volunteers and MINSA staff who were planning house-to-house mobilizations in the surrounding zonas.

Community meetings were not exactly rare by the time I started fieldwork, but in the years just after the revolution they were frequent and vibrant. Dr. David Werner, the author of the pioneering instructional text for community health workers *Where There Is No Doctor,* visited a health center in Ciudad Sandino in the early 1980s.[26] Werner had recently hosted a MINSA delegation at Project Piaxtla, the Mexican village health network out of which *Where There Is No Doctor* was born. Werner was in Ciudad Sandino to facilitate a multiday workshop involving physicians, MINSA bureaucrats, and health educators. Their goal was to implement a holistic, participatory primary care system. The system would address basic needs such as intestinal health, nutrition, and maternal health, and it would build social connections that could provide neighbors with immediate access to assistance if they needed it.

During his visit, Werner met a group of young community health workers who called themselves *brigadistas.* The brigadistas mostly came from local "base communities," the cells of revolutionary and social mobilization that formed the urban backbone of the FSLN.[27] The base communities' political and practical work featured house-to-house mobilization, in the form of dissident networks and *casas de seguridad,* and house-to-house infrastructure construction, in the form of movements like "Ten Yes, Twenty No!" By the time of Werner's visit, Ciudad Sandino was Managua's largest municipal sector, and with a population of seventy-two thousand, it was almost as large as León, Nicaragua's second largest city.[28] The purpose of the workshop was to train the brigadistas to become the front lines of primary care. Werner was there to help teach the brigadistas the basics of midwifery, oral rehydration, and other life-saving techniques, so that they could train others.

"After the first few days," Werner recalled in a 1992 essay, "a message arrived from ... MINSA ordering that the workshop be suspended so that the brigadistas could take part in a national campaign against measles."[29] Such national campaigns, often announced with little warning, were a hallmark of Sandinista public policy. They were intensive, high profile, and often quite successful, but Werner was worried, as were the leaders of the workshop, that the "emergency" order would undercut the progress being made in the meetings:

> The community group drafted a message back to the health ministry, reminding it that the ministry's responsibility was to advise and provide backup to the brigadistas ... not tell them what to do. The brigadistas pointed out that they were accountable to, and took their directives from, the community. ... they agreed that the national measles campaign was ... very important. Therefore they would continue the workshop, but with a

strong emphasis on community activities designed to inform residents and make possible the fullest participation in the campaign. I was astounded by the audacity of the brigadistas. . . . I was even more astounded when later a reply came back from the health ministry, apologizing for having given such paternalistic orders. It praised the community for keeping the ministry in line and endorsed the brigadistas' plan.[30]

Werner witnessed what other *internacionalistas* and solidarity workers would see in the early days of Nicaragua's revolutionary period: a government that, to a great extent, ceded the power to control the flow of knowledge about health to citizen groups.

Nicaragua's revolutionary government, especially in the period before the intensification of the CIA-backed contra war, in which young soldiers known as *cachorros* (or "cubs") manned the front lines, became noted for several innovations. Among these were the controversial redistribution of the lands that had been taken by coffee and fruit oligarchs over the previous century, the courting of the business elite in an effort to foment what they called "mixed socialism," and investment in grassroots, nongovernmental social groups like the base communities.[31] Brigadistas and other community workers were active even before the consolidation of revolutionary, religious, and grassroots groups under the FSLN flag. In 1984, the U.S. embassy estimated that about half of the country's adult population belonged to a grassroots social organization.[32]

Werner's story, like doña Josefina's account of the "Ten Yes, Twenty No!" campaign, recalls a unique moment not just in Nicaraguan history but in the history of public health. In the 1978 Alma Ata declaration on primary health care, in which the WHO famously aspired to "health for all by 2000," authorities put a new emphasis on health as a human right, mediated through states. The document explicitly identified a connection between health and socioeconomic development. The Alma Ata approach became something of a public health paradigm, and after the 1979 revolution Nicaragua became a site of innovation and experimentation in community-based primary care.

The Nicaraguan approach to public health in those years took lessons from Alma Ata, and it drew explicitly on the "problem-posing" philosophy of the Marxist pedagogue Paolo Freire.[33] Medical anthropologist John Donahue gives the example of a popular health brochure "in which the group is asked to link the two generative themes of 'diarrhea' and 'living conditions'" (figure 1). In the brochure, designed specifically for a Nicaraguan audience,

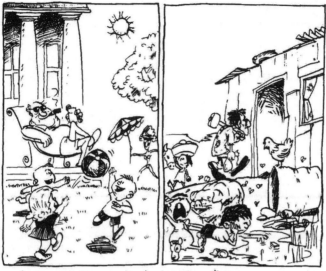

Analizar el dibujo y discutir las preguntas:

- ¿ Cuáles de estos niños se enfermarán más de diarrea?
  ¿ Por qué ?

- ¿ Por qué son diferentes las condiciones en que viven
  estos niños ?

FIGURE 1. Part of a MINSA diarrhea brochure, c. 1980. It pictures two households and asks the viewer to "analyze the drawing and discuss the questions: Which of these children are more apt to become ill from diarrhea? Why are the living conditions of these children different?" (Translation and picture from Donahue 1986: 71)

"conditions" and health are linked to "beliefs." The "healthy" children live with a portly, sunglass-wearing father and play in front of a (markedly un-Nicaraguan) columned house. (Its columns bear a remarkable resemblance to those of the U.S. White House.) The picture on the right would be more recognizable to a resident of Ciudad Sandino in the 1980s—and even in the 2000s—with chickens, water barrels, and mud surrounding a wood and sheet metal dwelling, into which an exhausted, skinny father trudges. Images such as these capture a particular moment, one in which the production of livable material conditions and the dissemination of knowledge about health were explicitly related. In the 1980s, brigadistas styled themselves as *multiplicadores* (multipliers). They were tasked with teaching their friends and neighbors about health problems *and* their structural origins, so that demands for improvement came from the grassroots to the centers of political power. Their job was to distribute brochures like this one, house-to-house. The house-to-house raising of *consciencia* was designed to lead to collective demands for improvements in roads, sewers, and other basic elements of infrastructure.

Dengue appeared at an inopportune time, and it may have disrupted this vision.[34] In the 1980s and 1990s, thanks in part to a collapse in the agricultural sector, urbanization skyrocketed across Central America. Amid this urbanization, the flow of people and consumer goods across regional borders actually increased. At the same time, government investments in sectors such as public health and urban infrastructure declined. By the time scientists recognized dengue's seriousness, *Ae. aegypti* and the dengue virus had taken advantage of infrastructural underdevelopment, intensified labor migration and trade, and the growth of cities to establish themselves from Paraguay to the Texas-Mexico border.[35] Dengue spread across the region, then, because changes in the large-scale flows of humans, nonhumans, and things collided with upheavals in local political economic orders.

When dengue was discovered in Nicaragua in 1984, during the heat of the contra war, the first reaction of the Sandinista government was to mount another grand campaign, this time centered on search-and-destroy efforts against the mosquito. At the time, President Daniel Ortega openly suspected the Americans of smuggling the virus to the country as a biological weapon.[36] In truth, the situation was a bit more complex. Previous eradication efforts, centered on the use of the pesticide DDT, had eliminated *Ae. Aegypti* from Nicaragua and the rest of Central America by the 1970s, but the mosquito continued to thrive in the United States. Slowly, it recolonized the American tropics, likely due to the increased importation of waste material—particularly car tires—from abroad. Managua, like most capitals in the region, was poor, but it had an airport, and Nicaragua had been an importer of garbage from North America for some time. As infected people moved in and out of the country by road and air, the dengue virus joined the mosquito.

Following an intensive model developed in the 1950s and 1960s under Somoza, the Sandinistas began sending vector-borne disease technicians from house to house spraying low-volume insecticides to kill adult mosquitoes, changing the water in storage barrels to kill larvae, and carting garbage and other potential breeding sites out of homes. Reporters profiling Ciudad Sandino at the time noted that these strategies had a participatory component, tied to the integration of community health committees through antidengue campaigns and Sunday "cleanups" known as Domingos Rojinegros (Red and Black Sundays), so named for the colors of the Sandinista flags its leaders, representatives of FSLN-affiliated base communities, draped over their windows.[37] The approach certainly had a lasting impact on Nicaraguan historical memory. Even years after these intense home visits had ended, former brigadistas like doña Josefina recalled them with nostalgia. MINSA's painstaking house-by-house mosquito control was costly, but it created immense goodwill between citizens and the state.

Amid such mass campaigns, brigadistas and base communities became absorbed into the revolutionary state and into a new, nationwide community organization, the Committees for the Defense of Sandinismo (CDS).[38] The CDS would become integral in literacy, urban agriculture, health projects, and other house-by-house mobilizations, or *luchas populares* ("popular struggles"). Over the course of the revolutionary period, the CDS stood at various points as both a hopeful model for state-civil society relations and a slightly disconcerting manifestation of popular revolution turned to vanguardism.[39] The CDS preserved order during the days of the contra war by informing on dissidents and reporting mothers who shielded their teenagers from military conscription.[40]

Eventually, the CIA-backed contra insurgency weakened the people's goodwill toward the FSLN, and in a 1990 election, the U.S.-friendly regime of Violeta Barrios de Chamorro came to power. Chamorro dissolved the CDS, imposed structural adjustment measures that effectively ended mixed socialism, and severely reduced the presence of the state in economic life and social welfare.[41] Bilateral aid to Nicaragua actually increased in the 1990s, thanks to the political neutralization of the Sandinistas, but the budget for public health was slashed. Per-capita health spending dropped by 12 percent from 1992 to 1996 alone.[42] In addition, Chamorro's government reorganized MINSA into seventeen regional offices, a Sistema Local de Atención Integral en Salud (Integrated Local Health System, or SILAIS).[43]

Meanwhile, dengue continued to spread, and international approaches to it began to reflect the logics that drove the Chamorro government's measures to reduce the active presence of the state in health care. In 1989, Duane Gubler, then the chief of the Dengue Branch of the U.S. Centers for Disease Control and Prevention (CDC), addressed the American Society of Tropical Medicine. State-led, house-to-house mosquito eradication, he argued, would not work in the long term. He argued that if *Ae. aegypti* mosquitoes were to be controlled, and if, by extension, the disease were to be controlled, people in affected communities could not rely on their governments to do it.

Gubler claimed that the elimination of breeding sites by government technicians was costly and "paternalistic." States were promising too much to their citizens, and "the result is an entire generation which blames government for a disease which exists, in part at least, because citizens refuse to participate in larval source reduction practices in the immediate vicinity of their home."[44] He added, "We want [people] to understand that most transmission occurs in and around the home by a mosquito that is there because of *their bad habits,* that the disease can be prevented, but that the *ultimate responsibility for prevention and control must be theirs, not the government's.*"[45] According to Gubler, a new sanitary ethic needed to take hold. Whereas the Alma Ata declaration called for an integration of citizens with strong states, in this new vision, primary "responsibility" for control of the domestic mosquito rested with individuals in their homes.[46]

Gubler ended his address by calling for a new suite of "horizontal" dengue control programs, in which intracommunity networks would be as important as "vertical" state ministries.[47] Social scientists (including medical anthropologists) were to be central in the horizontal approach, along with well-integrated laboratory diagnosticians, entomologists, and epidemiologists. Links between experts—not states—and communities would be most important. State ministries would play a role, but funding would come also from private business groups such as Rotary International and nongovernmental donors, especially the Rockefeller Foundation. From the late 1980s to the 1990s, Rockefeller was the lead funder on at least a dozen major community-based mosquito and dengue control programs, from Puerto Rico to Honduras to Mexico to Vietnam.[48]

Nicaragua followed suit. While per-capita spending on health dropped countrywide during the 1990s, Ciudad Sandino, which by the mid-1990s had expanded to include a three-kilometer portion of coastline along Lake Managua, saw its health centers grow in number and capacity. In 1996, a central hospital, complete with twenty-four-hour emergency ward, was established. The hospital was the central node in a network of four *puestos de salud,* or health posts. The *puestos,* smaller consulting clinics that operated each morning from Monday to Friday, were located in the outer zonas. In the new SILAIS model, it was their staff of doctors and nurses, rather than street-level community health workers, who acted as the front lines of care. Hospital directors used small daily stipends to call upon a new generation of brigadistas, often young women and students in search of extra cash, to aid in ad hoc antimalaria, hygiene, and vaccination campaigns. Though there remained a few older brigadistas with more advanced medical skills—midwifery, for example—the majority were foot soldiers in a drastically decentralized and biomedicalized community health system.

POWER LINES

In 1998, just as the Nicaraguan government was in the final stages of this decentralization, another environmental catastrophe struck the country. Hurricane Mitch devastated farms and small towns in Nicaragua's relatively remote central highlands and Atlantic coast, and it caused massive floods in the capital. Once again, Managua's poorest barrios—some of the same barrios on the lakeshore and near the city's dump that had been home to Ciudad Sandino's founding families—were inundated. International attention to the crisis was high, and aid poured into Nicaragua and other affected countries. Ciudad Sandino again became a destination for displaced people. Over the next year, nearly ten thousand refugees moved onto land just to the south of the city's hospital and market (see map in the front matter). With donor support, this settlement became Nueva Vida (literally, "New Life"), Ciudad Sandino's twelfth zona.

Nueva Vida, like the other marginal areas of Ciudad Sandino, is distinguished by a curious infrastructural feature. If you look up as you walk down the streets of these newer settlements, you will see a tangle of low-hanging power lines, often stapled or nailed to trees, or suspended on posts mounted to the edges of houses. The lines zig and zag over the narrow streets, splitting off to reach the scattered houses. While rolling blackouts (cortes de luz) were somewhat common across Managua in the early years of the new century, power in Nueva Vida was even more noticeably intermittent. Some said that this was because the residents of Nueva Vida were shameless electricity thieves. The webs of wire spliced and strung overhead were not the work of the Spanish energy firm Unión Fenosa, to which the liberal government had sold the grid in the 1990s. They were the work of Nueva Vida's residents. It was not uncommon to see a person perched in the trees, connectandose: connecting his house to the grid by running a new wire from the main line. Knowing of this clandestine activity, Unión Fenosa punished energy consumers in the barrios where these offenders lived with blackouts and aggressive collection practices.

For almost everyone in Ciudad Sandino, electricity was a nonnegotiable part of life. For example, my friend Felipe, whose father had sold sorbetes on the cotton haciendas, made his living as a metalworker. He fashioned scrap aluminum and other found items into pots, pans, spoons, and decorative items for sale on the local market. He depended on electricity to run the blowers in his homemade furnace, and like everyone else, he relied on electric power to run small appliances, from radios to water kettles to televisions.[49] "Even the water runs on electricity," he explained to me during a blackout. "The pumps are electric, so when they cut the lights, they cut the water. Every time Fenosa cuts the power or raises the rate, it is us—the poor—that pay more." He paused and shrugged. "So we just steal more," he laughed. Felipe didn't want to be a thief, but he didn't think he had much of a choice.

Felipe lived in a neighborhood called Pedro Joaquin Chamorro, an area with a reputation as a home to squatters and utility thieves. Residents who moved there were repeatedly denied the chance to connect to electricity, even through Unión Fenosa's official means. Company representatives claimed that building new lines was not worth the cost. The neighbors would either steal energy or neglect to pay their bills. The company's refusal came to the attention of the local branch of the Movimientos Comunales de Nicaragua (Nicaraguan Community Movements, or MCN). The MCN was formed after the 1990 electoral defeat of the FSLN, as a way to continue the community work of the CDS, which were disbanded under the Chamorro regime.[50] By the early years of the new century, the MCN had fallen on hard times, but it still held regular meetings at Los Cachorros.

For MCN activists, the lack of electricity in communities like Pedro Joaquin Chamorro was a health hazard. One of the MCN's local leaders, a MINSA employee called doña Jamaica, told her compatriots that she was tired of seeing her neighbors *conectandose* by dangerous, illegal means. Someone was going to get electrocuted. (Indeed, this happened on a fairly frequent basis around Managua.) Instead of decrying the informal connections as theft, however, doña Jamaica and the MCN managed, through a series of public demonstrations at Fenosa's office and the *alcaldía,* to establish the fire and electrocution risk of illegally connecting. They succeeded in turning Fenosa's own austerity against it and winning formal connection to the grid, subsidized by the government.

While Nicaragua's recent urban history is dotted with incidents like the MCN's uprising against Fenosa, and more traditional citizen actions such as labor unionization and women's movements, the political neutralization of grassroots groups, as well as of state agencies like MINSA, was a key part of the reforms undertaken by center-right governments in the 1990s and early

2000s.[51] But while community-based action was pushed outside the state sector, the brigadistas were pulled even more firmly into it. As anthropologist Laura Tesler explains,

> By the 1990s, *brigadistas* were still being recruited, trained and utilized, but the model had been co-opted and rendered a completely top-down hierarchy of relations. Whereas the Sandinistas had envisioned the community participation approach, complete with health action committees, to enable local community members to determine their needs and even help select personnel, now the health center administration primarily viewed *brigadistas* as a source of . . . labor that it could call upon to assist when needed. . . . there was no opportunity for *brigadistas* or other community members to launch their own health initiatives in conjunction with the government, participate in the hiring or evaluation of local health center personnel, or request particular types of health services in need.[52]

Effectively, brigadistas and other grassroots community groups were not only politically neutralized after the revolution but also deskilled. The brigadistas had ceased to be the *multiplicadores* that they had been in the 1980s, when trained health workers would train others, under the guiding philosophy of Frereian *conscienzao*. By the 2000s, MINSA saw them—and, thanks to a small monetary payment, brigadistas in Ciudad Sandino increasingly saw themselves—as lower-level cogs in a hierarchical health-delivery infrastructure.[53]

RESPONSIBILITY

When Daniel Ortega assumed the presidency for the second time, in 2007, MINSA was reformulated as a fount of state generosity and party mobilization. For sixteen years (1990–2006), the center-right governments of Chamorro, Arnoldo Alemán, and Enrique Bolaños had rolled back MINSA's public outreach programs. During the same period, dengue fever went from being a mild, episodic phenomenon to a severe and deadly challenge. The new FSLN promised more direct involvement in health, abolishing unpopular clinical consultation fees and deftly—if vaguely—using the language of democracy and "rights" to argue that MINSA should be accountable to a fourth branch of government, *el pueblo,* the people, or "Citizen Power."[54]

In late 2008, I asked a MINSA publicity officer about the dengue situation and the purpose of what she clumsily labeled the "popular struggle of

Citizen Power for the eradication of dengue" *(lucha popular del Poder Ciudadano para la eradicación del dengue)*. She explained that when the Ortega administration took office in January 2007, it confronted two "emergencies." One was the yearly outbreaks of dengue, diarrhea, and acute respiratory illness that the rainy season and the chilly temperatures left in their wake. The other was the deterioration of the universal health care system that the Sandinistas established in the 1980s. The reinstatement of this system required, in the *lucha popular* model, the return of old participants: doctors and nurses, of course, but also citizens. Rhetorically, at least, it seemed that the new FSLN wanted to return the power to address health issues to grassroots community groups, yet even among the most militant FSLN supporters in Ciudad Sandino, the years between Sandinista regimes raised difficult questions about which citizens were willing and capable of participating in *luchas populares*.

One of Hurricane Mitch's most palpable effects on Ciudad Sandino, according to many long-term residents, was an acceleration of neighborhood fracture. In my conversations with people who lived in Ciudad Sandino's more central zonas, it became clear that they perceived a divide between themselves and those who settled in Nueva Vida after the hurricane. People often employed the concept of *cultura* as the yardstick for this divide. *Cultura* is not equivalent to the idea of "culture" in the classic anthropological sense; rather, it is more akin to the notion of "cultural capital" or "bourgeois decorum."[55] To long-term residents, people in Nueva Vida did not know *how* to live properly in the landscape. In particular, they didn't dispose of garbage properly; they "stole" electricity; they failed to pay taxes. High incidences of violence, disease, and drug use in Nueva Vida seemed to indicate a rejection of the interhousehold ethic of cohesiveness that long-term residents of Ciudad Sandino celebrated in themselves.

In the years after Hurricane Mitch, many longtime residents began developing a narrative about the people of Nueva Vida and their houses. They noted with scorn that unlike in the OPEN III of the 1970s, nearly all the original houses in Nueva Vida were built by donors and *given* to refugee families. I was told over and over again how, in the first few months after the storm, thousands of families who had received free land and houses "selfishly" and "greedily" sold their plots and returned to the flood-prone Managua barrios from which they came. According to the narrative, Nueva Vida's original residents would always float back to lives of garbage scavenging, drug use, and crime, scheming to bilk a well-intentioned set of government, church, and nongovernmental aid groups out of goods and services when the next "emergency" arose.

This hostile narrative reappeared in daily conversations with brigadistas and other health center personnel. As Marianna, a MINSA hygienist, put it,

MARIANNA: People come with their ... ways, I'd say, of dirtiness, that although everything [sanitary resources] is in their reach, they don't use it. Sometimes it is as if the people don't do their part, I imagine ... the services are there, but the problem is that the people don't ... help.

ALEX: Don't help in what sense?

MARIANNA: Complying with the norms that one [hears] ... today [on] the radio, the television, [from] those of us that go around [house-to-house].

Though epidemiological numbers only partly bore out their suspicions, many felt that the rising problem of dengue, in particular, came from marginal barrios, of which Nueva Vida was the largest.

For Ciudad Sandino, Hurricane Mitch ushered in a new "geography of blame," a new way of spatially distributing responsibility for sickness.[56] The storm also fundamentally altered the city's physical makeup and political organization. At the time of the hurricane, Ciudad Sandino was still technically district 1, the largest municipal sector of Managua, but the storm came at a time when Chamorro's government and that of her successor, Arnoldo Alemán, were pushing for the decentralization of political power in the country. Managua's sprawl was seen by center-right politicians, as well as international lending organizations like the International Monetary Fund and Inter-American Development Bank, as an impediment to equitable economic development. Within a year of Hurricane Mitch, Ciudad Sandino was turned into an independent municipality. Starting in 2000, it had its own mayor *(alcalde)*, elected town council *(alcaldía)*, and—supporters of decentralization argued—a new sense of empowerment and solidarity among its population. An erstwhile "margin" would become a formal new "center."

Donors and multinational corporations showed immediate interest in investing in the new city's infrastructure. With the help of advisers from the European Union, the city became a beneficiary of a public-private development partnership called the Integrated Project for Peripheral Managua (PROMAPER). PROMAPER marked the single largest block of development aid in Ciudad Sandino's history, and it signaled a major change in city planning. Instead of being constructed by local residents, new public works would be designed and built by professionals, many of them from other countries. The city's political leaders managed to secure a loan from the European Union to design and install new water service, sewer, and water treatment facilities. PROMAPER's donations and its hardware, including earthmoving equipment, dump trucks, and land rovers, bore the E.U. logo. The European Union contracted much of the design work to EPTISA, a Spanish-based multinational engineering firm. EPTISA described its work for Ciudad Sandino in this way: "An action plan to assist reconstructing and contribute establishing bases to a sustainable development after the devastating effects of the Mitch hurricane."[57] The $20 million investment included six hundred house constructions or improvements, thousands of meters of pipe and sewage, and a water treatment plant.[58]

For people in Ciudad Sandino, PROMAPER was a bittersweet gift. It brought better roads, more reliable water, and houses, but it also seemed politically skewed in favor of the inner core of the city (zonas 1–8), which had arguably weathered Mitch in decent condition. Nueva Vida, which was not even founded until after the hurricane, saw few of PROMAPER's benefits. There, just one street was paved with Somoza stones, but no sewage was installed, while in zona 2, where I lived along with many of the other longtime residents, sewage and new pipes arrived, along with gutters and sidewalks. The major bus routes, which carried workers to and from Managua, were paved.[59]

The choices about *how* to install the infrastructure revealed as much about the changing times as the decision about *where* to place it. While grassroots infrastructure building was a strong part of local tradition, PROMAPER brought infrastructure to Ciudad Sandino in a different way. For example, under PROMAPER, if a family wanted to get rid of its pit latrine and install a flushing toilet that took wastewater out to the sewer line, that family had to pay to install its own pipes. The owner of my house had installed a flushing toilet just days before I moved in. My neighbors on both sides, however, had not, and their washbasin water would routinely flow in a yellowy sludge over the smooth new sidewalk. Pressure to "get connected" was rife throughout the community, but poorer families resented the stigma that the "modern" sewer created. Where there had once been generalized inadequacy in access to sanitary sewage, there were now cellularized gaps. Connecting was an individual responsibility, but failure to connect became a new form of antisocial, polluting behavior. Some were simply too poor to connect, but others didn't trust the new system. Backups were fairly common during the rainy season, and, as my neighbors pointed out, a pool of wastewater in a public street is much more offensive than a pit latrine in a hidden patio. A new form of social responsibility was emerging. Individual choice, rather than collective action, became the operative productive force in infrastructure. Houses were approached as individual units. They were nodes in a planned network, but that network depended on the rational decisions of self-interested actors to "get connected."

INFRASTRUCTURE IN AN "ERA OF VANITY"

When I asked him to compare the early days of the city to the present, an old Sandinista activist and doctor who lived in my neighborhood repeated a common nostalgic lament: "In those days [the years of the revolution and before], if we were cooking *baho* (a hearty beef stew) on Sundays, we would of course send a bit over to the neighbors, and of course they would send us food, too. Not just for a birthday or a funeral, but any time. Nowadays, it's each house for itself. What kind of *cultura* is that?" For the doctor this cellularization of households mirrored the kind of insulated existence favored by the wealthy of Managua, just a few miles away.

The difficulty of this shift was most apparent to older brigadistas and long-term residents of Ciudad Sandino, like doña Dora. When I met her, doña Dora lived with her teenage daughter in the *area verde* section of Nueva Vida. The *area verde* was the last section of Nueva Vida to be settled. Doña Dora received of a small plot of land from the city government around 2005 as part of a plan to formalize the land tenure of the squatters who lived there. She grew up in Managua in the 1960s, as she explained, "with everything." Her mother died young, but her father had owned three cars and a sizable house. She showed me a picture of her *quinceañera,* a faded color shot of a young woman in a pink, sixties-style dress and beehive hairdo. The photo was remarkable in its clarity, given its journey from the comfortable middle-class house of her father to the one-room metal shack in which she now lived. After the earthquake, doña Dora's father fell on hard times, and eventually she moved in with her aunt in zona 7 of OPEN III. (Her aunt's house was just across the road from where "El Gato" Aguilar hoisted the "Ciudad Sandino" sign in July 1979, and just a half-block more from what was then the city's sole health post.) By her mid-twenties, doña Dora was spending harvest seasons collecting peanuts on a farm just outside the OPEN, not far from present-day Nueva Vida. As a young woman she was poor, but after the revolution she was among the first in her neighborhood to be trained as a brigadista. She involved herself in Sandinista literacy and maternal health campaigns and, starting in the 1990s, in MINSA's antidengue campaigns. Doña Dora worked loyally for MINSA during the 1990s and 2000s, and she heartily embraced the new FSLN government's vision of social mobilization when Ortega was reelected. She remained a brigadista well into her fifties, even though, like many women of her age, type II diabetes was robbing her of her eyesight and her teeth and threatening her limbs.

Doña Dora was, self-consciously, an old-guard activist. When new health campaigns were announced, she was first in line at the health center to sign up. Frankly, she needed the small stipend she received for this work, but she also volunteered as a teacher of reading and as a cook at a local children's kitchen. Indeed, she was so dogged in her determination to participate that MINSA and *alcaldía* leaders would visibly roll their eyes when she lumbered into their offices, requesting medical care for herself or her neighbors, or demanding this improvement or that in the condition of the roads in Nueva Vida. She would organize groups of neighbors or children to accompany her on these ventures, but usually they fizzled. "The last sixteen years," she told me, "have been an era of vanity. People are out for themselves. It's un-Christian."

Things had changed so much that the health center's director, its head epidemiology nurse, and the director of city sanitation—two out of three of these avowed Sandinistas—routinely accused doña Dora of being "selfish." When she ran out of medication for her diabetes, she would arrive at the health center before it opened at 6:00 A.M., waiting all day for a consultation. When the government pharmacist would tell her that no medication was available, as he nearly always did, I would see her shuffling from office to office in search of the drugs that she knew must be available. "I've been a brigadista for twenty years," she would mutter. "I know they have *medicamentos* [medicines]. The ones on the INSS [those who received national health insurance, mostly those who were or had been formally employed] get *medicamentos*. We deserve them, too."[60]

Health center staff, mostly sympathetic, would have to turn her away, whispering to one another about the shameful "true story." Doña Dora, they alleged, was selling her medicine to feed her daughter. Early in my fieldwork, doña Dora, who knew of my connections in the sanitation department, asked me to follow up on her request for cement to repair her and her neighbors' fences. (The fences, slender wooden posts with strands of barbed wire, had been toppled by drunks and thieves.) When I mentioned doña Dora's name to the sanitation director, he chuckled, "That woman. . . . We've given that woman plenty of favors! And don't let her tell you she's working for the community. We're all working for the community, but we don't give out favors." Clearly, the director told me, doña Dora just wanted a nicer house.

Something had changed in the city in the years since doña Dora first became a brigadista. How did community-based social support become "favors?" In contemporary Ciudad Sandino, it was hard for city and ministry leaders to tell when old-style communitarian rhetoric was being used for personal gain. More striking, however, was the manner in which questions about the *reasons* for infrastructure deterioration or health problems were being omitted from official discourse. Homes and bodies were increasingly isolated as sites of responsible, individualized decisions and behaviors. Compare the diarrhea brochure from the 1980s (figure 1) to the dengue brochure in figure 2.

In figure 2, from a dengue campaign carried out during my fieldwork, many similar elements exist. There is a disease, posed as a problem, and a spatial and aesthetic rendering of that problem. Whereas the viewer in figure 1 is invited to "analyze the picture" and think about the questions it raises, in figure 2 the brochure answers its own questions. Dengue can be avoided through a series of steps, inspecting the house once a week to eliminate mosquito breeding spots. As in figure 1, the brochure in figure 2 presents an implicitly "healthy" house, but there is no interrogation of *why* the house is healthy. The implication is that the occupant is following hygienic recommendations.

The brochure's summarizing statement, "De nosotros depende evitar el dengue" ("It's up to us to prevent dengue") is telling. There is no mention of community leaders, brigadistas, or anything beyond the individual. Figure 2 offers a radically different view of citizenship from that posited in figure 1. There is no room in figure 2 for what Freire calls "critical intervention," a hallmark of revolutionary primary care in Nicaragua.[61] The authority of biomedicine is paramount. As in the PROMAPER model of infrastructure building, full citizenship is a given here—as it may not have been in the 1970s and 1980s—but the manner in which individuals can act as citizens is circumscribed. Infrastructure, once so integrally alive in discussions of health and social rights, becomes an individual responsibility to fulfill, rather than a social right to be seized. Indeed, to assert, as doña

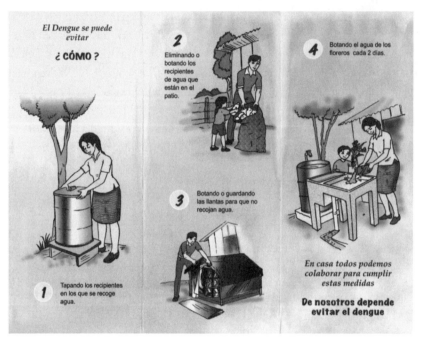

FIGURE 2. A MINSA brochure: "Dengue can be avoided. How?" (Author's archival collection)

Dora did, that one had the *right* to medicine or to cement for one's walls was to be unrealistic and selfish.[62]

ALL ROADS LEAD TO THE ZONA FRANCA

Infrastructures are both reflective and productive of the political economic contexts in which they emerge. The 1990s and 2000s were an era of rapid economic liberalization throughout Latin America, and in Ciudad Sandino the creation of zonas francas, or free trade zones, was the most obvious spatial manifestation of this. Around the time they were planning PROMAPER, the liberal governments of Alemán and his successor, Enrique Bolaños, signed a series of "free trade" agreements, culminating in the Central American Free Trade Agreement with the United States. These allowed Japanese, Korean, Taiwanese, and American multinationals to build apparel factories in and around Ciudad Sandino and the neighboring towns of Mateare and Los Brasiles and to operate them nearly tax-free. Beginning in the early years of the new century, employment opportunities, especially for young women, began to increase. Bus lines devoted to delivering labor to the zonas francas ran in and out of Ciudad Sandino nearly twenty-four hours a day, and new highways were built to carry eighteen-wheel trucks loaded with jeans, T-shirts, and other items from the factories to the airport in Managua. In 2007, the U.S.-based International Textile Group built a spur from the new León highway on Ciudad Sandino's east side purely for this purpose. Ironically, given the area's agricultural history, the inbound trucks came down that highway laden with bales of imported cotton, which workers from Ciudad Sandino spun into denim fabric. The effluent from the washing and dyeing process discharged into the city's network of *cauces*. The *cauces* and the proximity to the aquifer that fed the *tubos madres* were a major selling point in the government's campaign to bring the International Textile Group to Ciudad Sandino.

Spurs of highway and massive factories have replaced cotton fields as the most prominent landmarks in periurban Managua, but they have also come to symbolize an uncomfortable individualism. During my fieldwork, zona franca workers were among the highest paid in Ciudad Sandino, but they consistently failed to secure salary and benefits through labor unionization.[63] Changes in the physical organization of Ciudad Sandino, including the growth of highways and factories, the establishment of local government, and the founding of Nueva Vida, were paralleled at a national level by alterations in the organizational infrastructure of health care and health education. While urban Latin America's low-income and ethnically marginalized populations have seen their legal powers to vote, to assemble, and to control social services increase over the past two decades, they have had to devise new methods of converting these individual rights into meaningful forms of collective citizenship.

As anthropologist Julia Paley has argued, national elites and supranational organizations such as the International Monetary Fund, World Bank, and the Inter-American Development Bank have come to view the resurgence of democracy across Latin America as a vindication of their belief in the power of markets and individual entrepreneurship to solve social ills. In her ethnographic work on a community health organization in a Santiago shantytown, Paley shows that the demand among politicians, activists, and scholars for "participation" can effectively place responsibility for basic services such as health and sanitation in the hands of poor, underfunded citizen groups. Physical and social reforms precipitated new conceptions of the role of citizens in the building, maintenance, and transformation of health and the built environment.[64] Given Nicaragua's strong history of collective mobilization, it is perhaps not surprising that the move from collective solidarity to individual responsibility has been partial rather than totalizing.

The dengue prevention campaigns I describe in the following chapters took place in the context of this struggle between personal and communitarian models of responsibility for health and for space. Dengue seemed oddly appropriate as the disease of that moment, in that it brought state and nongovernmental attention to households, rather than to the material and institutional infrastructures that connected them. The particular behavior patterns of the mosquito—its adaptation to humans and the intimate, private spaces they occupied—made the house seem like the site at which biomedical knowledge should be developed and deployed. Despite the neutral rhetoric of contemporary MINSA brochures and educational materials, debates about the causes and mitigation of dengue are alive and well. What kinds of citizenship are possible in the age of dengue? What happens when houses—and not roads, pipes, and electrical wires—become sites of participation and knowledge? Finally, is it the case—at it seems in Ciudad Sandino—that when infrastructure makes "sustainable peripheries" of erstwhile slums and shantytowns, solidarity and collective capacities for healing really diminish?[65] Chapter 2 returns to Nueva Vida and the question of differential habits, with a contemporary story about the entanglement of infrastructure and public health.

TWO

Patrons, Clients, and Parasites

SOURCE REDUCTION

I am trudging slowly behind a garbage truck as it winds through zona 10. The streets here are mostly short alleys *(callejones)* that all spur off of a main central artery. These *callejones* are not just short but perilously narrow. This means that after we've tossed just five or six houses' worth of garbage sacks up to the bed of the truck, don Gilberto has to effect a multipoint turn to get us headed back to the main road. At first, the process of collection seems familiar and tedious. *Recolectores* (they are all men) pick up bags of refuse in each house, transfer their contents to a truck or trailer bed, and walk off to the next house. Things get more interesting when the bed fills up. That is when we load up and drive to the municipal dump.

Ciudad Sandino's dump is a disused farm field that the city leases from a large landholder. There are two ways in and out. One is by municipal vehicle: usually a white Toyota dump truck whose doors are adorned with weatherworn stickers that read "DONATED BY JAPAN." Drivers like don Gilberto prefer to go in and out rapidly. In the dry season, this means that the *recolectores* who ride atop the mounds of refuse in the exposed bed become shrouded in a fine red dust. In the rainy season, the trucks splash through mud puddles, garbage gets heavy with moisture, and chances are high that the vehicles will become stuck in the furrows of the dump, which sits adjacent to Nueva Vida.

Before unloading the garbage, most crews make a quick stop on the entrance road that divides the field from Nueva Vida. There, the *recolectores* in the bed jump out and jog into a nearby house, a structure made of wood and sheet metal surrounded by a flimsy fence of immature tree trunks and a few

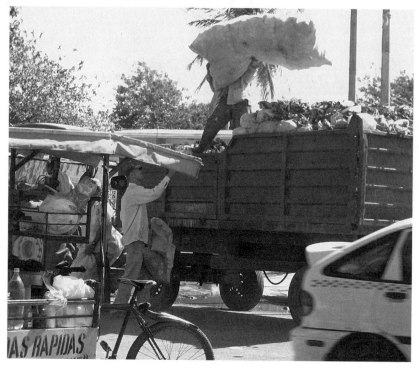

FIGURE 3. City garbage collectors unload a large sack of plastic bottles for sale at a chatarrero. (Photo by the author, 2008)

strands of rusty barbed wire, spilling into the *cauce* that separates the barrio from the entrance road. The *recolectores* haul massive plastic grain sacks filled with their day's catch of *chatarra*. (*Chatarra,* literally "junk," is the omnibus term in Nicaragua for recyclable materials, from plastic bottles to cans, copper wiring, scrap iron, and paper.) A woman in the house will weigh and buy these items. While awaiting payment from the buyer (or *chatarrero*), the *recolectores* might cross paths with garbage scavengers like doña Flor, a fiftyish-year-old woman who works in the dump picking out the recyclables that the crews leave behind (see figures 3 and 4).

On this day, I decide to say goodbye to don Gilberto and his crew and accompany doña Flor to her house. She leads me on the other route out of the dump, by foot over the *cauce* and down the narrow road into Nueva Vida. She walks slowly, a spiked metal prod for sifting through rubbish piles balanced on her shoulder. For me, her pace through the barrio, shaded from the sun that scorches the treeless dump, is as refreshing in its ease as the rides on

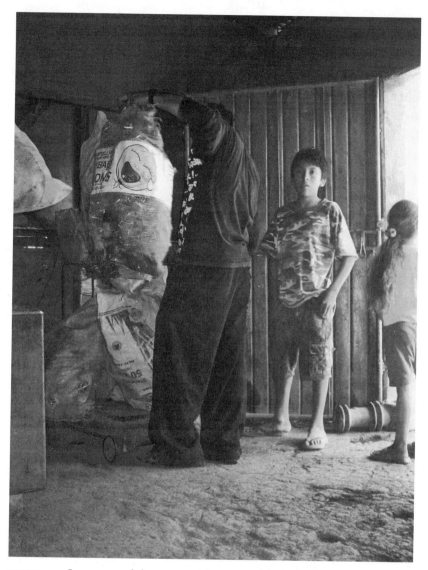

FIGURE 4. Scavengers and chatarrero weighing items. (Photo by the author, 2008)

the garbage trucks were in their briskness. She shares her house with two sons and a few grandchildren. The house, too, has a flimsy barbed wire fence enclosing piles of recyclables. The piles grow and shrink inversely with the market prices of the materials they contain.

Over the weeks and months, recyclables move in and out of her house and in and out of Ciudad Sandino in a waste stream that flows from scavengers to small buyers, on to large brokers in Managua, and ultimately to faraway ports on other continents.[1] The stream bears money, people, and product brand identities. Insects also ride along. The mosquitoes that carry dengue sometimes lay eggs in the things doña Flor and others collect. When those things fill with water, the eggs hatch into larvae, mature into pupae, and emerge as mosquitoes, poised to feed on the blood of infected people and spread the virus.

Unlike the arguably more famous *Anopheles* mosquito, the genus that breeds in large bodies of water and transmits malaria, *Ae. aegypti* breeds in small places, from used car tires to the overturned tops of soda bottles. *Ae. aegypti* is more difficult to control than its distant cousins in genus *Anopheles* because it occupies the intimate, private spaces people call home. Given its adaptability to households and their surroundings, controlling *Ae. aegypti*—and thus controlling dengue fever—requires, first, that communities have effective water and waste management. Second, someone must inform individuals about the mosquito and its breeding habits and convince them that they should be on the lookout for potential breeding sites. In the early years of the twenty-first century, these two priorities, waste/water management and communication, have led MINSA to undertake a house-to-house "source reduction" strategy against *Ae. aegypti*. The goal of this strategy is to make the urban environment unwelcoming to the mosquito by encouraging people, through a combination of insecticide application, public education, and law enforcement, to rid their homes of potential breeding sites, or "sources," including waste.[2]

SANITARY CITIZENSHIP

The growing number of dengue epidemics across the globe has caused experts and citizens to contemplate anew an idea that dates back for centuries. That idea is that bodily and environmental conditions are connected. As I write, the Intergovernmental Panel on Climate Change is reaffirming the scientific consensus that global warming puts some people, particularly residents of low-income cities like Ciudad Sandino, at higher risk for infectious diseases such as cholera, malaria, and dengue.[3] The body's connection to its surroundings may seem self-evident, but in the context of public health governance, such a recognition produces new kinds of risks and new kinds of obligations. From a liberal economic point of view, all citizens share some blame for climate change because each person's behavioral choices—for example, driving in lieu of walking, using too much electricity—contribute to the problem. As "global" citizens, we are told, we all must contemplate and act upon the collective health burden of global climate change.[4] Of course, this calculus makes some "more responsible" than others, and disputes over degrees of accountability have been central to governments' refusals to act on the issue.

Disputes about the links between collective risk and personal responsibility, like ideas about the connection between health and the environment, are nothing new in Ciudad Sandino. Indeed, such disputes are a key part of public health across Latin America. As Charles Briggs suggests, ideas about who is capable of contemplating and acting on environmental health risk and who, by dint of racial, ethnic, or gendered discrimination, is doomed to be victimized or demonized constitute a domain of "sanitary citizenship."[5] In the case of dengue, the making of sanitary citizens means fostering a recognition that things, people, and mosquitoes are entangled and determining differing levels of responsibility for managing that entanglement.

From my earliest visits to Ciudad Sandino, concerns about the proliferation of mosquitoes seemed to parallel concerns about the proliferation of garbage. Discarded containers, tires, and other items make good breeding grounds for mosquitoes, but how, exactly, did the movements of these inanimate things connect to the movements of insects and people? Were sanitary citizens emerging amid Nicaragua's dengue epidemics?

Sanitation has been a central element in Nicaraguan dengue control since the 1980s. Tied to a shifting set of governments, health-oriented hygiene efforts produced new anxieties about collective and personal responsibility for public health. These were on display during my first visit to Nicaragua in 2006, when MINSA began using dump trucks and megaphones to stop the spread of dengue fever. In weekend-long campaigns, doctors, garbage collectors, and brigadistas exhorted homeowners to discard the plastic, rubber, and scrap metal piled in their homes. Brigadistas walked alongside the garbage trucks, reminding residents that mosquitoes lay eggs in the pools of rainwater that form in those piles, and that there was neither a cure nor an effective vaccine for dengue. The legacies of an earlier era of Sandinista-inspired collective action were apparent in these campaigns. Doctors and other health workers spoke vividly about the consequences of inaction: the spread of a virus that causes hemorrhagic fevers, physical impairment, and even death. But the campaigns failed to create a consensus among residents about how to stop dengue from spreading. Instead, they aggravated social divisions among health workers, city garbage collectors, and the garbage scavengers who survived by collecting items in streets and neighborhood dumps and selling them to recycling companies. These divisions arose not over how to define the disease (no one disputed that dengue was a problem) but over how to foster community participation in public health, how to manage space, and how to balance resources and hazards in the landscape. In short, they were about the limits to sanitary citizenship.

Managing waste is easier said than done, especially when, for people like doña Flor, waste is often not actually waste at all. Waste is itself an entanglement of relationships. Consider this story, taken from my field notes for December 22, 2008, after a visit to the house of a group of scavengers:

> The patio of the . . . house was empty of almost all stuff, evidence that they had sold their stored plastic, etc. for Christmas. Their five-year-old son . . . mentioned to me after spotting a stray electrical plug on the ground that they had a bit of copper wire indoors. He then volunteered that "they [chatarreros] buy steel, scrap metal, aluminum, and copper." I asked him if he could tell the difference between these, and he said yes. So I asked him what his little bicycle was made of. "Hierro [Steel]," he said. So how much would that be worth on the market? He studied the bike carefully, stroking the handlebars, flicking the chain, and spinning the plastic tires (not "hierro," he reminded me). "Cinco pesos," he said.
>
> Not much, then, I commented.
>
> He said that the price was fair, considering how light the bike was, picking it up with his right hand to demonstrate. A bigger bike would fetch more, naturally. Then he got back on it, and as he drove around me in a tight circle, he told me that THIS bike was a gift from his aunt, who got it from his grandmother in Las Torres (a barrio in Managua). She had brought it to him "like new," and it was still a "good bicycle." I agreed and let him continue his little sprints back and forth across the dry strip of street that ran along the muddy gutter running from the front of his house.

At five, the boy was starting to see things both for their base material contents and as items of sentimental or personal value. Thus, this little bicycle, purple with white hard-plastic wheels, a loose chain, and one pedal missing—as standard a child's toy as existed in Ciudad Sandino—could be distinguished from "a bicycle" in the abstract. The boy could break it into its constituent parts and raw materials, just as when he saw the plug on the ground. When he saw the plug, he thought of copper, but he also told me about the TV and stereo set that had been stolen from his family's house, and about the DVD player they now had, which worked, but not if it heated up too much and not unless the discs it played were clean before you put them in. That equipment, too, was both potential raw material and a personal possession with a "social life."[6]

I heard often about the multiple identities of things from brigadistas, who worked from house to house carrying out the source reduction strategy, telling people like doña Flor and this boy's parents about *Ae. aegypti* and trying to convince them it was their responsibility to control it. The boy didn't balk at the thought of his bicycle both as a personal gift and as potential chatarra. He saw it both ways, at the same time, with a different toolkit of emotions. Breaking the bike into its valuable parts placed him in a social category, that of the garbage scavenger, but talking about his aunt's generosity did not. Seen through dengue control models based on source reduction, the presence of recyclables in homes like the boy's or doña Flor's indicated a deficiency in the garbage service and a breakdown in people's relationships to waste. The point of a modern waste service and public health program was to get such items *out* of houses. But doña Flor and the boy's parents were providing for their families. Garbage, as scavengers and brigadistas alike would often half-joke, was "gold." And mosquitoes, for their part, lived not only in garbage but in items of material culture that were more permanent features of household landscapes: flower pots, gutters, and cisterns, for example. The oscillation of material from refuse to resource occurred alongside an oscillation in perceptions of household space, from safe human habitat to pathological insect harbor, and of householders, from potential dengue victims to potential dengue spreaders. Changes in the process by which garbage was traded in the city and beyond had particular impacts on the ways in which people experienced dengue, as well as on the ecology of the disease itself.

GARBAGE ECONOMIES, DISEASE ECOLOGIES

The year 2008 saw two turning points in the relationships between Ciudad Sandino's garbage scavengers, its mosquitoes, and the Nicaraguan state. The first turning point came in March, when scavengers organized blockades of the dumps in Ciudad Sandino and nearby Managua. Until 2006, the scavengers had a nearly uncontested claim to garbage of value, but persistent poverty and a spike in global demand for recyclables changed both the geography and the demography of scavenging. From late 2005 to mid-2008, worldwide prices for recyclable materials soared. City garbage collectors like don Gilberto and his crew, whose work gave them easy access to the waste stream, took special advantage of the boom, picking up large amounts of plastic, metal, and aluminum on their daily routes. This on-route recycling sparked the scavengers' protests. For several days they lobbed rocks at city vehicles that dared to enter the dumps. They demanded that city leaders order garbage collectors to stop selecting and selling plastic, aluminum, paper, and scrap metal during their work routes.

Both scavengers and garbage collectors recognized not only that without their labor, recyclables could not realize their market value, but also that without their efforts, the city could not come close to being clean. Although both groups tried to secure exclusive access to garbage of value, neither found a satisfying way to convince the city government that it deserved rights to collect. Both groups were trying to secure their positions as what scholars of Latin American politics call "clients" to powerful "patrons" in the city government.[7] Elaborated in the postindependence period, the concept of patron-clientelism helps explain how wealth and power become distributed systematically across spaces that government institutions cannot reach. In the ideal-typical version, "patrons" use wealth and generosity to mobilize the labor of poorer clients, who reciprocate with political loyalty. Importantly, individuals may play the role of both patron and client simultaneously. A small-time patron may in turn be the client of an even more powerful person. At each level, people sacrifice their individual rights as citizens for material goods. Thus, a system based on patron-clientelism—as Ciudad Sandino's garbage economy largely was—is somewhat at odds with the goal of free, individual "sanitary" citizenship, as well as with a free and open market.[8] The scavengers saw city leaders' tacit approval of the garbage collectors' actions as a violation of an implied moral contract. They, not the collectors, deserved to pick up the city's valuable wastes.

But the situation was not that simple. Though the garbage collectors appeared to hold familiar, modern public works jobs, they depended on strong relationships with political bosses for their job security. Civic leaders, likewise, needed someone to keep the city minimally clean. Their patronage was not simple generosity. They, too, depended on formal and informal garbage collectors to validate their own political legitimacy.

If the dump conflict marked the first turning point in the relationships between garbage scavengers, mosquitoes, and the state, then the Plan Chatarra, a nationwide campaign devised by MINSA in 2008 to ban scavenging and garbage trading from city centers and relegate it to areas far from homes and shops, marked the second. The implication of the Plan Chatarra was clear: trash was dirty; dirt bred bugs and rodents; bugs and rodents carried disease to people; concentrations of trash must also lead to concentrations of sickness. One official emphasized in the conservative daily newspaper *La Prensa* that "chatarreras are sites of large mosquito breeding areas. . . . [These] businesses have exposed more of the population to . . . dengue."[9] Patron-client relations were central to the chatarra business as well. Large, well-capitalized chatarra buyers in Managua would routinely sponsor smaller buyers. These smaller buyers, in turn, would work to develop reputations among scavengers as fair-minded and generous in their payouts.

Both the disputes at the dump and the Plan Chatarra reveal how persons and things and creatures that look singular can have multiple identities. The work of collecting and circulating garbage was a mode of *personal* survival that, paradoxically, threatened *population* health. Garbage scavengers were alternately the cause of and the solution to the dengue crisis. The state and the health ministry seemed to be acting both to promote the welfare of the city's poorest residents and to undermine it.

In Ciudad Sandino, as in other places, waste has long been a focus of mosquito source reduction efforts, whether in organized, one-off cleaning campaigns or in more routine house-to-house mosquito source reduction visits. While some have posited links between inadequate solid waste control and dengue, those links tend to be simplified. Studies tend to characterize the wastes that can become mosquito-breeding sites as problems typical of "consumer societies."[10] An emphasis on such problems as consumptive mischaracterizes them as deficiencies in local political will and local peoples' desires to eliminate waste. Discourses about the "choice" to scavenge or otherwise harbor garbage that might play host to mosquitoes spin an "apolitical" narrative of dengue ecology.[11] What is missing is an investigation of how economic pressures and social relationships entangle the social lives of mosquitoes and people with those of nonliving materials, making the ideal of sanitary citizenship impossible to achieve.

In late 2008, I interviewed don Dionisio, who had been a chatarrero in Ciudad Sandino for just under two years. At the peak of his business, he had a fleet of pickup trucks and a staff of employees plying the streets of Ciudad Sandino, buying chatarra directly from people's homes. Don Dionisio would then sell this chatarra to a larger broker in Managua. When I asked him to tell me who owned the newly valuable garbage, he answered with a riddle:

"The fish in the sea could be anyone's, right? But the owner of the fish is the one who goes fishing." Did he mean that garbage was common property?

It is certainly not news that some city dwellers, from North Carolina to Nicaragua to Nairobi, survive by scavenging for garbage of value, but from late 2005 until the global financial meltdown of 2008, the world market for recyclables reached unprecedented heights.[12] As market prices for recyclables went up, the number of scavengers also increased, and scavengers, a group that included families that had been collecting and selling recyclable waste for generations, saw their claims to that material deteriorate rather than improve. From just ten licensed chatarreras in 2005, the city counted twenty-six by the end of 2008. Scavengers I interviewed in 2008 told me that increased competition during the price boom caused their earnings for an eight-hour workday to drop to a low of just thirty córdobas (roughly $1.50) from a high of more than one hundred córdobas. The average adult supported at least three family members.[13] The entanglement of human bodies with mosquitoes and garbage was thus mediated by economic volatility. Just as dengue epidemics can spike rapidly in unexpected places due to circulation of people, viruses, and materials and then recede with little warning, global prices for aluminum, steel, plastics, and paper rise and fall with impressive speed. Over the course of 2008, Nicaragua's garbage trade reached a climax, producing up to forty million dollars for the national economy.[14] Later that year, in the wake of the global economic crisis, the business crashed. It was during the boom, however, that the protest in the dumps occurred and the Plan Chatarra was put into action.

GARBAGE, ABJECTION, AND CONFLICT

A scavenger-turned-chatarrera gave me a brief history of the garbage trade in Ciudad Sandino. Around 1998, after rains from Hurricane Mitch flooded homes on the shores of Lake Managua, government resettlement plans moved some scavengers to Nueva Vida. "We kept scavenging," she said of the move. "Back then there was lots of garbage coming in, and no one else bothered with it." Like other displaced families, hers had been scavenging since the opening of Managua's large open-air dump in 1972. (The Nicaraguan term for "garbage scavenger," *churequero,* comes from the nickname for Managua's dump, "La Chureca.") She told me that after the hurricane she and her husband had been able to salvage their horse cart, into which they would pack material from Ciudad Sandino and drive from Nueva Vida to Managua, where buyers paid better prices. In 2007, they were approached by one of these buyers, who helped them finance a pickup truck, scales, and a small storage lot. By the time of our interview, she and her husband were patronized by an even larger broker. They weighed and bought recyclables from both churequeros and city garbage collectors.

Everyone involved in the trade kept up with the prices for different materials, from plastic and paper on the cheaper end to copper and bronze on the higher end. The key to being a good chatarrero and cultivating a base of client churequeros was a reputation not just for prices that matched the accepted daily rate but for fair weights and measures. Churequeros quickly turned on patrons whom they considered dishonest with scales, and chatarreros were careful to inspect sacks of material before payment, looking for rocks and sand hidden within to increase their weight and value.

As these checks and balances developed, a steady supply of waste streamed into Ciudad Sandino. Trucks from nearby apparel factories established in zonas francas carted scrap shoe soles, shredded fabric, and giant plastic packing sacks—all recyclable, all valuable—into the dump. In the early years of the new century, the number of zonas francas was growing. During the same period, noted Adán, who worked as a churequero, municipal solid waste was becoming more saturated with valuable items. Consumption patterns among his neighbors were changing along with the economy. He gave a convenient example. "Before, nobody drank Agua Pura [a local bottled water brand]. Now you see plastic water bottles, plastic coke bottles . . . before it was all glass bottles." Adán grew up in the Americas Dos barrio of Managua and also moved to Nueva Vida after the 1998 hurricane. His wife and brothers-in-law were also churequeros. He and others tried several times to formally organize the churequeros, but some suspected him of working to benefit himself politically—to tap into aid money or resources and redistribute them as a kind of petty political patron, or *caudillo*.

A labor organization of sorts finally did emerge—albeit with no clear leader—when the churequeros started to come to the consensus that the city garbage collectors' poaching of the waste stream had become intolerable. When I asked Adán why the scavengers had protested, he couched their action in moral terms, arguing that going into the dump every day and collecting for eight to ten hours was preferable to working on the streets. He told me that this hard work, in a recognizable workplace, helped keep people away from drugs and crime. In a city where formal employment was difficult to find, *chureque-*

ando was a morally acceptable alternative to other "underground" methods of making a living. Adán did not understand why city leaders should undermine this by allowing city collectors, who already had paying jobs, to scavenge. He added that workmates who ventured into the streets to look for chatarra were seen as "delinquents," "thieves," and "vagrants." Like most churequeros, Adán recognized that as either undereducated young people or "older" (i.e., older than thirty) adults, churequeros' chances of securing formal employment in places like the zonas francas were small. Churequeros, in other words, were cut out of a new system of trade and work that had allowed cheap, recyclable materials to proliferate in Nicaragua. Recalling the older form of trade and work, based on patron-clientage, they framed their blockade of the dump as the effort of a group of maligned clients to press their patrons to treat them fairly. They asserted that their work in the dump was a contribution to the city. "Put it this way," another churequero told me after the strike: "How would it be if we *didn't* live this way? We'd really be the worst city in Nicaragua."

In negotiations with the garbage collectors and the churequeros, city supervisors tried to remain neutral. Drawing on a liberal market logic, they maintained (at least publicly) that the streets were a free range. The garbage in them was an open resource. Once waste hit the sidewalk, anyone could sort through it. Those who might profit from its circulation should not be stopped. Still, when we spoke, Ciudad Sandino's municipal services director, Licenciado Felipe Lopez, acknowledged the poor public image that garbage collectors' participation in recycling gave the city. The thirty-five-year-old Lopez usually put the title *Licenciado* in front of his name because he was a university-educated engineer. (In this, he was not unusual. All higher-education degrees in Nicaragua tend to come with titles.) He grew up in Ciudad Sandino, and his family had long been active in politics. Aside from running municipal services, he was a political secretary for the FSLN in his barrio. Lic. Lopez was responsible for hiring the city's sanitation supervisor, a high managerial position that tended to go to a person who was strongly connected to the party. The sanitation supervisor coordinated all garbage collection activities and was the de facto manager of the city dump. While Lic. Lopez recognized the churequeros' complaints about the collectors as legitimate, he reminded me that the city had limited power to govern the dump. His priority was to keep the peace there and to keep garbage trucks flowing in and out.

The garbage collectors all belonged to a labor union, which was affiliated with the national federation of municipal workers, also a historically FSLN-dominated organization. Shortly after I arrived in Ciudad Sandino, the union successfully pressured Lic. Lopez to fire the city sanitation supervisor, partly on suspicion that he had a financial interest in backing a move by churequeros to organize themselves. Moreover, as garbage collectors told me, the supervisor was intentionally divisive, reassigning routes and rearranging crews without notice, and even hiring someone to take time-stamped, digital photographs of collectors selling recyclable materials to chatarreros. The collectors suggested in meetings with Lic. Lopez that the supervisor was taking these actions in order to turn the churequeros into a loyal and personally accountable "work force."[15] This was a violation of the collectors' understanding of their moral relationship to the city government. Twinges of the early Sandinista ethos of community-state solidarity ran through their protests. Collectors claimed that when crews switched routes, for example, moving from a neighborhood where they were well known to one where they were relative strangers, cooperation from the public suffered. Each crew had its own timing and its own method of plying the streets. Even if they were steadily paid city employees, the gregarious, smelly, and sweaty male garbage crews had to be careful to seem courteous and honest to the people whose waste they collected. Good work was rewarded, particularly at Christmastime, with tips of food and cash from grateful neighbors. In cultivating the loyalty of the churequeros, the supervisor was costing the collectors. Lic. Lopez eventually replaced that supervisor with the president of the local municipal workers' union.

Don Gilberto was one of the garbage collectors' most passionate spokesmen. He could recall the early days of the city's collection service, when he and others drove through the muddied barrios in tractors, carts, and borrowed half-ton pickup trucks picking up the garbage. A rugged, long-haired man who had spent much of his youth on a relative's cattle farm, his views on health were unique: he was a self-described *naturalista* who avoided doctors and pharmaceutical medicines whenever possible. (He used to claim that dengue was curable with herbal remedies.) His particular interest in health made him unusual, perhaps, but like most collectors, he viewed the churequeros as unwelcome refugees who should not benefit from the work that the community's founders had done.

Though collectors acknowledged that the churequeros made a living from scavenging, don Gilberto and other union activists argued that what churequeros did was not really "work." During the March 2008 blockades, those who opposed the churequeros argued against the possibility that scavengers could collectively bargain. As Ulrich Schilz, Managua's sanitation supervisor, declared in an editorial published in the normally left-leaning newspaper *El Nuevo Diario,* "The churequeros are not workers; they are informal businesspeople who sell their labor to no one. They exploit themselves, a few with great success. . . . The only one who gives value to a product is the worker. . . . In this case, the product is the organization and cleaning of garbage. . . . The agents of the informal, opportunistic economy don't add any value to this product."[16] The opinion of Ciudad Sandino's garbage collectors' union approximated that of Sr. Schilz. From the union's point of view, the churequeros were not working in cooperation with a party or a government. They were parasites, living on the margins of the city. Collectors represented themselves more positively, as underpaid and overworked providers of a "service." The city could never pay collectors enough in cash for the service they rendered. It owed them the chance to make extra money by recycling.

Yet senses of moral obligation among city collectors were more complex. Don Nelson, another garbage truck driver, confessed in an interview: "I don't really think we should be doing it, and we didn't do it so much before. The churequeros are poor and they live on the garbage. But I . . . let the others [the *recolectores,* who put garbage into the truck] recycle. They don't earn as much money as I do; they also need the income." Don Nelson had lived in Ciudad Sandino since 1980 and worked for the city since it became an independent municipality in 2000. He was a Shell gasoline attendant in Managua during the 1970s and helped organize a clandestine station workers' union with a group of fellow Sandinistas. When the revolution became violent, he continued his involvement and was injured in the *repliegue,* the tactical retreat of militants from Managua to Masaya in 1979 in the run-up to the final Sandinista takeover of Managua. He still walked with a limp and had kidney problems that came from that injury. In the past he had been a union leader, but he had surrendered his position due to "exhaustion" with local politics. He left negotiations to more powerful and better-educated men like Lic. Lopez and younger colleagues like don Gilberto, but he was ambivalent about the union's defense of scavenging. As a necessary but reviled outgrowth of consumption, garbage was a stain on the entire community, but as an economic resource, it was, at least intuitively, "for" those really in need.

Garbage collectors' relationships to the city government and to churequeros were both moral and economic.[17] If don Gilberto was correct that his former supervisor was favoring the churequeros over the city collectors, he had a moral reason to be outraged. But don Nelson was also correct: the churequeros were precisely the kinds of people that the Sandinista revolution was supposed to bring into the community of citizens. The churequeros were not simply economic adversaries, and the government patrons were not simply distributors of resources.

The dump protests ended in a partial victory for the garbage collectors' union. Each collecting crew, led by a truck driver like don Gilberto or don Nelson, negotiated with the churequeros about which materials it would salvage and sell and which it would leave for those in the dump. Even before dengue entered the picture, the politics of chatarra in Ciudad Sandino centered on a set of contradictions. Was waste a collective nuisance or a privatizable resource? Could it be both? If waste was a nuisance or, worse, a threat to public health, what would best control it, state regulation or a more streamlined market?[18] The Plan Chatarra, which went into effect just weeks after the settlement of the dump strike, only piled on the paradoxes.

THE PLAN CHATARRA

Chatarreros saw the Plan Chatarra as scapegoating. In a June 2008 meeting at Ciudad Sandino's main health center, they asked repeatedly for "proof" that their businesses were sites of mosquito propagation. "We fumigate," they said. "We have sanitary licenses from the city, from MINSA." "Why this sudden change in the rules?" "How come we are being held responsible *now* if we know dengue affects us every year?"

The health center's director, wielding a dry erase marker, tried to explain the health implications of Nicaragua's garbage economy for his audience. "You see," he began, "there are large brokerages, medium brokerages, and small—we say 'family'—brokerages." He drew parallel horizontal lines on the board to schematically indicate the large, medium, and small brokerages. As he descended, each line became longer, forming a pyramid. Then, below the last line, which indicated the "family" brokerages, he began making vertical, slashing hash marks, indicating that they were more numerous than the large and medium ones. "What's the problem with all these small brokerages?" he asked, not waiting for a response. "They are inside the barrios, inside the . . . center of the city." He circled one of his hash marks, making dots around it. "There are houses, businesses, schools." He paused, almost like a preacher or a schoolteacher giving a scolding. "And what happens when an infected mosquito or an infected rodent [i.e., a rodent infected with the disease leptospirosis, also a concern of MINSA] lives there?" He paused again. Having temporarily silenced the room, he went on to give an extensive recap of the life cycle of the *Ae. aegypti* mosquito, explaining how it might propagate from a chatarrera.

I attended this meeting expecting this sort of interaction: defensiveness from the chatarreros, loquacious scientific speechifying from the MINSA authorities. What I did not expect was the candid appeal to environmental stewardship on the part of the chatarreros that followed. One by one, the chatarreros—mostly men, but a few women—stood to explain to the director that they were "responsible" businesspeople. They were quite aware of the stigma of dealing in garbage, but, they repeated over and over again, "If we did not have this business, where would the garbage go? Who would you blame then?" The chatarreros, they argued, were "cleaning up" the city. Moreover, they were providing employment to a needy population of scavengers. The director's pyramid had yet another rung, even lower and even wider, made up of churequeros, for whom wealthy Nicaraguans also had an entomological nickname: *hormigas* (ants), presumably because a churequero carrying a giant sack of empty bottles or cans resembles an ant lugging an improbably large morsel of food.

"Who are our clients?" One man asked, impatiently. "They are the old, the children, the most poor. If you move us out of the city, where will they go? Are you going to ask an old man to walk five, six kilometers out of town so he can survive? This is their survival!" The brokers left the meeting resolved to make a direct appeal for "evidence" of the mosquito problem from MINSA. I left impressed at they way in which they turned their "dirty business" into a civic contribution. They were styling themselves less as sanitary citizens than as responsible patrons.

To don Eliseo Ordoñez, it was not surprising that MINSA launched the Plan Chatarra when it did, in April 2008. Don Eliseo was the owner and manager of one of Nicaragua's four to five large *centros de acopio,* a patron to many small family chatarreros, and a leader in the Association of Recyclers of Nicaragua (Asociación de Recicladores de Nicaragua, or ASORENIC). He was bilingual, and he had traveled and worked extensively in the United States. His business was one of collection and export. He and a handful of other large chatarreros bought aluminum, plastic, paper, and assorted metals in bulk, loaded them onto shipping containers, and sent them abroad. In the first part of the new century, the destinations of these shipments tended to be in Asia, particularly China, where a boom in construction meant high demand for cheap raw material. In Nicaragua, don Eliseo was politically and socially active. Among other things, he had been involved in the years before the FSLN returned to power with an effort to lobby the Association of Nicaraguan Municipalities to replace municipal garbage collection services with private firms such as his. Starting in 2002, ASORENIC began to style itself as a proenvironment, prohealth organization. In that year, it generated a press release promoting the recycling business as a way to connect Managua to a world of business and wealth, asking, "If they can do it in Miami, in Los Angeles, in Mexico, in Guatemala, in Costa Rica, or in any other country in the world, why NOT in NICARAGUA?" When MINSA initiated the Plan Chatarra, ASORENIC again began making the case that the private sector—not the state—could best handle urban hygiene problems. The firms would pay the cities for the right to collect valuable garbage and profit by selling the vastly increased volume they would yield. Given that projects like the rebuilding of Ciudad Sandino's infrastructure in the days after Hurricane Mitch relied upon private enterprise, such a proposal might not have seemed so far-fetched.

Don Eliseo had no doubt that MINSA had hatched the Plan Chatarra as a response to a political opportunity created by the churequeros' protests. The protests had been covered extensively in the national television and print media. Managua's dump, "La Chureca," was already a high-profile stain on the government's reputation. It was the largest open-air waste facility in Central America, and it had become a regular tour stop for photographers and church and NGO activists looking either to expose the environmental damage it was causing or to alleviate the poverty of its residents. Ciudad Sandino's "chureca" was a similar if less well-known site. Located just a few steps away from a large, private charity health clinic, Ciudad Sandino's dump was also regularly visited by volunteer and aid groups, mostly from the United States and Europe. Given the proliferation of painful images of these dumps and their inhabitants on television, the Internet, and in newspapers, don Eliseo explained, the new FSLN government was under pressure to do something. The protests against garbage collectors who seemed to be skimming resources from their needy residents could not have come at a worse time. They had further undermined the public's trust in city services.[19]

As a result of the protests, don Eliseo told me, with the zeal of a muckraker, "the government realized how lucrative the business is, and they are setting up these restrictions on us so that they can take it over." To don Eliseo, the Plan Chatarra was nothing more than thinly veiled socialism or, better yet, parasitism. The government was using the pretense of dengue to disrupt a long-standing and productive set of reciprocal patron-client relationships that linked large buyers like himself to street-level churequeros. For the business-minded leaders of ASORENIC, the solution to the health and economic problems posed by garbage was not a crackdown on scavenging but a formalization of it. Such a formalization would modernize Nicaragua, improve conditions in the churecas, and—presumably—allow private businesses to handle a problem that the corrupt state was clearly ill-equipped to address. When the Plan Chatarra was put into action, "family" chatarreros cited their role in "cleaning" the city and giving the poorest of the poor a chance to make a living. Large chatarreros like don Eliseo took this narrative of environmental stewardship one step further, playing on the struggles of the poor and trumpeting the market to frame the garbage trade as a "comedy of the commons," in which harvesting waste seemed like a solution to, rather than a symptom of, the ravages of poverty.[20]

Don Eliseo's suspicions about a vast socialist conspiracy notwithstanding, the significance of the timing of the dump conflict and the Plan Chatarra cannot be understated. In mid-2008, Ciudad Sandino and the rest of Managua *were* facing the onset of another dengue epidemic, and traders *were* seeing record highs in the prices of recyclable materials. The number of chatarreras and churequeros was swelling, it seemed, alongside the number of dengue cases. The correlation between this market surge and the epidemic surge was circumstantial rather than causal, but it had power nonetheless.

There is little doubt that the spaces where garbage changes from waste to commodity do sometimes overlap with the spaces where mosquitoes reproduce and spread disease. Mosquitoes, therefore, actively mediated the conflict of economic and environmental management that was occurring at the height of Ciudad Sandino's garbage boom. Waste and mosquitoes "explained each other."[21] The city garbage collection service, however partial, reinforced the idea that the solution to environmental problems began in homes. For people like most residents in my zona, who had access to regular curbside pickup, a failure to dump signaled a glaring absence of social responsibility. Those neighbors who insisted on harboring garbage in their homes were named and shamed by their neighbors. A similar discourse surrounded the management of mosquitoes. Mosquitoes were a public problem that originated in private space. People who refused to have their homes purged of insects faced public rebuke. In the more marginal barrios where scavengers like doña Flor resided, however, the division of space and responsibility into stark categories of public and private did not make as much sense. Houses on Ciudad Sandino's margins were much more tenuously private. Many people in Nueva Vida, including a significant number of churequeros, had constructed their homes out of donated material, on land they did not own. Others were deep in debt to private electrical and water companies. Churequeros who had no legal title to their own houses showed me power bills that reached into the tens of thousands of córdobas. In the face of aggressive bill collectors, house abandonments were a fairly common occurrence. Residents thus had trouble seeing the upkeep of their homes as a long-term private interest, much less a public one.

The idea that dengue "hot spots" can be localized by identifying "high-risk" zones like chatarreras or the homes of churequeros is more easily postulated than proven.[22] *Ae. aegypti* are highly adapted to human movements, breed in small colonies, and are difficult to isolate. In addition, the majority of dengue cases are asymptomatic. Absent a massive sample of human blood for evidence of latent dengue antibodies, there was no practical way that MINSA could have proven that hot spots existed around chatarreros. The Plan Chatarra raised still more pressing questions about how to regulate a disease with no cure or effective prophylactic, in an environment where overcoming poverty often trumped other collective priorities, including health and sanitation.

HYGIENE AND THE MORAL ECONOMY OF MOSQUITO CONTROL

The Plan Chatarra linked the unruliness and uncleanliness of the recycling business to disease, but it was more than the fact that chatarreros traded in garbage that bothered MINSA officials. After all, as don Eliseo, don Dionisio, and other chatarreros reminded me, "We are helping to clean up Nicaragua." The problem was the manner in which they traded. More insidious still, as was noted both in published press accounts and in the June meeting between the director of Ciudad Sandino's health center and the local brokers, was the proximity of "small," "family" recycling brokerages to private homes.[23] Chatarreros were bad neighbors. But MINSA's efforts to regulate them failed to change the system just as completely as did the churequeros' efforts to secure rights to scavenge. That failure stemmed in part from the sheer ambition of the Plan Chatarra. Ending garbage scavenging once and for all would have been nearly impossible. The plan did nevertheless strain the relationship of "client" chatarreros to large "patron" brokers like don Eliseo.

In early summer 2008, the small chatarreros of Ciudad Sandino learned that an advocacy alliance was being formed. An environmental NGO that also claimed to represent banana plantation workers injured by the pesticide Nemagon was being financed by ASORENIC, the consortium of Managua's largest garbage brokers, to organize opposition to the Plan Chatarra. By paying a membership fee to the NGO, Ciudad Sandino's chatarreros would receive a card that identified them as "recyclers," along with a small diploma, and a blue-green, earth-themed sticker to place on their front doors. The sticker read, "We the Chatarreros of Nicaragua demand that the government respect us and allow us to work for the daily bread of our children. God bless this nation. Yes to work! No to unemployment!" Like the churequeros, these normally independent actors would band together, making a moral case for their rights to collect and sell waste.

Doña Nubia was one of the first to join. She opened up a chatarrera in her small house near the main entrance to Ciudad Sandino around 2007. She had lived in the house since the 1980s, when the revolutionary government gave her land as compensation for her husband's death in an industrial accident. For most of her life, she had been a street vendor, selling juices and *sorbetes* at the bus stop near the barrio's entrance. As she got older, that work became a strain on her knees and back, and her grown son, who owned a small pickup truck, suggested that she begin work as a chatarrera. Doña Nubia's chatarrera was typical of the cottage industry that blossomed and withered in the space of a few short "boom" years in the late 2000s. Her main tool was a heavy-duty scale, of the kind that was common in meat or grain stalls in Managua's markets. It was a bronze, spring-calibrated mechanism with a sharp hook attached to one end and an eye attached to the other. Doña Nubia had it nailed to a rafter overhanging her small front porch, which was set a few feet down from street level. On a large piece of scrap roofing metal, her son had fashioned a sign, in black paint, that read SE COMPRA CHATARRA. Churequeros, local schoolchildren, and neighbors would arrive with sacks of plastic, aluminum, steel, copper, or other items (usually presorted), and doña Nubia would weigh them and pay the going per-pound rate, which she set by taking a small reduction from the rate she would receive from a buyer in Managua. Then she would empty the bag into one of the piles of like materials that dotted her patio. When the piles became large enough (or the price spiked high enough), her son would load them into the pickup, take them to the capital, and sell them to a trusted patron.

Like most of the twenty-six other chatarreros in Ciudad Sandino, doña Nubia was visited by representatives of ASORENIC's environmental NGO. The NGO representatives convinced her to pay and join. As they explained, dengue was a danger, but the real problem was that the government was over-regulating the garbage, a nuisance to be sure, but also an "inexhaustible resource." If they would let the chatarreros and businesspeople treat it for what it was, health and wealth would both improve. During the interview at his office, don Eliseo showed me a PowerPoint presentation he had prepared for municipal governments interested in privatizing their garbage services. Its concluding slide contained green words on a gray background: *Basura = $* (Garbage equals money). As one of his own business circulars noted, "Chatarra represents a great source of income, not just for its owner, but for the country, if we just take advantage of it." Don Eliseo was linking the commoditization of garbage to the achievement of health and wealth. MINSA's renewed zeal for regulating recycling, he insisted, had little to do with health.

This, as it turned out, wasn't don Eliseo's first fight against the health ministry. ASORENIC, the chatarra industry's lobby group, had been confronted by MINSA in 2002 over accusations that the industry's dependence on informal collection networks was bad for public health. That year, they sent MINSA an open letter, but they did not directly involve the small-time brokers. In the letter, ASORENIC instead portrayed itself as a group of petty patrons, "Recycling businesspeople, the vast majority of whom are humble, honest, hardworking people, have found a way to make a living, improve their economic situation, and PROVIDE WORK TO THOU-SANDS OF NICARAGUANS." In 2002, MINSA and the rest of the Nicaraguan government were run by a largely probusiness, center-right regime. This message had a supply-side tint that was missing from the "bottom-up" flavor of the 2008 response to MINSA sanctions. The 2008 response was built not around talk of trickle-down economics but around the colorful, earth-themed environmental logo. Though the environmental alliance ASO-RENIC formed was shaky, and its ultimate motives unclear, the quick organization of patron and client chatarreros against MINSA proved somewhat effective. The literally and metaphorically "green" logo started popping up on the walls of chatarreros all around town.

Then September came, and everything changed. The bottom fell out of the scrap metal industry, as the global financial crisis slowed world trade to a crawl. Indeed, in the words of Hilario Zepeda, a chatarrero who was elected to Ciudad Sandino's municipal council on the FSLN ticket earlier in 2008, once the prices went down and the churequeros' dump protests were out of the news, MINSA seemed to forget about them. But Zepeda and every other chatarrero I met in Ciudad Sandino also reported that the environmental NGO ASORENIC had found to represent the industry had also disappeared.

"I think [the NGO] just wanted us to pay our inscription fees, to buy our little ID cards and be done with us," said doña Nubia, whose business failed to survive the price crash. "They won't be back. MINSA won't be back."

Doña Lesbia, a chatarrera who lived in zona 8, concurred. In hindsight, she couldn't understand why the NGO identification card said "recycler" and not chatarrera. Recycling seemed like the act of a conscientious consumer, not a trader. The work of a chatarrera tended to be quite different. She didn't think of herself in any particular way as an environmentalist. The truth was, "chatarra is a dirty thing. It's something that dirties you." A younger woman with little experience in the trade, doña Lesbia was approached by a large buyer in Managua who wanted to make an inroad in zona 8. He loaned her a scale and taught her about how to weigh and value copper, aluminum, bronze, steel, and plastic. When the crash ended her relationship with that patron, she, like doña Nubia, had to diversify. When I met her, she was in the process of starting a door-to-door tortilla business. She kept the "recycler" sticker on the wall of her patio (she liked its bright colors), but as a small chatarrera, she no longer mattered, either as an object of state scrutiny or as a symbol of "sustainable" capitalism.[24]

Doña Lesbia's ambivalence about being called a "recycler" was telling. Perhaps she was aware of her status as a vulnerable "middle person," a parasitic figure in a pyramid scheme dominated by large interests like don Eliseo's. She had come to see what the churequeros in Nueva Vida were seeing: in a commoditized landscape, the kinds of rights a poor person could assert—including the rights that come with clientage—began to shrink.[25] Chatarra was part of a survival strategy, but it was hard to turn it into a civil action. "Rights" to collect were not given.

MINSA lacked the power to convince people in greater Managua that the junk business as it was—an open range where technological, political, and monetary might determined who had resource rights—might be dangerous enough to public health to be regulated. The more garbage circulated, the less it seemed to be a common concern. Or perhaps don Eliseo was onto something—perhaps the Ortega government wanted to add chatarra to the list of industries in which it had a major stake and from which it could provide a lucrative outlet for loyalists.[26] In an ecological sense, mosquitoes and the virus had taken advantage of the situation, thriving in a set of spaces (dumps, streets, parks, and gutters) that were neither public nor private, neither common nor collective.

"Dirtiness," as doña Lesbia reminded me, was "part of the business."

PATRONS, CLIENTS, AND PARASITES

The last time we spoke, shortly before she closed the chatarrera, doña Nubia told me the story of how her neighbor's child was stricken with dengue. "The child got sick, and soon MINSA and the neighbors were coming here telling me that the mosquitoes came from me." She paused. "Do you think that's possible?" she asked, "that a mosquito from here made her sick? There are clouds of mosquitoes in Ciudad Sandino."

She paused again and looked pensively in the direction of her neighbors' house. Neighborhood FSLN activists eager to carry out the dictates of the Plan Chatarra had fueled the accusation that the child's sickness was her fault. "They'll be happy now because now I'm not buying anything anymore. So now they'll be happy." She threw her hands up in the direction of the last pile of scrap metal in the corner of her porch. By the time of our last conversation, in November 2008, few people were coming by to sell chatarra. In any case, doña Nubia could rarely afford to buy it, given the depth to which prices had fallen. So the material sat there, rusting and collecting the last of the seasonal rains. And doña Nubia sat beside it, pondering the lives of mosquitoes, of the little girl—now, thankfully, fully recovered from her bout with dengue—and of rumors from her fellow chatarreros about the prospect of a market recovery: a recovery that might make her solvent once again, but might also, once again, make her the object of neighborly and state scorn.

In the Plan Chatarra, it was small operators like doña Nubia who received the bulk of MINSA's attention. In an antidengue crusade built on a hygienic premise, that clean homes harbored few mosquitoes while "dirty" ones were potential breeding spots, this made perfect sense. It also makes sense that the connection between chatarra and dengue became strongest when the market was strongest. Intuitively, it would appear that a strong market for recyclables *could* produce a cleaner and maybe even "healthier" city. What better incentive to clean than money? Yet the market could do little to produce a sense of ethical or social connection. Indeed, combined with a mounting series of dengue epidemics, the growth in the garbage market actually turned certain spaces and the bodies that occupied them into dangerous internal threats. Along the way, it destabilized the patron-client system that regulated the circulation of garbage. Under stable circumstances, chatarreros and churequeros, even as "dirty workers," could rightfully claim to be improving public space. The soaring market, however, brought the details of the trade to broader attention. All of a sudden, churequeros and chatarreros appeared dangerously unconcerned with the quality of the private spaces of their own homes and bodies. It was their seeming disregard for the interior worlds they shared with mosquitoes that made them suitable objects of scorn.

The churequeros and chatarreros certainly made easy targets as public health officials in Nicaragua searched for someone to blame for the ever-mounting number of dengue cases. Scavenging disrupts standard narratives about the proper relationship between people and the things they buy, sell, and consume. People tend to characterize waste as polluting and dangerous material, and turning it into value seems to violate basic norms about the proper way to make a living.[27] The economic lives of the chatarrero and the churequero seem somehow "parasitic." They thrive by milking the dark underside of a larger system of trade and consumption. In another sense, however, chatarreros and churequeros were themselves beset by parasites. As clients, the churequeros and chatarreros of Ciudad Sandino depended upon the buying power of large patrons in Managua and beyond. Chatarreros and churequeros provided cheap, free labor for these well-capitalized entities, as well as for the city planners who—whether they openly admitted it or not—depended upon an army of *hormigas* to keep the streets minimally clean. The assignment of blame rested not only on ideas about the ethics of seeking profit from the refuse that was so prominent in the urban landscape but also on normative ideas about ecology. The spaces that brigadistas and MINSA officials called *focos* (or what English-speaking entomologists sometimes call mosquito "hot spots"), from doña Flor's piles of garbage to the flower pots in my neighbors' patios, were essential for the reproduction of life in the city. The mosquito, too, seemed to behave in a parasitic fashion, feeding and breeding opportunistically among humans in these same spots.

Parasitic relationships tend to complement and build upon one another. It is impossible to disaggregate the parasitic relationships between scavengers and large brokers from those between mosquitoes and people. Householders in poor cities cannot survive without scavenging. The global consumer economy arguably cannot thrive without the work of informal scavengers. It goes without saying that mosquitoes cannot spread without the help of the human garbage trade. Mosquitoes and garbage do something more than make people sick; they are productive of political and social relationships. Their role in human affairs is thus far from incidental or disruptive.

Seeing human and insect lives as entangled makes it difficult to argue that a will to sanitary citizenship—the kind of will that mosquito control programs are meant to instill—inevitably results from membership in a "consumer society." One of the lessons of both studies of parasitic relations in nature and those of patron-client relations in Latin American social life is that the terms of such relations are interchangeable. Beyond anthropocentrism, there is no necessary reason to see viruses or mosquitoes (both of which are much more abundant on Earth than are human beings) as thriving parasitically upon humans. It seems just as reasonable to say that epidemics of dengue, avian influenza, and the like are the result of human parasitism: exploitation of global resources, excess consumption, and global warming. Likewise, in the patron-client relationship, who is behaving parasitically and who is being preyed upon depend upon one's point of view. Are garbage scavengers milking the city's material excess, or is the city milking the labor of scavengers to keep those excesses out of sight and out of mind? Power resides among those who can identify and neutralize parasites and clients.[28] The local conflict masked the global contradiction that increased consumption of disposable goods, even among the poor, makes parasites of almost everyone. Cities and certain groups within them become both reviled for their association with waste and indispensable to the reproduction of the waste-driven economy.

Parasitism happened at both a material and a symbolic level. At the material level, the fact that dengue mosquitoes could potentially find a harbor in otherwise valuable waste made these wastes even more abject. At a symbolic level, the circulation of wastes and mosquitoes through urban space—private, public, collective, and in-between—altered the social meanings of those spaces. From a free-market point of view, for-profit recycling might be seen as a cure to the environmental ravages of urban life, and the chatarrera might be a site of a kind of "green capitalism," while from MINSA's point of view, the same space could be one of risk and danger, or a threat to Sandinista "socialism." The connections between waste and dengue are far from direct, but so are those between scavenging and sustainability. The absence of clear rights, whether those of churequeros to make a living from the dump, of the city government to regulate and resell refuse in the name of the public interest, or of MINSA to make the health implications of the postconsumer economy a point of public consideration, ultimately benefited large operators like don Eliseo—and small ones, like *Ae. aegypti.*

PART TWO

Bodies

Sometimes one needs to overcome . . . so what I did was clean up.

XOCHITL, *December 2008*

Dengue mosquitoes are single mothers.

—MINSA EPIDEMIOLOGIST, *January 2009*

THREE

Householding and Evangelical Ecology

ONE DAY IN 2008, I went with Morena Sanchez, my closest brigadista confidante, to visit a friend of hers who lived in Nueva Vida. Morena knew Karen from their days as coworkers on a zona franca shop floor. Karen's job was to cut pieces of denim fabric into short strips, which Morena then sewed onto blue jeans to make belt loops. The work was repetitive, hot, and often humiliating. The predominantly female zona franca workforce was closely monitored by a group of Taiwanese managers, who zealously enforced production quotas. Karen and Morena worked side by side in the factory, but they had few chances to socialize there. Gossip and talking were frowned upon. Instead, they got to know each other on the bus trip from Ciudad Sandino to the zona franca, which was located in Los Brasiles, a few kilometers to the north. Karen had been glad to leave the zona franca once she had made enough money to start payments on a small house in Nueva Vida, just as Morena had been glad to find part-time work as a brigadista. When we visited, Karen's mother also happened to be in the house, visiting from the northern city of Chinandega. As we sat down and greeted one another, Morena asked Karen's mother how she liked Ciudad Sandino.

Morena answered her own question, only half-jokingly, "Ugly, right? I've lived here ten years, and I still don't like it." As she often did, Morena identified herself as *really* being from León, Nicaragua's charming colonial capital, two hours' drive to the north of Ciudad Sandino. She had come to Ciudad Sandino when she met her current partner *(marido),* a sporadically employed construction worker whose family had a house in zona 5. The three women chatted for a while about Karen's three small children and her problems with an ex-husband, against whom she had taken out the equivalent of a restraining order. Karen talked about having to fight the ex-husband, who was often drunk and violent, off of her property and about how her current marido was in prison due to a spat of violence for which "the other guy" got no punishment. At the time of our interview, Karen was supporting her children by selling tortillas and beans to her neighbors, but running a business from home was difficult. In Nueva Vida, water service had been cut for the past month (no one was entirely sure why, but the alcaldía blamed the heavy rains). Men were going from house to house in a pickup truck, offering to fill fifty-five-gallon barrels of water at a nearby farmhouse for fifty córdobas ($2.50) apiece. Karen managed to avoid paying too often by not washing her family's white clothes. (Whites were normally soaked in bleach for long periods of time and then rinsed, requiring more than double the water it takes to wash colors.)

Karen suspected that she knew why water service had been cut, and it came down to irresponsibility. "Because here in Nueva Vida, nobody pays! For *guaro* [cheap liquor], there's always money; for rice and beans, there's *usually* money; for *pega* [glue, the most popular street drug in the barrio], the addicts always find the money; but for water, nothing!" Karen paid her bills, but she sometimes felt silly doing so.[1] She struggled to cope with the tension between personal responsibility for cleanliness and hygiene and structural limits to it (the price of water, the failure of the legal system to protect her from violent partners).

In the Ciudad Sandino of the early twenty-first century, these kinds of negotiations between knowledge and action were key elements both of householding and of health. Anthropologists are sometimes thought of as collectors of phrases or idioms that crystallize a moment of change, upheaval, or shared value. In two years of fieldwork, however, there was just one expression that I heard repeated in all three countries where I researched the dengue pandemic. The saying is common in Latin America, and in Nicaragua it usually went something like, *En casa del herrero, cuchillo de palo*, which loosely translates to "In the blacksmith's house there's a wooden knife." Brigadistas found the phrase apt for describing the irony that the hospitals and health centers in which they worked routinely failed mosquito control inspections. More broadly, it applied in the discourses of entomological technicians, when they tried to explain the distance between knowledge and practice in regard to dengue. By most measurements, knowledge about dengue transmission is high in countries where health ministries have implemented community interventions, yet translating knowledge into preventative action remains difficult.[2]

Stories like Karen's, about responsibility and its structural limits, speak to the difficulty of building and maintaining attachments, even in the tight spaces of home and barrio. Brigadistas experienced this difficulty in a particularly acute way. The conflicts over sanitary citizenship that arose so starkly in the context of the Plan Chatarra percolated throughout Ciudad Sandino. These conflicts came along with questions about how people should identify "home." People in Ciudad Sandino had never known quite how to refer to themselves. For such a major city, it struggled to come up even with a single name. Older residents often slipped and called it by its old name, "OPEN III," a bureaucratic moniker that hardly inspired civic pride. In 2007, more than thirty-seven years after the community's founding, and eight years after its establishment as an independent municipality, a journalist from the city wrote that he and others had grown tired of being known as residents of the "Ciudad Dormitorio," even though other nicknames for local people, like *citasadinenses* or *sadineños* or *sandinistas,* seemed awkward, or partisan, or both.[3] In my experience, few people had time to contemplate this as much as this journalist had. Instead, I heard people identify with natal rural towns or suburban neighborhoods. Within Ciudad Sandino, local gangs *(pandillas)* would paint tags on buildings and park walls, using their gang names and their zone numbers. (A typical tag would read, "Los Junior, x 2" [The Juniors—Zona 2].) This meant that for many residents, the name of "home" was not Ciudad Sandino but something more specific, like zona 5 or Nueva Vida.

The journalist was ambivalent about his city's "partisan" name, but for brigadistas, political parties were only one of several fracturing social devices. Morena and the majority of the other brigadistas with whom I worked remembered the heady days of the revolution either from their childhoods or not at all. Their understanding of the connections between households, blocks, and barrios, and between personal and social responsibility, was therefore quite different from that of older residents. Even if they became disillusioned (and Morena certainly sometimes did), brigadistas worked fervently to develop an attachment to the place they lived. Such senses of place were key to developing senses of health.[4]

Though dominant public health narratives about dengue suggest that bodies in a given endemic environment may be differently exposed to the risk of infection, the concept of "exposure" normally hinges upon rather straightforward links between geography and risk. Exposure narratives in epidemiology reify rather than historicize racial and gendered identities, asking nothing about the web of relationships that produces health differences.[5] By this logic, by *being in* Nicaragua, anyone—resident, anthropologist, tourist, or journalist—is exposed to dengue. Such language tells nothing of the divergent historical, political, and economic pathways by which people mingle with diseases and disease vectors. In the case of dengue, the language of risk prompts us to think in terms of the body's proximity to mosquitoes and viruses, rather than the body's entanglement with those things. A shift from exposure to entanglement reframes dengue as a set of ongoing relationships among species and objects. As the brigadistas knew well, dengue was as much a problem of householding as of embodiment. In Ciudad Sandino, people didn't just live in houses. They built them, and as best they could, they "held" them. Amid social and spatial fracture, disease, deprivation, and domestic violence, holding onto houses was a moral and a technical project. God and science were both integral to it.

TRANSFORMING BODIES

Dengue epidemics and evangelical Christianity were both in their ascendancy in Ciudad Sandino during the first part of the new century. The city's population was by most accounts split roughly in half, between those who maintained affiliation with the Roman Catholic Church and those who had joined one of the more than one hundred evangelical congregations in the city. Indeed, as the journalist who complained about the city's lack of identity noted, the split between evangelical and Catholic residents had deepened the community's sense of fracture.[6] The *católicos* attended mass at a large, modern-looking cathedral, an open-air structure situated on a large plot of land that was surrounded by an imposing metal and concrete wall. The services of the *evangélicos* took place in ten- by thirty-meter lots tucked directly into neighborhoods. In fact, most evangelical churches were converted houses, or even the living rooms of homes. Charismatic preachers (mostly male *pastores* but also a few female *pastoras*) sermonized—over long hours punctuated by breaks for sing-alongs set to upbeat contemporary Latin gospel—about the need to expunge the presence of evil from everyday life. These intense services were contrasted to the ostentatious but programmatic services of *católicos*. Unlike most *católicos*, *evangélicos* vocally (and, according to some non-*evangélicos*, obnoxiously) renounced alcohol and extramarital sex, which they saw as signs of moral decay.[7]

The *evangélicos* spread a message of individual bodily and spiritual transformation. Anyone could be reborn as a *cristiano*. (In Nicaragua, as elsewhere, evangelicals referred to themselves as *cristianos*, and Roman Catholics self-identified as *católicos*.) Yet these individual transformations afforded membership in a larger and seemingly more cohesive community. Singing and oral testimony were common features of churches like the Iglesia de los Actos, a small but growing congregation headed by a pastora who had had her personal conversion during a short period of time in which she lived in the United States.[8] Her message—like that of many pastors in town—was that a communion with Jesus and the Holy Ghost would cleanse and purify even the most tainted bodies. She liked to include the stories of converted gang members, prostitutes, and homosexuals in her sermons. Once that purification happened in individuals, it could happen in couples, then in families, then in entire households. Her congregation gathered three nights a week in an empty building with a few plastic chairs and a boom box on which her assistants played Christian pop songs, to which the assembled sang or hummed along between sermons and *testimonios*. The building was unadorned, except for a purple banner hanging from one wall that read "IGLESIA DE LOS ACTOS: CIUDAD 'SANTA'." The pastora insisted on calling Ciudad Sandino *Ciudad Santa*, or "Holy City." Moving from a worldly revolutionary referent to a godly one, her objective was to build a new social order, house by house. Messages like the pastora's, centered on a "restoration of the family," were especially common among *evangélicos*. The Iglesia de Los Actos was one of several near my house, and on frequent evenings I would see congregants swaying and humming rhythmically, their hands outstretched and their eyes gently closed. As the meetings went on, some might speak in tongues; others might be struck down in rapture. Women dominated the ranks of the Iglesia de Los Actos congregation and most others.

Evangelism is not simply about individual conversion. It means spreading the message of salvation with single-minded purpose. One's rebirth is only as good as one's ability to spread the "good news" to others. Thus, in Ciudad Sandino, it did not take long for the *cristianos* in a given street or neighborhood to identify themselves. One could expect on most nights of the week to hear the sounds of Latin gospel emanating from giant speakers and echoing off of the concrete walls and metal roofs of houses, and on frequent occasions to be visited, stopped at work, or approached on a bus with an invitation to *conocer a Jesucristo* in the house of a local pastor. House by house, body by body, the *cristianos* were spreading their message.

There was a significant number of *cristianos* among the brigadistas and other MINSA staff with whom I worked. In clinics and in public health interventions, questions about the biomedical discipline of the body blended with questions about other kinds of bodily discipline. Depending on the messenger, public health interventions about HIV-AIDS, nutrition, or dengue might take on a religious tone. Messages about the dangers of alcohol, about domestic violence, about the hidden forces of infection, and about one's responsibility to children crossed back and forth between the religious and the medical spheres.[9]

Those brigadistas who had not become *cristianos* sometimes resented the sanctimonious attitudes of their evangelical coworkers. Morena, in particular, was resistant to the idea that she should deny herself the chance—rare though it was—to go dancing with her marido or to enjoy a glass of rum or a bottle of beer. She disputed the implication that as a non-*cristiana* she was somehow self-polluting or, worse, jeopardizing the lives of her children and husband. As she said, her loyalty was to God, not to a pastor or pastora. But dangers to the body *did* abound in Ciudad Sandino. Dengue was one of them. As members of a predominantly female workforce, the brigadistas were particularly sensitive to this. But whether Morena liked it or not, the work of tracking dengue epidemics and educating the public about the disease was also, in a sense, "evangelical." The discourse of dengue prevention, like that of evangelical Christianity, was one of aggregated transformation, house by house and body by body.

DENGUE AT THE THRESHOLD

Dengue is a miserable disease, even on first exposure. What sparks fear in the minds of public health experts and epidemiologists, however, is the fact that second and third infections can cause even more severe complications. Dengue, properly speaking, comprises four distinct viral serotypes (known as dengue 1, 2, 3, and 4). Each, on its own, can cause a form of "dengue fever," including nausea, eye pain, and the extreme muscle and joint aches that give dengue its colloquial English name, "breakbone fever." Together, however, the serotypes are capable of playing an insidious trick on the human immune system. In a phenomenon immunologists call "original antigenic sin," bodies exposed to a single serotype (e.g., to dengue 1) develop antibodies and immunological "memory" of the antigens dominant in that particular serotype. Problems arise when the same body confronts another serotype. Dengue 2, 3, or 4 may contain some of the same antigens as dengue 1, but the antigens that were dominant in dengue 1 are often recessive in the other serotypes. Immune systems equipped to deal with dengue 1 engage the new serotype, only to be thwarted when their preprogrammed antibodies are insufficient to engage unfamiliar dominant antigens.[10] In a process called antibody-dependent enhancement, preexisting antibodies produced to neutralize a previous dengue serotype bind to the antigens of the new serotype but cannot neutralize the virus. Instead, the antibodies actually bind to receptors on the viral monocytes that help the virus replicate *more* quickly than it otherwise would.[11] Such systems have "sinned," metaphorically speaking, in that they have lulled themselves into complacency, treating one dengue serotype as identical to the next. Bodies pay a hefty price for original antigenic sin.

Though all of the dengue deaths that occurred in Nicaragua during the period of my fieldwork were attributed to severe dengue, likely due to antibody-dependent enhancement, agreement among scientists about the veracity of claims about dengue and original antigenic sin theory has never been uniform. Some findings suggest that "sin" may in some cases be protective rather than negative.[12] Nevertheless, brigadistas, *católicos* and *cristianos* alike, told a version of the original antigenic sin fable over and over again. They repeated it among one another and in visits to their neighbors during prevention campaigns. Their message boiled down to the mantra that dengue "makes you sick the first time, but it kills you the second."

In a classic anthropological study, Emily Martin tracked shifts in metaphorical understandings of the body and the immune system. Once characterized by scientists as a fortified military complex, securing rigid borders against invasion by pathogens, as immunology has become more sophisticated the body has become revisioned. In the age of complex viral diseases (Martin discusses AIDS) with unpredictable effects on the body, scientists have begun to see the immune system as a "flexible" one. Rather than a military complex, the revised body is more akin to a modern workforce, with different types of immune cells adapting to the reality of porous bodily borders, much as laborers adapt to the realities of modern capital accumulation. Those bodies that thrive—like those workers who survive in the global economy—are not the most rigid and set in their laboring ways, but the most flexible. Scientists recognize healthy bodies as those that are capable of adapting to new antigenic realities.[13]

The antigenic sin fable draws on some of these same tropes about flexibility, but it also couches the immune system as an inherently flawed and even lazy character. To do this, it uses moral, rather than military or economic, overtones. The solution to original antigenic sin may be technical (scientists have worked for decades to perfect a "tetravalent" dengue vaccine that would protect people against all four dengue serotypes at once), but it is most often social. People cannot change the terms of original antigenic sin, which like biblical original sin is an irrevocable given, but they can, according to public health logic, protect their bodies by guarding the borders of the spaces they inhabit. In dengue prevention discourse, a person's failure to create distance between the self and mosquitoes is also "sinful."[14] In the houses where dengue strikes, the discourse of original antigenic sin has not led to a return to the "military" vision of immunity based on defense and aggression. Instead, it has produced a particular set of caring practices.

In Ciudad Sandino's antidengue campaigns, as in the city's evangelical discourse, the work of hedging against original antigenic sin began at home. Late in 2007, MINSA officials in Ciudad Sandino hung a cloth sign outside the health center. To the right of the blood-red words "De vos depende . . . Prevenir el dengue" (Dengue prevention depends on you), the sign featured a drawing of a menacing mosquito (figure 5). The sign summarized Nicaragua's dengue strategy: household control of *Ae. aegypti*. The female *Ae. aegypti* lays eggs in small, usually anthropogenic bodies of water and feeds exclusively on human blood. It is *females* that transmit the dengue virus (and only females), and only among humans. In educational messages from MINSA, these mosquitoes were poised to do harm, unless citizens agreed to rid their homes of potential breeding sites. At each doorstep, and in each home, brigadistas exhorted their neighbors to recognize viral/insect/human entanglement and to act against it.

This "evangelical ecology"—this call to recognize and repent for original antigenic sin by taking action in the home—was not only moral; it was, like the story of original sin in the book of Genesis, gendered. Bodies faced with multiple serotypes often fail to recognize their own vulnerability, much as Eve failed to curb her own inherent curiosity in the Garden of Eden. Descriptions of women as moral guardians of household space are nearly cliché in the anthropology of Latin America, and Nicaragua in particular. But brigadistas were not simply guardians of the private sphere of the household. They were monitors of the boundary between private and public space.[15] Brigadistas were asked by medical authorities, who could do nothing to undo original antigenic sin, to be evangelical ecologists, working to curtail its effects by recognizing not just the porosity of their bodies but the "permeability" of their homes.[16]

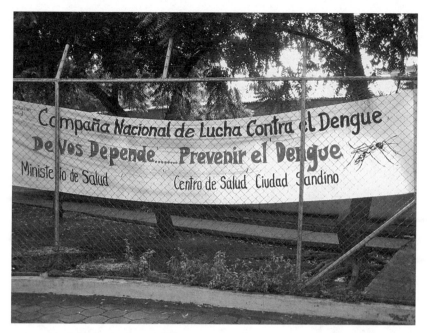

FIGURE 5. "Dengue prevention depends on you!" A sign in front of the Ciudad Sandino Health Center. (Photo by the author, 2007)

For Morena and many other brigadistas, however, the porosity and pre-cariousness of household space was not just a problem to be managed—it was a defining feature of social life. Morena had had her troubles with sub-stance abuse, and she knew that her marido was not always faithful. But her choices were limited. She and her marido shared a home with his parents and a sister who also had children. Morena had little choice but to live in her marido's family's house. The two of them together did not earn enough money to buy their own land, and when both of them did work, the large family provided much-needed childcare. Morena was sensitive about the risk of dengue precisely because she, like so many others, lived in close proximity to her family and her neighbors. Just as an alcoholic or physically abusive family member could profoundly destabilize these precarious arrangements, a contagious pathogen could threaten everyone. As those responsible for transmitting biomedical and ecological messages about dengue, brigadistas worked to reconcile the discourses of scientific and other kinds of authority about the goings-on in bodies with the realities of everyday life in home environments.[17]

Brigadistas and others confronted the problems of the city in houses where pipes emptied into sinks—or didn't—and where garbage was disposed of—or sold. When infrastructure broke down in this way, questions about the politics of entanglement arose. Whom should they blame for a lack of water, the presence of an infected mosquito, or the piles of refuse in a neighbor's yard? Some of the possible answers were structural. Blame the political class. Blame the volatile garbage economy. Blame the tropical environment for harboring tiny mosquitoes. These structural explanations were always available, but I noted an ambivalence on the part of brigadistas to use structure to explain problems of sickness and hygiene. Instead, their explanations oscillated between passive submission to big forces, and active engagement—along evangelical lines—with those forces. Houses were the spaces where relationships between people, things, mosquitoes, and microbes got "knotted up" and assigned value.[18] Given that so much of public health work, political organizing, and garbage economics was acted out on a house-to-house basis, houses were also the spaces in which people encountered "structured" power systems: state, church, and economy.

The MINSA dengue program's focus on households and bodies was understandable, given the realities of mosquito and viral ecologies. The house has been a standard (and standardized) site in epidemiological approaches to mosquito-borne disease from the earliest hygienic interventions against it.[19] The assumption that houses, like bodies, can be approached as undifferentiated "natural units" runs through many kinds of public health and social development interventions.[20] Likewise, state and nongovernmental authorities have turned adherence to particular ways of managing them into a key moral and ethical responsibility.[21] Instilling this responsibility requires the articulation of people's relationships to viruses and mosquitoes not just in globally standardized terms but in contingent "local" terms. Anthropologist Erin Koch has adopted the metaphor of the "threshold" to describe this kind of articulation. Brigadistas worked to filter standard meanings of pathogenesis through their own experiences of place: "to navigate and negotiate precisely what [was] for them social" about dengue.[22] Importantly, Koch notes, the threshold is both a *gateway* to a social engagement with biology (as in the doorway of a house) and a *limit* to such engagement—the point at which the realities of social life interfere with the standard practices of public health.[23]

As material and symbolic artifacts, houses were models *of* the communities around them, as well as models *for* those communities. Clifford Geertz developed the twin concept of the model-of and model-for to describe the operations of religious orders in social life.[24] *Evangélicos* worked house-to-house to encourage individual repentance in response to social ills, working to help people overcome the fracture of life in contemporary urban Nicaragua through intensive bodily transformation. By teetotaling, speaking in tongues, and being sexually faithful, they demonstrated that transformation. Individual conversion would produce membership in a universal community.[25] This discourse of individual transformation resonated with the work of brigadistas, who—like door-to-door Christian evangelists—were using their gendered knowledge of intimate spaces to deliver messages about personal responsibility.

HOUSEHOLDING

In the world of dengue, houses are key nodes of exchange and adaptation.

Houses are very much alive. They are "held" by attachments that are as much material as emotional. They are "worlded" by the work of people, mosquitoes, and other things, acting, wittingly or not, together.[26] Houses and their construction, breakdown, and maintenance were favorite topics of conversation for the brigadistas and me, perhaps because we spent so much time visiting and discussing one another's dwellings. Brigadista work was, essentially, about reconciling two life cycles *(ciclos de vida):* those of mosquitoes and those of people. The brigadistas knew them both well. The mosquito would develop from egg to larva to pupa to adult in just over a week. This meant that, in order to stop mosquitoes, people needed to get rid of garbage, scrub sinks, and barrels and tend to the gutters and hidden puddles around their homes once a week. The limitations were clear. Brigadistas could visit only once every other month, at most, and only if someone was there to receive them. They could apply organophosphate larvicides to buckets and barrels, but people might toss the chemically treated water out for fear of being poisoned. Of course, in places like Nueva Vida, water was often considered too precious to toss out and change, even if poisoning was a risk. Houses were vital, if also dangerous.

In Ciudad Sandino and Managua more generally, houses are virtually inseparable from other kinds of spaces. Shops, offices, churches, and private health clinics all double as houses. The possible exceptions to this would be hospitals, schools, and government buildings, although, as in other cities

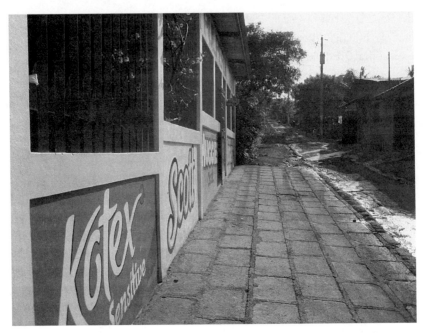

FIGURE 6. Walls and entrances: a street in zona 7 of Ciudad Sandino. (Photo by the author, 2006)

around the world, these were permanently occupied by both official "residents," such as guards and caretakers, by unofficial occupiers, such as dogs and cats, and by human street dwellers.[27] Though Ciudad Sandino had a few parks and one plaza for ball games, performances, and youthful gatherings, the urban landscape was for the most part a spatial monoculture of houses. With very few exceptions, each house sat on a lot of ten by thirty meters. Some were made of wood or metal, but by 2007 most were of concrete. Generally the entrances were gates or metal doors, positioned flush with the street, creating a series of walls and alcoves along the thoroughfare (see figure 6).

Ciudad Sandino was, like much of Managua, a "city of walls," a series of little "fortresses" where doors were nearly always locked, even in businesses and shops.[28] At corner stores *(pulperías)*, customers had to approach a set of iron bars and holler, "Buenas!" in order to get the attention of the owners. There was no window-shopping, because there were very few windows. Despite the closed doors and the imposing walls, people constantly circulated from house to house. Nearly everyone had something to sell: cellular phone recharge cards, clothes, dry goods, beans, bread, cheese, haircuts, washing and ironing services, and pirated CDs and DVDs.

These sales usually took place in the front rooms of houses *(los porches)*, and most houses had inner doors, also of metal or hardwood, leading to private areas. Inside, houses were typically divided into a single large living and dining room, often with a television and/or minicomponent stereo system, and one or two satellite rooms for sleeping. Loud music, a gumbo of Nicaraguan folk, Caribbean-Atlantic *costeño, reggaetón*, Latin gospel, American hip-hop, and 1980s European/American rock of the "Total Eclipse of the Heart" variety, was de rigueur at any social occasion, and dancing was popular. Kitchens were occasionally located in separate rooms, but usually there was a thin partition, if any, between the living/dining area and the cooking area of the house. Many families used open fires for cooking, especially when preparing large amounts of beans and rice or making corn tortillas, but propane gas cookers were also fairly common. Bedrooms were often collective, divided again by plywood or cloth partitions from the main areas of the house. In back of most houses was an open patio, where families kept sinks and washbasins for clothes and dishes (see figure 7).

It was the patios that the brigadistas inspected, looking for evidence of mosquito larvae in plants, garbage, and the water dishes of the animals most families kept there. Chickens and dogs were present in nearly all houses, and in a great many, one would encounter horses, pigs, turkeys, and geese. Ciudad Sandino's patios were also home to the majority of the city's fruit trees, from mangoes, with their long, invasive, coarse falling leaves, to coconut palms and bananas, to limes and oranges. Sitting on my quiet patio in the morning and afternoon, I could hear the faint thud and roll of fruits falling from the trees on to the hot galvanized roofs.

Garbage usually flowed, along with food, water, and clothing, from the front of the house to the patio and back again, through the hands of women. Women performed most cooking and cleaning duties, and most of the brigadistas would awake before dawn to begin washing clothes and preparing meals. Children who went to school were expected to arrive in clean, pressed school uniforms: navy blue skirts or slacks with bleached-white shirts. Ciudad Sandino's sandy soil, a reddish black substance that flew through the air in the dry season and clung to shoes in the form of mud in the rainy season, made uniform washing a daily chore. Care of the body was important not just for schoolchildren. On my block, the teenage boys from the local *pandilla* would stalk the streets in alarmingly

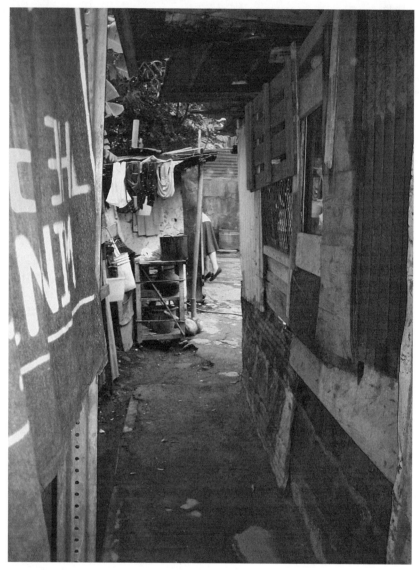

FIGURE 7. A patio in the Bello Amanecer neighborhood. (Photo by the author, 2008)

white socks and gleaming American basketball jerseys or T-shirts. The brigadistas, who made a point of arriving to work each morning with clean hair, makeup, and perfume (women), or carefully styled, gelled hair and cologne (men), regularly chastised me for the disrepair of my own clothing.

The gendered cultivation of bodies was mirrored in the care and cultivation of household space. Sweeping, mopping, and "watering" *(regando)* floors and patios was a semidiurnal task that, again, fell to women and young girls. The practice of *regando* was seasonal. Women would flit water from buckets or hoses onto dirt floors and onto the dirt streets in front of their houses in order to tamp down flying dust. In the rainy season, this was not necessary. In those periods, people would work to stave off houseflies, commonly recognized as sources of diarrhea and respiratory sickness. Women would hang bags full of water—or, increasingly, old compact discs—from trees and eaves. As they explained to me, the purpose of these shiny adornments was to confuse the flies and drive them away. The patios brigadistas visited, whether they were paved or made of bare dirt, were so reliably free of leaves and debris that comparing the relative disrepair of "dirty" ones became something of a pastime. Women counted as garbage *(basura)* everything from plastic food wrappers to the fallen leaves of trees. *Basura* was anything that got in the way of a clean patio, and it was either swept into piles and burned in the street or collected in large hundred-pound grain sacks for the passing garbage men.[29] Recyclable material, on the other hand, was separated in many families, often in a dedicated area of the patio or a separate grain sack.

Given the regularity of house size and style across Ciudad Sandino, it is reasonable to describe the city as a residential landscape. The house, rather than the market or the square, is its defining spatial form. When people arrived in new sectors, they built houses, roughly in the same proportions as those in the older, more recognized zones of the city. The ten- by thirty-meter form, repeated, demolished, rebuilt, elaborated, abandoned, and reclaimed, was dispersed across the landscape. Infrastructure projects such as water pipes served the collective by serving these individual cells. Water was for houses, not streets or parks. As the space where infrastructure mattered most, the house was not only a physical container for people, animals, and possessions—a private, domestic space, or *oikos*. It was also a key point of communication to the outside world—a part of public space, or *polis*. Though houses were often the legal property of men, they were in local discourse almost always associated with their senior female occupants (e.g., "La casa de doña Julia" [Doña Julia's house]). In the remainder of this chapter, I use the examples of two of Morena's brigadista cohorts to examine the different ways in which brigadistas drew on personal experiences of householding to make dengue social.

Xochitl was about my age. She was born in the Managua barrio of Manchester, not far from Lake Managua, where she lived with her mother and sisters until 1998, when floods resulting from Hurricane Mitch destroyed their home. After the hurricane, she, her mother, and her sisters were relocated by a government disaster relief program to Nueva Vida. When Xochitl's family arrived, Nueva Vida was little more than an empty field, dotted with the remnants of anemic wheat and peanut crops, the last vestiges of what had been the Blandón hacienda. The families from the flooded barrios spent their first few nights under donated plastic sheets, using whatever they could find to dig out the plant stalks and tall grasses that punched through the volcanic soil and into their weary backs.

When she arrived, Xochitl was pregnant with her first child, a boy, and her relationship with her mother was already quite strained. She told me how in those first months the government and relief organizations provided Nueva Vida's displaced families with supplies to build new houses. In fact, she said, she could still identify the donor organizations that helped build houses in the different areas of Nueva Vida, just by looking at the construction materials they contained. A special kind of doorway might have come from a Spanish Rotary Club, a certain cement brick from a North American-Nicaraguan relief organization. When she came to Nueva Vida, Xochitl was eighteen years old, with a steady boyfriend. Though not legally married, she considered herself an adult. (Most women of her generation did not get legally married.) Despite this, the relief agencies, designated community leaders, and city officials who were in charge of giving out housing plots refused to give her land apart from her mother.

"They told me I had to have a husband, had to have a family," she explained, "There were lots of us, lots of women without houses. Some people got them and some didn't."

Xochitl spent the next three years moving with her infant son between the house of her mother in Nueva Vida and those of her boyfriend and her other relatives back in barrio Manchester, which was rebuilt despite the government's efforts to move flood victims to Nueva Vida. Finally, she managed to secure a small piece of land on the edge of the deeply cut old farm road that separated what residents referred to as stage 1 of Nueva Vida from stage 2. The road lay in a ten-foot ditch between the two stages, and Xochitl's house was one of about two dozen perched on its edge. To build her house, she saved money she had earned while working as an ambulatory seller of food and clothing near the Roberto Huembes Market and bus depot, in a middle-class section of Managua. She also did a short stint in a zona franca, sewing apparel, but she found the work demeaning. She was fired, she said, for talking back to the floor managers and for chewing gum.

When I met her in 2008, Xochitl was supporting herself by taking in washing and ironing and working as a brigadista. We got to know each other during the brigadistas' house-to-house mosquito control inspections. The day we met was hotter than usual. It was June, a time of year when the rains would come quickly to the Pacific coastal plain and then depart, permitting the sun to create a steamy vapor in their wake.

As Xochitl and I settled for a rest in front of a house, under the shade of a *roble* tree, I told her I was tired, exhausted: *rendido,* in the local Spanish phrase. I remember watching the sweat seep through the leather on the tops of my shoes and then looking to Xochitl's feet, protected by flimsy plastic sandals. They were dry and cracked despite the heat and the miles we had already walked.

"I've been up since 5:30 this morning," I told her. "My neighbor was celebrating his wife's birthday and started playing music on his stereo for the whole street to hear!" (On birthdays, family members liked to wake the *cumpleañero* with music, often played from a compilation CD sold in nearly every corner shop. It had several versions of "Happy Birthday" in Spanish, English, and other languages; the traditional Mexican birthday song "Las Mañanitas"; and even one that I think was performed by Maurice Chevalier.)

"5:30?" Xochitl answered in a tone of gentle mocking. "So late! I'm up every day at 3:00 A.M."

"Why so early?" I asked.

"Oh, I like to work early in the morning, before it gets too hot. I've got to do the ironing, cook breakfast, take the children to school, and take my little one"—by this time, she also had a daughter that was less than two years old—"to my sister before I come to the health center. I love getting up early. By now, I'm tired, too, but then at night I can't sleep. Once the children are asleep, I like to do the *ropa gena* [piecework washing and ironing for paying customers]. It's nice and cool then." She was matter of fact about her routine, and as I later found out, nearly all the women brigadistas with whom I worked operated on similar schedules.

I recorded an interview with Xochitl around Christmastime in 2008. We sat in the patio of her house. The house was made of wood and sheet metal and contained a set of curtains that partitioned the kitchen from the bed in which she slept and the smaller one in which her children slept. The patio surrounded the small structure, and a barbed wire fence hemmed in the property. Xochitl was planning to dig a pit latrine but had not yet saved enough money. When she or the children had necessities, they went into the bushes or to a friend's house down the road.

Still, obtaining the house was a proud moment for Xochitl, as it was for many of the women I met over the course of my fieldwork. Men, including Xochitl's marido at the time, tended to have lots of options for room and board, but for women, a house of one's own was essential to security. The physical and emotional attachments between women and their houses ran deep, even if the political and practical implications of domesticity were sometimes ambiguous. Xochitl's personal narrative frames the house not only as a symbolic reference point for women's experience but also as the basic material node of social and ecological life in Ciudad Sandino. It is worth quoting at length.

We were discussing the relationship between garbage scavenging and dengue. Nueva Vida abutted the city's dump, and it was home to most of the city's full-time garbage scavengers. Over the previous six months, I had heard Xochitl and the other brigadistas complain about the difficulty of communicating MINSA's message about household hygiene. I asked her to explain why it was so difficult to convince garbage scavengers, people who knew about dengue (and had perhaps even had it once) but also harbored items in which mosquitoes could breed, to "clean" their houses properly:

ALEX: But do you think that . . . the people who, let's say, don't clean their houses. . . . Do you think that it's because they don't know where diseases come from?

XOCHITL: Sometimes it's ignorance, sometimes it's poverty, sometimes it's a lack of will, sometimes for lots of things, there are lots . . .

ALEX: Lots of what?

XOCHITL: Lots of reasons—

ALEX: Lots of, like, barriers?

XOCHITL: Yes, and all these barriers, sometimes you get . . . look, there was a time I was depressed. With the pregnancy of [Eliza], I was depressed. I left the house, but I didn't want to go or stay. I'd go to Managua and come back crying. And I think that even—now I think I'm okay, but I think . . . there are moments that . . . I cry and I don't know why. And I don't want to come back to this house. . . . Even when I would come into the barrio . . . I would come here and just cry and cry and I didn't maintain the house. It was abandoned: weeds over there, weeds over here, the dishes stacked there. I didn't cook. Nothing. My mother gave me some food, but she wouldn't come here. My kids stayed with her [in another part of Nueva Vida], and I'd go over there and she'd cook and I'd just come back to sleep. And horrible. I felt bad, bad, bad. I felt better not being here. I would go to my friend's house and the same thing. . . . But I said to myself I can't go on like that.

Sometimes . . . my mind gets hard, difficult, horrible. But I say, "No. I can't go on like this." I have problems, I don't know what to do. But I say I'm not going to go on like this . . . sometimes one has to give oneself something because sometimes—I ask myself, "Why live? So that, for what?" Sometimes . . . one needs to fight for one's children. When . . . I had given birth to my daughter, I remember that I suddenly was sitting there and I started to tremble. To tremble, like this [shaking her hands and shoulders], like I couldn't control it . . . I remember that I had the girl in the hospital, and when I had her, the first, the first thing I said when she fell asleep . . . was, "I'm not going to go on like this. I'm not going to go on like this. I've got to . . . change. I have to look out for her. It's not her fault I'm suffering."

I remember that from there I began to live my life another way. . . . In my life, I look after my children. I don't need anybody's help. . . . But nobody knows how I feel. Nobody knows what I need. How I felt this morning, how I slept, how work was, how I feel. Nobody asks me, not even my mother . . . and if I maybe didn't have my kids, what would my life be? Sometimes one needs to overcome . . . now with all this depression and the birth of my girl, I came back and I cleaned all of this. I cleaned here, there, everything, the street, out front. I started to take care of the street, as you can see. At least I've got it clean now, no more spider webs. . . . A house with spider webs looks abandoned. . . . So I came back and what I did . . . was clean up.

The purpose of my question was twofold: I wanted, first, to find out how Xochitl weighed the relative importance of personal and shared responsibility for sanitation and health and, second, to find out the extent to which she thought forces of poverty and oppression hindered people's ability to comply with health regulations, which were based upon household-level sanitation. At the time, I considered Xochitl's lengthy confession a digression. She had seized my inquiry about the practical limits of household hygiene to recount her own struggle. She located her problems in her mind, but given that it was overlaid on the space of her house, her depression also had an embodied element. The move was subtle, but Xochitl routed her emotional angst through the state of her house. The house was a communicated space. The story Xochitl told was one of personal overcoming, yet it remains tinged with social suffering. Even after deciding to "change," she lamented that no one knew how she "felt" or what she "needed." Even within the victory over sadness came a pointed reminder of isolation. Stories of *personal* rather than communal overcoming—the kinds of stories one was apt to hear between sermons at the Iglesia de Los Actos—were common in my interviews and conversations with brigadistas and others in Ciudad Sandino, even if, like Xochitl's, those stories didn't actually come along with a religious conversion. These narratives of personal transformation often took bodily form, but just as often they were routed through talk about the physical state, construction, or deterioration of houses. They were about people who were searching for routines that might forge attachments to home, and how those routines were disrupted and reinitiated.[30]

The context in which Xochitl's narrative of routines and disruptions arose was important. She was a woman, living precariously in the most marginal barrio of a marginal city, but she was also a brigadista. Her experience of the home "reverberated," such that "movement between the person and the house" obliterated "any clear distinction between the two."[31] She thought of her own emotional well-being through the state of her house and through the relationship between her house and the others in her barrio. As a brigadista, her job was to deliver services, information, and policy from the institution to her neighbors, house-to-house. As a washerwoman and an ambulatory vendor, her job was, again, to move goods, services, and value, house-to-house. In both cases—the economic exchanges and the community health work—Xochitl experienced the precariousness of household routines firsthand. As sociologist Harry Ferguson suggests, "We need to start looking... not just from the direction of the public into the private but from the 'private'—or 'intimate'—outwards and from the vantage point of embodied experience." Viewed as nonlinear, reverberating, "it is then possible to see how... power ebbs and flows as laws and bureaucratic rules are turned into practice in the context of people's lives."[32] Put in the language of dengue prevention campaigns, the power of hygienic norms about the state of households reverberated in and out of Xochitl's household practice. The suggestion that social norms were received and contested at the level of the body is nothing new to anthropologists.[33] Putting that embodiment into motion, however, requires attention to entanglement. It requires close attention to the spatial formations that reverberate through embodiment: the house, the street, the barrio.

YAMILETH'S STORY: EVANGELICAL ECOLOGY AND EMBODIED ENTANGLEMENT

Yamileth also told me her story through the story of her house. "It's under construction, you see, but we always have plans, and then we change the plan." She laughed. We were sitting in the main room of her home, which was on the edge of zona 5, near the line that separated Ciudad Sandino from the neighboring municipality of Mateare. Actually, Yamileth began the story of her home by telling me how she became home*less*. She had become estranged from her mother and father around the time she became sexually active, bouncing between her home and those of friends and family members in Ciudad Sandino. When she became pregnant by the boy with whom she first "fell in love," she moved into the house of his parents.

She explained:

> At his house sometimes I had to eat in the bathroom, hidden, because his father said, "Don't give that woman anything to eat." You see, and so I had to eat in hiding in the bathroom. And someone had to spy for me to see if the old man was coming, because if he came then I would go through the other door, inside, and jump next door so he wouldn't see me eating. And if I didn't put in money for the water, the lights, they wouldn't wash my clothes, or they'd leave them wet. Twice they shut off the water and left me covered in soap in the bathroom. . . . I went to finish my bath at the neighbors and they said "*Muchacha,* don't be stupid! Go home! Why suffer?" But I was in love. . . . Later they started locking me out of the house, and I'd have to jump the wall to get in, two or three times they left me to sleep in the street. So eventually I returned to my mother.

Yamileth used this painful memory to explain why she had made the construction of her own home a central goal in her life. Like many other brigadistas, Yamileth suffered through years in which the space of the home had been a confining, repressive one. Paradoxically, however, the home—or the ideal of a self-built home—was also a space of creativity and liberation.

A few years after she finally left her first *pareja* and his tyrannical parents, Yamileth met another man and had three more children. She managed to buy a small plot of land with savings from her work selling refurbished shoes, and soon after moving into the modest shack she had built there, she was introduced to an American evangelical preacher who helped her buy materials to construct a larger house. As she told it, the preacher, a Nicaraguan by birth, was caught in a rainstorm during a visit to a church on her block. Yamileth invited the preacher and his wife inside and began a friendly relationship with them, explaining her husband's endless search for work and her own struggle to keep house while running a small business from the front of her house. The preacher promised to help, and within a few months Yamileth had the money to begin an improvement on the wood and sheet plastic structure she shared with her partner and four children.

But things quickly went wrong. The workman they hired was slow, and he failed to maintain the existing structure while he was building the new one. The modest house Yamileth and her husband had built was falling down, and the new one she dreamed of was slipping away. Worse still,

> a man from the church in Miami came and told me that he had heard complaints that we were selling the construction material. I began to cry and said, "Brother, we're with God, we're not selling our material." So I became angry . . . and then people in the neighborhood began to talk. They were saying that we sold drugs, that we had begged for the material, when we never asked for anything. God touches your heart, right? And they were the ones helping! They had a church there in Miami, and I still remember them fondly, right? I don't know what they heard, but in the end the blessing stopped, and there the project stayed. But the . . . the house project was . . . grand! It was beautiful. Windows, doors. . . . I imagined what it was going to be . . . but everything was in the plan.

Yamileth told this story in hushed tones, shaken by the memory of being accused of begging or selling drugs. Unbeknownst to her, she had violated a connective ethic. Her success in securing what all of her neighbors wanted, a livable space, became a sign of selfishness.[34] Her connection to an evangelical network that spanned a continent had actually weakened her connection to her closest neighbors. Yamileth understood that her neighbors might be suspicious of her success, but she couldn't move. No matter what state of repair it was in, this was *her home*. She held the deed and would be foolish to relinquish it. Instead of leaving zona 5, she and her husband completed the reconstruction of the house as best they could. Yamileth also thrust herself wholeheartedly into barrio activities. She worked as a preschool teacher, helped organize food and aid for families with recently deceased relatives, and with the help of MINSA opened her house as a *casa base,* a site for basic health triage, the distribution of condoms, bandages, Tylenol, or advice about how to navigate the health center's maze of clinics. As a model-of and model-for the community, Yamileth's home would become an expression of her good citizenship.

Yamileth understood her house-to-house brigadista work explicitly as that of a mother and homemaker. When we talked, she told me how two of her young sons contracted dengue at the same time. This happened after she had already become a brigadista. Once again, the events inside her house caused her to feel embarrassed and ashamed at the glances of neighbors. This time, she worried that she had endangered the barrio. In the interview, she detailed the experience of carrying her children to the hospital, waiting for them to be diagnosed, and coming home to watch MINSA's vector-borne disease technicians comb through her home and those of her neighbors with insecticide fogging machines. Soon after her children started showing symptoms, she, too, began to show signs of dengue. As the three of them convalesced, she began to wonder if she had contracted dengue because her work as a brigadista brought her into contact with an infected mosquito. The thought troubled her deeply. She committed herself to spending more time at home, citing the "exploitation" of brigadista work.

"What they pay us," she explained, "they don't call a salary *(salario)*. They call it a *refrigerio* [literally, "refreshment"—brigadistas were supposed to use the money to supplement the cost of food and drink during work]. So they don't treat us like real workers." Moreover, working in the streets required a great sacrifice of time. "When I go out on the campaigns," she said, "I don't eat breakfast. And then I get home at three or four in the afternoon, and I eat breakfast, lunch, and dinner all at once!" Yamileth had had enough. She decided that if the "real" hospital workers, such as the doctors who supervised the brigadistas, could take a day off to care for their families, so could she. In 2008, when it came to the attention of the head epidemiologist that Yamileth had skipped a day of brigadista work to care for her children—a son sick with a cold, a daughter who had been beaten up by an abusive boyfriend, and another son who had been in a street fight—she was fired.

Yamileth was fired because she was caught in a paradoxical situation. She was trying to make her home physically and socially more secure—keeping infection away, being present to watch after her children—but in order to do this, she felt the need to work as a brigadista, doing the evangelical ecology of teaching others how to keep their homes safe. She could not do both to her satisfaction, and she lost work completely. FSLN billboards promoted solidarity between the state and the poor, even quoting the "Internationale": *Arriba los pobres del mundo!* (Arise ye wretched of the earth!). The FSLN routinely blended the moral economic rhetoric of socialism with messages familiar to the increasingly evangelical population. "The Bible also says we should love the poor," Yamileth remarked, making implicit comparison to the FSLN messages, "but not everyone has this attitude." Like other brigadistas, Yamileth was unsure why her government had forsaken her, or why many of her neighbors refused to follow the recommendations she made on her home visits: to clean water barrels and rid them of larvae, to take out garbage and trim weeds to keep adult mosquitoes from biting their children, to keep pests out of the house. The messages of the brigadistas seemed so simple, yet so hard to convert into practice.

DENGUE AS ATTACHMENT

An understanding of dengue as a primarily somatic phenomenon would be somewhat misleading. Yamileth was a one-time dengue victim. Xochitl and Morena claimed that they had never had dengue at all. Yet as brigadistas, as homemakers, and as people whose flawed immune systems (whether they had had dengue or not) made them fellow original antigenic sinners, all three nonetheless experienced the disease in a bodily way. Geographers Ian Shaw, Paul Robbins, and John Paul Jones have compared the "transduction" by which mosquitoes navigate their amazingly complex flight patterns and the similarly iterative process by which an Arizona entomological technician stalked them. Mosquitoes do not "see" the world; they react to it.[35] As transducers, they know what they know based on the fit of information to already-recognizable patterns. Mosquitoes do not just live in their environments. Like householders, they make their environments by forming patterns of attachment, participating in the collective work of entanglement.[36]

For brigadistas, the meanings of original antigenic sin were to be found in their interactions within and around the houses they coinhabited with viruses, mosquitoes, and one another.[37] As these women's commentaries on the precarious practices of householding show, the construction of the home environment was a public act, forming both symbolic expressions of conformity to an outside world and individualized statements about the future of that world. If Ciudad Sandino was a fortress, its entrances were as multiple as its houses. It had a history, an origin, but geographically it had no single beginning. The brigadistas entered Ciudad Sandino anew each time they entered one of its houses.

In Ciudad Sandino's houses, the tension between social norms about hygiene and structural limits to hygiene became collapsed. In Ciudad Sandino's houses, a globally circulating disease made punctuated and painful appearances in human bodies. In Ciudad Sandino's houses, a change in the global price of aluminum could mean the difference between nutrition and privation. In Ciudad Sandino, being in and holding a house was, paradoxically, an expression of independence and a realization of vulnerability. Houses were places where pastors attempted to rebuild and revive "the family," even though the nuclear ideal type seemed hard to find in most of the ten- by thirty-meter lots in town. Houses were where brigadistas circulated, negotiated, and sometimes subverted the mapping and epidemiological techniques promoted by state and global health organizations.

In evangelical ecology, as in evangelical Christianity, the line between "public" and "private" space, and public and private life, is not rigidly drawn at any particular threshold: not the door to the house, or the living room, or the bedroom. Rather, the public and the private are constantly "articulated" in bodily and linguistic practices.[38] The house is a space in which borders between *polis* and *oikos,* between production and reproduction, and between human and nonhuman, are constantly under negotiation. Women tend to do most of this work of "dwelling," of reproducing and sustaining family and social orders, as well as the microenvironments of home.[39]

Metaphorical ideas about sin (antigenic and otherwise) induced reflection among brigadistas about the worlds they were creating. They were not repressed by metaphors, laden though they were with gendered implications. Nor were they exactly empowered by them. They were, however, engaged by them. The metaphor enabled them to reflect about what it would mean to live well in an environment where adaptation in the vulgar sense was not possible, due to (among other things) economic inequality and political division. Ideas about immunity to disease as moral and gendered emerged not in a social vacuum but in an already moral and gendered landscape, within which brigadistas were in the active process of becoming. It was through the moral metaphor that immunity—the actual immune system of the body—ramified out into the world around them. Metaphor was not just about perception but about engagement, not just about taking in but about going out.

Brigadistas' desires to be known, to be safe, and to be *related* were played out in material and symbolic interhousehold connections. Think again of the tension in Xochitl's story between *independence*—building a home of her own—and *interdependence*—her reliance on friends and neighbors, and subsequent melancholy at the idea that they might not care "how she feels."[40] As I discuss in the next chapter, brigadistas saw themselves as belonging *in* and caring *for* a particular "biological community," which included their neighbors as well as the dengue virus and the *Ae. aegypti* mosquito.[41] Houses were spaces in which it was difficult not only to parse *polis* from *oikos* but also to classify human lives and human bodies apart from other-than-human lives and bodies.[42] Controlling mosquitoes—and dengue viruses—involved the regulation of interactions between several forms of life (human, mosquito, microbial).[43] This meant not only that the classificatory distinction between *polis* and *oikos* came under question but also that the normative assumption that mosquitoes were *anti*social was also under question. *Ae. aegypti* is a uniquely domestic creature. Undoing this domesticity, or making mosquitoes "killable," was more complex work than planners might first have imagined.

FOUR

Mosquitos, Madres, y Moradores

DOÑA JAMAICA was a vector-borne disease technician, one of half a dozen employed full-time by MINSA's Ciudad Sandino health center. MINSA colleagues referred to technicians like doña Jamaica as *celestes,* in reference to the sky-blue polyester uniforms they wore, set off by navy blue caps and shiny black military boots. One of the main jobs of the celestes was to train brigadistas to search out the breeding spaces of *Ae. aegypti.* Doña Jamaica was, in other words, a professional mosquito tracker. On a warm morning in 2008, she led a group of brigadistas through a neighborhood near the health center. Her walk was interrupted by regular pauses, during which she would point out new breeding spots *(focos).* In just a few minutes, doña Jamaica found larvae in an eggshell, a soda bottle cap, and a water bucket.

"The mosquito will lay her eggs wherever she can," she explained, "but you won't find focos in mud puddles or streams. She likes clean water. Just here"—she pointed out another bottle cap—"she can lay dozens of eggs!" She overturned the cap with a black-booted toe, and we all crouched to watch the gray larvae wriggle on the dusty ground. Soon, the brigadistas and I found ourselves examining the dark corners of house lots, crooking our heads into piles of garbage and over abandoned car tires. We delighted in the discovery *and killing* of this intimate insect other.

The brigadistas saw another benefit in this work. "The brigadista has the opportunity to visit all the barrios of the city," a brigadista called Fillermina told me, "because the mosquito colonizes all parts of the household, all parts of the city. Being a brigadista, you get to learn all about her habits." Many women brigadistas had worked at other jobs, notably in zonas francas, but they had few opportunities to explore the city.

Another brigadista elaborated, "For me, it's out of the routine. I get to learn, and I like to walk . . . because normally there's nowhere for you to go, you know?" The work of following mosquitoes opened up the landscape in exciting ways.

A rather simple observation thus became a persistent element of my notes on work with brigadistas. The gist of it was, "Looking for mosquitoes is not just learning. It is *fun*." My June 2008 field notes include the following passage: "When I look now on a pile of soda bottles, mouths to the sky, full of greenish water, I [anticipate] the satisfaction of throwing out that water . . . a big part of me WANTS to find larvae." *Ae. aegypti* breed most often in household water supplies, both formal (sinks, barrels, buckets) and impromptu (crooks of trees, garbage, coconut shells). Once we learned to find these things, the impulse to continue was compelling. Our fascination with the human-insect world was renewed with every upturned palm frond and discarded CD jewel case.

A kind of fascination is also identifiable among entomologists. An entomologist from the CDC's Dengue Branch told me in an interview that the more he studied *Ae. aegypti,* the "more respect" he had for her: her ability to find new places to breed, and her ability to feed on his blood—in his apartment, the apartment of a professional entomologist!—with seeming impunity. Grasshopper expert Jeffrey Lockwood puts it another way. His studies, normally focused on learning *about* grasshoppers (to find better ways to kill them), also permitted him to learn ethical lessons *from* grasshoppers, specifically the power of stillness and resignation.[1] Such learning occurred in the process of what he calls "dancing," that is, movement *with* grasshoppers.[2] Entomologists like Lockwood claim that ethical engagements with landscapes, like bioethics, must be "anthropocentric."[3] I disagree. In this chapter, I use accounts of brigadistas' day-to-day activities to show how experiences of learning and care exist recursively with transformations in biophysical ecology, resulting in a particular kind of pleasure.[4]

This combination of exploratory learning and pleasure has entanglement among people, mosquitoes, and their habitats at its core. Brigadista work afforded a "transformative" recognition of this entanglement.[5] Brigadistas were practiced at contemplating the material and semiotic connections between people and mosquitoes. In this way, their work went beyond even the evangelical practice that MINSA's dengue control strategists envisioned. Dengue thrived amid economic and political conflict. Indeed, dengue may have contributed to social breakdown. But that is not the whole story. Entanglements could also be productive. Women brigadistas learned more about who they were by inviting themselves into the lifeworlds of mosquitoes and viruses. Mosquitoes and viruses became what they were by disrupting an anthropogenic landscape. In Ciudad Sandino, brigadista work was thus part of a collective process of becoming.[6]

AESTHETICS OF CARE AND CONTROL

MINSA's mosquito control strategy emphasized that good housekeeping was the only way to stem the threat mosquitoes posed to public health. As they shared information about mosquitoes and their habitats, the brigadistas also treated water receptacles with an organophosphate larvicide, usually temephos, which Nicaraguans called *abate,* modifying one of its trade names. The need to collect data on mosquito populations meant that the brigadistas also had to document the focos in each house. MINSA provided them with official worksheets for recording each type of foco.

Brigadistas had to count and record the focos on the worksheet; apply larvicide and note the quantity on the worksheet; and explain the mosquito life cycle to householders (*moradores*) and, again, mark the worksheet. The worksheet rendered life into bureaucratic form: boxes ticked, larvicide accounted for, habits corrected. It placed organisms, discreet and knowable, into precise relation to the similarly static objects that constituted their environment.[7] The worksheet made of human-insect relations a prescriptive metaphor for human-human relations. It promoted a particular aesthetic vision: a tidy household in which humans were insulated from dangerous insect others. The orderly home environment symbolized the orderly *habitus* of the human *morador.*[8]

So far, this strategy seems to make sense. Why should controlling household mosquitoes in the name of public health *not* give good citizens pleasure? Although sanitary discipline and order have long been central to the discourse of dengue control, ambivalence about dengue mosquitoes has been documented. In Villavicencio, Colombia, an anthropological research group found an urban population that was pointedly *un*willing to see the vector as a "tropical Godzilla." For householders in Villavicencio, *Ae. aegypti* was "part of . . . everyday life." For them, its presence evoked neither fear nor, it must be said, fascination.[9] For the brigadistas, on the other hand, who actively rather than passively encountered *Ae. aegypti,* the mosquito's appearance was not quite so unremarkable. Brigadistas' searches were more akin to adventure than to exorcism.

While brigadistas' pleasure in those searches might affirm the rationality of the enterprise, it also suggests another possibility. Regimes for the management of urban spaces hinge on the alienation of people—and in the case of dengue, women in particular—from urban natures.[10] By taking pleasure in the search, Nicaragua's brigadistas uncovered an open-ended, "ecologically aesthetic" alternative to this alienation. The "ecological aesthetic" originates in the anthropologist and philosopher Gregory Bateson's thoughts about the ethical implications of human entanglements with the nonhuman. In her ethnography of whale hunters turned whale watchers in the Azores, Katja Neves found pleasure and fascination wholly commensurate with hunting and killing. "Chasing whales" yielded a recognition of what Bateson called the "pattern that connects" humans and cetaceans—a pattern perceivable only in the *event* of hunting.[11] Neves contrasts the classical aesthetics found in the ordering of home or landscape with Bateson's ecological aesthetics, the senses of beauty and pleasure that emerge in the realization of our entanglement in the world. The difference between classical aesthetics and ecological aesthetics is one between knowing *about* the world and knowing *in* the world. While classical aesthetics has human control *over* life at its core, ecological aesthetics privileges a relational knowledge *of* life.[12]

The dominant discourse among brigadistas and global health policy makers during my fieldwork was not one of mosquito "eradication" but one of "control." Brigadistas used the terms *control de focos* or *abatización* (lit. application of *abate*) to describe their work. This linguistic nuance points to a specific relationship between technique and experience, allowing for different kinds of pleasure. While it is conceivable that eradication, or what previous generations of mosquito hunters called "species sanitation," would induce pleasure or mania (participation in mass killing must surely interpellate the killer in some meaningful way), control allows different emotions to come into play. The work of control involves constant movement, along well-worn paths, from house to house.

Moving through these paths, brigadistas seemed motivated by something other than a desire merely to order their world. In their search for mosquitoes (even dangerous ones) they displayed a capacity to respond to the environment in an open fashion, with "judgment and sensitivity." As Tim Ingold has argued, *enjoyment of* and *care for* the environment are most elusive when we try to categorize and order it.[13] Brigadistas felt a tension between the need to collect data and the process of caring engagement—one that was much more experiential than informational—in which the search for data enrolled them.[14] Neves applies the concept of aesthetics to the practice of community gardening. Viewed as an aesthetic practice, gardening affords a "recognition of degrees of shared ontology between humans and . . . other biological entities," which may lead to more relational views of health.[15] While gardener-plant relationships are rather peaceful, relations between humans and mosquitoes are usually antagonistic. Still, human-insect relations are more similar to gardening projects than they might first seem. Both involve a combination of control over collective bodies (or "multiplicities on the move"), with an ethic of care and an open sense of fascination with the world.[16]

BIOLOGICAL WARS

Three of the dengue prevention campaigns in which I participated were led by don Francisco, Ciudad Sandino's lead celeste. Don Francisco took time each week to brief the brigadistas. He would stand before them, clipboard in hand, carefully explaining their progress on a map of the city. Through what he called a *guerra biológica* (biological war), he hoped to "chase" the mosquitoes from the barrios on the shores of Lake Managua, into the countryside west of the city, and over the ridgeline that led into the Pacific, systematically driving them out of town. The militarism of the strategy was matched by the daily ritual of *pasando revista,* in which don Francisco examined each brigadista's equipment: pencil, worksheet, *abate,* and chalk for marking the outsides of each house inspected. Every morning, each brigadista stood ready with this equipment, well dressed, with walking shoes, cap, and a satchel for carrying it all (figure 8).

Don Francisco liked to remind the brigadistas of their dual responsibilities as "technical" and as "social" workers. "Muchachos," he said, one week into a 2008 campaign, "we're starting off badly. Three more dengue cases this week." He let this sink in. "If we start off badly, we end badly. And I don't understand it." He paused again. Then he asked them all, rhetorically, what they would think if one of those cases was one of their relatives. The brigadistas shifted on their feet, not daring to talk back.

Don Francisco asked, rhetorically again, how each of the brigadistas started her day. "I, as a Catholic, pray each morning, then I greet my wife

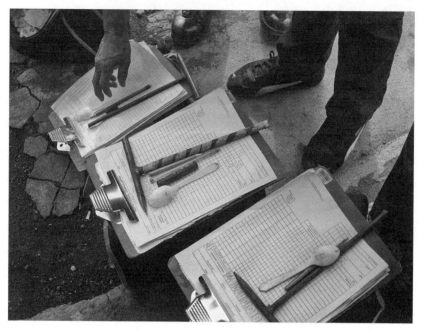

FIGURE 8. Brigadistas *pasando revista,* with worksheets, pens, *abate* spoons, and small hammers *(piquetas)* for making holes in cans and bottles. (Photo by the author, 2008)

and my children," he said. "And when I leave the house and I see my neighbor on the corner, do I pass on my way like an animal *[como un animal]*? [*Animal* is colloquial Spanish for insect.] NO! I greet him. 'Good morning, how are you, have a nice day.' Right? We greet each other because we're not animals, and because greeting others is good for your health." This was the kind of behavior he expected of brigadistas: rigid techniques for mosquito abatement had to be supplemented by sociality. Even if they had to invent something to say in the way of small talk, don Francisco wanted the visits to be social, believing that this would foment more concern for health. It came down to self-esteem *(autoestima):* people feeling wanted and appreciated. In the ideal case, "we can congratulate the people because their patio, their water barrels, are clean."

This semimilitary, semicommunitarian rhetoric has its roots in the history of global mosquito control programs. Dengue prevention strategies based on household sanitation are nearly as old as modern public health itself; indeed, well before scientists knew that diseases like dengue, malaria, and yellow fever were spread by mosquitoes, ideas about the risk of contracting those diseases were attached to ideas about hygiene.[17] Since the discovery of the connection between mosquitoes and diseases, the linkage between hygiene and mosquito control has tightened and loosened. This tightening and loosening has occurred for a variety of reasons. While changing technologies for fighting mosquito-borne disease have rearranged the ways viruses, mosquitoes, and people interact, the reverse is also the case. The movements and actions of mosquitoes, viruses, and people have also been integral to the development of those same technologies.[18]

Today's casual student of the history of mosquito-borne disease probably knows a few key names: Ronald Ross, who gets credit for discovering the symbiosis between mosquitoes and the malaria parasite; or Walter Reed, who did the same for *Ae. aegypti* and the yellow fever virus; or William Gorgas, famous for successfully demonstrating that *Ae. aegypti* and various *Anopheles* species could be controlled through manipulation of their habitats in Havana, Cuba.[19] These were public health pioneers, but they were also scientists of empire. Ross was part of the British Imperial medical complex; Reed and Gorgas were U.S. military men whose early work took place in the context of the Spanish-American War.[20]

Ross pushed his colleagues in the British academy and colonial administration to adopt a strategy of "species sanitation," a concept he developed in an 1899 lecture. As he argued, "We may expect to find ourselves in possession of a cheap and effective means of *extirpating* malaria, at least from the more civilized and therefore more important areas."[21] Gorgas's success in Havana led to more notable work in the Panama Canal Zone, where control of malaria and yellow fever mosquitoes through control of the water, forests, and grasses that surrounded workers' quarters was integral to the successful construction of the canal. But like Ross, Gorgas had no illusions about who he was protecting. For Gorgas, "species sanitation" was not for all people. Imperial powers until well into the twentieth century operated under a hygienic and therapeutic apartheid, which separated soldiers, administrators, and settlers from polluting "natives."[22] The environment itself was a source of impurity, and "rational" bodies were those that could reasonably be insulated from that environment.[23] The work of Ross and Gorgas was predicated on a limited understanding of people's capacity for sanitary citizenship.

In the early twentieth century, the linkage between sanitation and mosquito control shifted. Along with a wave of progressive politics and optimistic modernization programs across the Americas, the idea that people could control mosquitoes not just in certain key places like the Canal Zone but in *any* environment began to take hold. Programs for environmental "improvement" in disease-ridden areas were expanded in this period, particularly in Latin America. In the early 1900s, Dr. Oswaldo Cruz, a Brazilian scientist and sanitarian working in the crowded cities on that country's coast and Amazonian frontier, began to devise "interventions against mosquitoes [that] were accompanied by the systematic collection of garbage, the provision of drinking water systems, the paving of streets, and general urban cleanup measures."[24] Cruz's intuition was that both diseased and healthy environments were always *human* creations. He was less concerned with the relative biological capability of "whites" and "others" to resist infectious diseases.[25] In Latin America, this inclusive approach to mosquito control quickly became part of grander political strategies for nation building. The notion that the places in which malaria was most prominent were in need of drainage, clear-cutting, piping, and other interventions led to the creation of what geographer Eric Carter calls "state spaces," such as mosquito control districts, clinics, and hospitals.[26] A combination of paternalism and modernist zeal inflected this expanded "environmental sanitation" approach.[27]

As the science of insect ecology became more fine-tuned, however, control of mosquitoes became disaggregated in the minds of public health experts from wider social development agendas.[28] By the mid-twentieth century, "species sanitation" began to mean drawing a sharp divide between mosquito and human living conditions.[29] From this revised standpoint, poverty didn't promote mosquitoes and disease; mosquitoes and disease caused poverty. Control of *Ae. aegypti* still involved intensive house-to-house intervention, but entomologists in the mold of the American Fred Soper (who used the quasi-military term "brigade" to label the teams of eradication specialists he assembled) focused their efforts on the microhabitats of insects (water containers, drainage ditches, swamps), to the exclusion of infrastructure conditions and other "hygienic" concerns. The development of this more precise mosquito ecology came alongside the development of more powerful technological tools and strategies. Early international health organizations like the Rockefeller Foundation favored an approach that turned disease control from a social into a technical and scientific project.[30]

This approach showed some success, especially after the introduction of the insecticide dichloro-diphenyl-trichloroethane, or DDT.[31] After the end of World War II, the WHO made a DDT-driven mosquito control program one of its first priorities. The WHO's strategy was designed and executed largely around the ecology of *Anopheles gambiae,* the malaria vector that had colonized the Middle East and the Mediterranean. DDT, mixed with kerosene and sprayed on the walls of houses and other buildings, seemed particularly effective at killing the unusually anthropophagic *A. gambiae*. It was not as effective against other malaria-carrying mosquitoes, but it did prove to be an efficient killer of *Ae. aegypti,* another domestic mosquito, known as the yellow fever and dengue vector.

The WHO's western arm, the Pan American Sanitary Bureau, launched a massive campaign against *Ae. aegypti* and *Anopheles* mosquitoes across Latin America in the years after the war, with DDT as its centerpiece.[32] The campaign came with resources and training, and nearly every country in the region, including the Somozas' Nicaragua, participated. Nicaragua's national vector-borne disease program celebrated its fiftieth anniversary in 2008. This dating makes the program, which employed celestes like don Francisco, one of the only institutions in the country to date itself back to the Somoza era. By the middle of the 1960s, intensive house-to-house operations featuring DDT had spelled the demise of *Ae. aegypti* in Nicaragua and nearly all of the Americas. The fight against *Ae. aegypti* was one of the first—and seemingly first successful—international, nonmilitary, noncolonial public health projects in history.[33] While DDT is often seen as the driving force in this success, *Ae. aegypti* eradication went along with a suite of nonchemical methods. *Ae. aegypti,* even at the height of the DDT era, was recognized as a social insect.

Don Francisco was old enough to remember when DDT was the ministry's preferred tool against mosquitoes. Indeed, his talk about socializing the "biological" war would have been familiar to his celeste predecessors in the 1960s. When the use of DDT for *Ae. aegypti* eradication became standard practice, the U.S. Communicable Disease Center (later to become the Centers for Disease Control and Prevention) produced several manuals for entomological technicians. These manuals took a great deal more space to discuss "community involvement" and "esthetics" than they did to discuss the technique of applying DDT (see figure 9). Making DDT operational against an insect enemy as intimately attached to humans as *Ae. aegypti,* it seemed, required reliance on the older, "sanitary" approaches that DDT's champions saw the chemical as replacing.

The CDC's *Ae. aegypti* control techniques were gleaned explicitly from successful programs in Latin America.[34] The approach centered not just on the deployment of professional DDT applicators but on the involvement of the community in eliminating mosquito habitats. As the U.S. Department of Health, Education, and Welfare's 1965 *Ae. aegypti* control manual explained,

Working With
The Community

Public cooperation is essential in the eradication program. But it can be assured only if people are knowledgeable about Aedes aegypti and the method of attack in use against the species. To this end, pertinent knowledge is provided to the community through meetings with community leaders, through the newspapers, over radio and television, and by every other practical means. The people are encouraged...

To permit inspections, and insecticidal treatment when needed;

To remove all unnecessary containers and junk that can breed Aedes aegypti;

To care for needed water containers in a way that prevents aedes aegypti breeding.

Special community-sponsored cleanup campaigns are desirable. They may be limited to portions of a city with particularly heavy breeding, or they may be conducted city-wide. These cleanup activities are carried on by existing official and voluntary agencies of the community, working cooperatively with the program's area offices. Thus, improvements need not be restricted to elimination of Aedes aegypti breeding containers, but can also include the removal of breeding and feeding accommodations of other mosquitoes and of rodents and flies, as well as improved esthetic considerations in portions of the community where such values are often neglected.

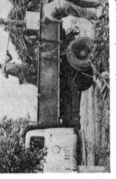

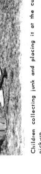

Children collecting junk and placing it at the curb for pick-up.

Community-owned equipment and personnel removing junk.

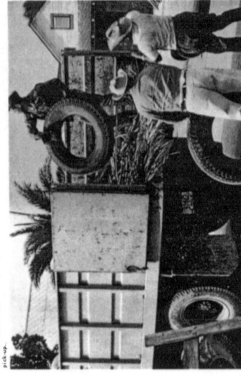

Citizens participating in the clean-up drive.

FIGURE 9. From a 1960s CDC *Ae. aegypti* eradication manual. The text to the left reads, in part, "Public cooperation is essential in the eradication program. But it can be assured only if people are knowledgeable about *Aedes aegypti* and the method of attack in use against the species." It then speaks of "improvements" that come from cooperation, including "improved esthetic considerations in portions of the community where such values are often neglected." (From the archives of the David J. Sencer CDC Museum)

"Source reduction produces a more beautiful community, better utilization of living space, and a more pleasant way of life."[35] A CDC manual for home inspectors from the same year spent considerable time on the importance of communication, in terms that don Francisco might recognize: "A person may be reached to a degree, as a member of a group, but is reached most effectively at his home where he is the master [sic], and has interest in any fact, good or bad, relating to the home environment. Considerable care must be taken to establish an effective and friendly relationship, or much harm will result."[36] These manuals individualized and *humanized* the dengue problem.

Alongside technical rules for mosquito treatment lay a discourse about the unanimal nature of the household. The CDC encouraged its mosquito technicians to work with local sanitarians to identify "poor," "lower middle-class," and "good" housing. Tellingly, the manuals warned that "good" housekeepers with seemingly "clean" houses could be most resistant to public health intervention.[37] The resistance of "clean" householders to home visits was replicated in Nicaragua, and don Francisco's emphasis on "socializing" the work—complimenting "clean" *moradores* to secure their cooperation—was a way to combat this. Brigadistas were sensitive to the outward appearances of houses and of homeowners, and many manipulated their language in order to gain entry, crossing thresholds by identifying with householders, sometimes as good, "clean" citizens and sometimes as simply overburdened fellow homemakers.

SOCIALIZING *LA TÉCNICA*

But once inside, what made a good household visit? Brigadistas' work was social in the sense that the CDC manuals and don Francisco encouraged, but it was highly regulated. To turn the contents of a private home into public knowledge required a certain degree of routinized authority. Indeed, the work had a ritualistic, if not industrial, quality. In trainings, old brigadistas could recite *la técnica* like a prayer. "From right to left, inspect all the flower pots and all the barrels, counting how many spoonfuls of *abate* you use, and don't forget to look up, on the roof, on the shelves, because they also breed there!" Again, the parallels with CDC rhetoric in the DDT era are striking.

Brigadistas came to houses with the goal of simultaneously changing behavior and garnering evidence of behavioral change. Don Francisco's speech embedded the notion of "cleanliness" into the technique. The "social" reward was being able to "congratulate" a homeowner for being "clean." Don

Francisco presented this sociality as pointedly *un*animal. As he said, if it was intrusive and brutish, the routine could be negative. The intervention had to seem caring and empathetic, not wild and capricious. In practice, much more went into *la técnica* than merely repeating a script.

After *pasando revista,* the brigadistas would fan out into teams of four or five, each headed by a celeste. They would walk to a barrio, where the celeste would assign each brigadista specific blocks for inspection. With every home came an environmental challenge. As the brigadistas were at pains to explain, *Ae. aegypti* could "colonize" the most unexpected places: the crooks of trees, drainpipes, plastic soda bottle tops, dog dishes, and car engines, in addition to water barrels, buckets, and wash sinks. Brigadistas knew that don Francisco and the other celestes would be checking their work, and that if they missed a foco, they would risk reprimand.

Despite the pressure, the brigadistas relished the opportunity to hunt for mosquitoes. Morena was known for being a wily inspector. On a normal day, she could expect at least 10 percent of the households she visited to be either "closed" or *renuente* ("unwilling," refusing to let the brigadista inside). The protocol was to mark the "closed" houses with a chalk "C" and the *renuentes* with an "R." Morena knew, though, that she needed to visit as many houses as possible, and she was willing to wiggle her way across barriers. Often, she could charm her way into the house of a *renuente* by complementing its occupant on a fruit tree or an adornment, or starting a conversation about the telenovela that was on at the moment. If a house was closed, chances were she could get herself in next door. Ciudad Sandino's urban landscape was marked by a peculiarly cellular construction. Each house lot measured ten meters wide by thirty meters deep, and many had slim partitions between them. This meant that if Morena crossed the threshold of one house and reached its back patio, she could peer into the patio next door, scanning for untended barrels, sinks, and *calaches* ("stuff" lying on the ground exposed to rain).

When we found ourselves behind a house that was divided from its neighbor only by barbed wire, Morena would turn to me, handing me her clipboard and satchel. "*Toma.* I'm going to jump." Then, making a pincer with her fingers, she would bend the wire low enough to swing her leg into the neighboring patio, bucking the fence and slapping the rust off of her thigh as she reached the other side. With a flourish, she would tour the empty yard, calling out what she found: "Two chicken troughs. One tire. A sink. Two barrels. Two focos." Finding and eliminating focos made it worthwhile. Soon, I found myself with my eyes pegged to the ground, peering into the cavities of the broken bottles cemented to the tops of patio walls, delighting in the sound of crunching eggshells and coconuts under my feet.

When they gathered for lunch, the brigadistas would trade stories. As Morena told of subverting property lines, others would chastise her.

"One day someone's going to come at you with a machete," the celeste scolded.

"I don't care. I don't like to leave houses behind," Morena responded.

The story wheel went on.

"I found a foco on a roof today!" Nereida exclaimed. "But when I was climbing up there, the dog got loose, and there I was, standing on top of this broken chair, while the old man in the house tried to pull away this crazy dog, barking and barking! And here I am swatting at him with my clipboard and my bag of *abate!*" Nereida stood up and mimed the action. Everyone laughed and hollered, breaking into a litany of similar stories. Encounters with aggressive dogs *(perros bravos)* were a known hazard of the trade.

Génesis countered with her own story. "Well, I got into this house with a beautiful patio. Fruit trees everywhere, mangoes, limes, passion fruits. *Gente gruesa.*" She held her thumb and forefinger in front of her nose, miming a wad of cash. (*Gruesa* means "thick.") "In the middle, the *señora* had this big pool.... I said to myself, 'What a huge *foco!*' So then I start tossing in bags of *abate*. Three, four of them." She mimed the tosses. "And as I'm turning around, here comes the lady screaming, 'No! My turtles! You'll kill my turtles!'"

Everyone gasped.

"*'Ay, dios mio,'* I said. So we started fishing through the pool pulling out all the sachets and all the turtles, washing them off."

"Well, did they survive?"

"Yes, and I'm glad they did, because the lady was kind. She gave me this bag of mangoes." The brigadistas swarmed.

As they traded stories of such encounters, they would trade food and advice about children and relationships. Conversation turned from the ripe fruits of the season to the beans, meat, or cheese we had brought for lunch. Sharing stories and food during lunch—what the brigadistas called the "sacred hour"—was an indispensable part of the work routine. "How can I say it?" Xochitl asked rhetorically in an interview. "I had the *honor* of meeting these people, and getting to know the barrios.... I felt *fulfilled* [satisfecha]." The lunchtime meetings, like the conflicts with *perros bravos* and the emergency rescue of reptilian pets, were valued parts of the social practice of dengue prevention. As homemakers, brigadistas understood houses as occupied by many other than human cohabitants. Cultivating fruit trees and aggressive dogs (as well as hoarding water in barrels as a hedge against Ciudad Sandino's routine stoppages in supply) were all part of the unfolding process of household reproduction. Women undertook such activities to produce "livable" spaces.[38] Though these activities took place outside of (or even in spite of) the dengue control program, they were, in the "social" vision outlined by don Francisco and elaborated by the brigadistas, also productive of health.

Every campaign reached a point, however, at which the social side of the endeavor had to be sacrificed to the bureaucratic and the paramilitary.[39] The work of don Francisco's brigadistas and their celeste supervisors was itself supervised by higher-ranking celestes, and three to four weeks into the campaigns, don Francisco found himself having to retract his recommendations to the brigadistas that they "socialize" with the neighbors they visited. Eventually, as he put it in August 2008, "we have to balance *quality* with *quantity*. If we can't complete all the barrios efficiently, the director will call in the Army to do the job." The brigadistas had seen this before. During a 2007 outbreak, soldiers had joined them. The soldiers efficiently visited every house to which they were assigned, but there was no small talk, no socializing, and certainly no exchange of fruits. Each campaign was marked by a familiar trajectory: excitement and engaged inquiry in the beginning, followed by increased regimentation and calls for speed and "quantity" near the end.[40]

MAKING MOSQUITOES "KILLABLE"

The goal of the global DDT programs in the 1960s was not to eradicate mosquitoes per se but to eradicate malaria and yellow fever by killing enough mosquitoes to interrupt pathogen transmission. Nevertheless, the effort ended up leading to a disappearance of *Ae. aegypti* throughout much of the Americas, including Central America.[41] The exceptions were the Southern United States and a few parts of the Caribbean.

During *Ae. aegypti*'s short hiatus from Central and South America, the region became more connected to routes of global transportation and trade. In the 1980s, dengue reemerged as a serious health problem in the Western Hemisphere.[42] By this time, thanks to concerns about its effects on the health of humans and other animals, DDT had fallen out of favor as a public health tool. It had been banned in most countries and abandoned by the WHO.[43]

In the absence of DDT, increased transnational movements of people and goods allowed carriers of the four viral serotypes of dengue to meet in new places, joined by a population of *Ae. aegypti* that likely spread in shipments of used car tires from the United States. All the while, increases in the numbers and concentrations of the urban poor benefited the mosquito, which thrives off of the physical proximity of breeding sites (garbage piles and small water containers) and what entomologists call "blood meals."[44] In this context, health policy makers and governments in places like Nicaragua began revisiting their approaches to dengue. The Sandinista regime, eager to establish its credentials as a propoor, activist government, organized regular Sunday cleaning campaigns called Domingos Rojinegros (Red and Black Sundays), and they sent technicians into neighborhoods armed with a suite of chemical alternatives to DDT.[45]

As the Sandinistas were beginning to lose political power, public health policy makers in the Americas began to lose faith in state-led models for mosquito control.[46] By the early 1990s, "participatory" dengue programs, run by community groups and NGOs, were lauded as more "sustainable" replacements for state-run interventions. In places where governments seemed incapable or unwilling to devote the time and resources to abatement, citizen "participants" were seen as a potential solution.[47] Frustratingly for scientists and policy makers, however, evidence of the long-term effectiveness of this approach has been hard to find, largely because of the problem of balancing what don Francisco glossed as "quantity" and "quality."[48] In 2009, I began attending dengue prevention conferences and visiting research centers in Nicaragua, Puerto Rico, and Cuba. In interviews and impromptu conversations, I asked fourteen experts to explain the "failure" of the participatory model. I received three types of explanations.

"There was never any science behind it," said a CDC official. One of his colleagues identified the problem as "assigning a great deal of agency to very strapped people." A prominent microbiologist and early proponent of participation concluded that the problem was that "people always want to cheat their governments." The assessments were thus that experts could not manage community contributions (meaning that "participatory" interventions were unscientific), that they had expected too much of them, or that people—by nature—tended to willingly defy authorities.[49]

An entomologist, however, suggested that participation was simply underdeveloped: "I would kill more mosquitoes if I had a social facilitator in each community than if I had an exterminator." The discourse of "failure" elided deep social entanglements that continue to exist between people, viruses, *Ae. aegypti,* and the landscapes they inhabit. Most participatory models presume a predictable, linear connection between the "rational" decisions of people and the "natural" habitats of mosquitoes. In other words, they presume a world of discernable separations and discrete species.[50] By this logic, the mosquito and the virus are "matter out of place": matter that, once identified, will be consensually removed by the participant.[51] This implies separations between humans and things, humans and insects, and humans, insects, and the other elements of their habitat. Such separations ignore the entangled history of people and insect vectors.

That history was well understood by the dengue experts with whom I carried out fieldwork. The CDC, for example, breeds an *Ae. aegypti* control colony, known as the "Rockefeller Colony," which for over fifty years and countless generations has had a population identical in behavior and reactivity to insecticides as its ancestors. Colonies like this have been bred to *stop* adapting. Their homogeneity provides statistical control for entomologists. "Field-derived" *Ae. aegypti,* on the other hand, have adapted to altitudes, temperatures, and environments previously believed to be inhospitable. In the mid-2000s, CDC scientists in Puerto Rico found them breeding in old septic tanks. It took months of retesting to "prove" that this adaptation had taken place. For dengue scientists I interviewed (though not necessarily for entomologists), adaptations such as these were further signs of the "failure" of mosquito control. Chemical, environmental, or participatory approaches might have worked with standardized strains, but standardized strains were patently unnatural.

Or were they, in their isolation, unsocial? To an entomologist, *Ae. aegypti* is a "domestic" creature. The "field" is the barrio.

Dengue emerged as a disease and as a scientific object alongside processes of war and colonialism.[52] To explain changes in the pattern of dengue's spread, including mosquito adaptations, entomologists routinely point to processes of economic, political, and social change. The dengue virus probably originated in Southeast Asia, as a "sylvatic" pathogen circulated among primates by *Ae. albopictus* mosquitoes (commonly known today as "Asian tigers").[53] As human settlements encroached on the forest, perisylvatic transmission, in which humans could acquire the virus from apes but weren't particularly good at passing it to one another, became more common.[54] Because *Ae. albopictus* was not a house dweller, cases of dengue in humans were probably isolated, rarely resulting in widespread transmission.[55]

Meanwhile, in eastern Africa, another perisylvatic mosquito, *Ae. aegypti*, slowly began to change its habits, settling in villages and towns and feeding exclusively on humans. As people moved from place to place, *Ae. aegypti* moved, too. Already accustomed to laying eggs in gourds and ceramic bowls, it moved along caravans and trade routes, stowing away on slave ships, traveling from Africa to the Indies and the Americas.[56] Trade in and out of Southeast Asia brought more people to ports, and as the region urbanized, *Ae. aegypti* thrived. As it turned out, the African *Ae. aegypti* was a highly competent carrier of Southeast Asian dengue—even more competent than its cousin *Ae. albopictus*. By the mid-eighteenth century, at the height of the slave trade, dengue epidemics were occurring regularly in port cities.[57]

Through the nineteenth and twentieth centuries, dengue remained a relatively minor epidemiological problem. Compared with yellow fever and malaria, it was, to use the parlance of contemporary global health, a "neglected tropical disease." With hindsight, we now know that the reason for this lay in the geographic distribution of dengue's four serotypes. All four most likely originated in Southeast Asian forests, and though global trade and transport helped transmit the virus and *Ae. aegypti* around the world, it took centuries for all four serotypes to become endemic around the globe.[58] When one serotype circulates, patients can usually recover from fevers quickly. In order for *multiple* serotypes to circulate with regularity in a specific place, a few conditions must be met. The human population must expand fast enough to produce a reliable number of new, immunologically ignorant members, usually children or immigrants. People must be able to move from place to place with enough speed to carry live viruses and/or mosquitoes with them, and finally, people must create new mosquito breeding habitats as they move.

In the period before, during, and immediately after the DDT era, the development of roads, shipping lines, and other technologies for moving people and goods—the rudiments of global infrastructure—combined with the *under*development of technology for housing, feeding, and watering people—the rudiments of local infrastructure. This combination was vital to the emergence of multiple serotypes in single places, what doctors call "hyperendemicity." During World War II, the Pacific Theater was the site of unprecedented road building, airstrip construction, shipping, troop movement, and human displacement. Soldiers and civilians in the war years became global travelers, and the bombing, clear-cutting, and industrialization of the Southeast Asian landscape in the period during and after the war allowed dengue's four serotypes to spread like never before. Just a few years after the war, dengue hemorrhagic fever was first described in the Philippines.

Although dengue is certainly an example of how political and economic processes demolish species borders, contemporary global health has centered on a compulsion to *redraw* the lines between people, bugs, viruses, and other life forms, often in the name of biosecurity.[59] Seen from a different point of view, however, life is not a result of exclusion, negation, or even ordering. Rather, as Ingold has suggested, life is something that happens *within* an environment where things—animate and inanimate—mingle.[60] This reverses a view of living beings (including people) as locked in competition, divided by "boundaries of exclusion," and prompts us to question a view of health that has the *dis*entanglement of people, things, vectors, and pathogens as its primary objective.[61]

Like the DDT protocols their predecessors used, technical tools like the worksheets and the *abate* gave brigadistas straightforward patterns for observing and recognizing the causes and effects of disease, but they also required that brigadistas learn about the disease through intimate interaction with insects and other people.[62] Brigadistas neither refused to kill mosquitoes nor denied that dengue was a serious disease.[63] To be ethical, however, killing had to be a *creative* rather than a *repressive* act. The question for brigadistas was how to make mosquitoes, dangerous but "significant" others, "killable." Considering this conundrum, geographer Uli Beisel notes that "the interesting question is not so much if we should or should not kill. The more relevant questions are rather concerned with *how* do we kill, *who* is the we, and how do we react to the *mosquito's response?*"[64] A link between caring for nonhumans and killing them has a long anthropological heritage. As Paul Nadasdy indicates in a critical reassessment of this scholarship, relations between Kluane hunters and their quarry in the Southwest Yukon resemble competitive "gift" exchanges. Nadasdy argues that hunter-quarry relationships can be respectful and unequal—even antagonistic—at the same time.[65] The difference in the case of dengue is that mosquito killing takes place not in the context of an exchange between partners but in an inhabited world that includes mosquitoes, peoples, viruses, and other living and nonliving things. Vector-borne epidemics demonstrate that conflict is part of "becoming."[66] The answer to the question of how to kill mosquitoes lay not in *separating* species from people from things but in navigating a household environment, a "zone of entanglement," where life was collective.[67]

To live a healthful life was not to order the world but to be entangled well within it.

DENGUE MOSQUITOES ARE SINGLE MOTHERS

Brigadistas who could engage householders long enough might tell them about what they saw as the insect's peculiar characteristics. For example, the mosquitoes that carried diseases were female *Ae. aegypti,* so the colloquial Nicaraguan word for mosquito, *zancudo,* was incorrect—technically, she was a *zancuda.* The brigadistas liked to correct one another on this. They also loved to talk about what a prolific breeder she could be, and they routinely parroted doña Jamaica: "In one of those little soda bottle caps, she could lay tens, *hundreds* of eggs!" Yet when they hatched, *Ae. aegypti* wouldn't swarm like another common Nicaraguan household mosquito, *Culex nigripalpus. Ae. aegypti* took refuge for most of the day in dark corners. Unlike the *Anopheles* that carried malaria, she would feed mostly during daylight, in the early morning hours and at twilight, when members of the household— especially women—were about the home cooking and washing. This meant that, unless you were already sick and in bed, a mosquito net wouldn't do any good. Finally, there was the question of flight. This little mosquito might travel a hundred meters for a blood meal. "And she doesn't respect the boundaries of your house," another Nicaraguan entomological technician liked to remind us. "She goes, she colonizes, she bites where she wants to."

Her ecology was disarmingly congruent with our own, but could you *follow Ae. aegypti?* During the 2007 epidemic, a group of neighbors from zona 8, outraged that a "dirty" neighbor was harboring mosquitoes, registered an official *denuncia* with the health center's department of hygiene, which arranged a meeting with the city's epidemiologist. The epidemiologist listened as the neighbors described the piles of garbage in the offending family's home and the "clouds" of mosquitoes that would emanate from the patio at all hours. They demanded that someone fumigate, someone send in the brigadistas, someone send in the police. The epidemiologist might have entertained their demands, but he told them, as he was fond of saying to people who brought in these kinds of complaints, "We all live with mosquitoes as if they were pets."

The epidemiologist couldn't agree with the idea of singling out one family for punishment. You never knew where you'd find *Ae. aegypti* next. After

DDT, the idea of "eradicating" the insect was passé. Mosquitoes were uncannily persistent. I was reminded of this when the CDC entomologist confided to me that his work had given him "more respect" for *Ae aegypti*, especially its ability to avoid human defensive responses to bites. This adaptation developed over a thousand years, as the African mosquito migrated to the ports of Southeast Asia, where it became entangled with the dengue virus. The unpredictability of "field" mosquitoes—the unpredictability to which the Rockefeller Colony stood in opposition—provoked both fascination and fear. *Ae. aegypti* was hardly wild. She was "other," but also, in the parlance of entomology, "domestic." For the Nicaraguan epidemiologist, pests were not too distant from pets. He assumed the gaze of one whose "habits" (and those of his animals) are under his "control." The brigadistas in Ciudad Sandino knew that *perros bravos,* for instance, were desirable pets. Indeed, brigadistas who could afford it had a *perro bravo* or two chained in their own patios to ward off intruders. Being attacked during a mosquito inspection was normal, and it didn't necessarily reflect badly on a householder.

But mosquitoes were not pets. For the largely female corps of brigadistas, the appropriate metaphor for describing them was more feminine.

"The mosquito is a *madre soltera* [single mother]," another Nicaraguan epidemiologist (this one female) told a group of brigadistas at the start of a training session. The epidemiologist was doing a round of introductions in advance of an upcoming dengue campaign. She introduced herself, too, as a *madre soltera.* She was speaking about mosquito life cycles, trying to explain the female mosquito's need for blood as a part of reproduction, but she was also attempting to shorten the social distance between herself (a slightly more economically comfortable, white-collar professional who lived in Managua) and the brigadistas, all semiemployed residents of Ciudad Sandino and many *madres solteras* themselves. *Ae. aegypti*'s preference for laying eggs in houses was something brigadistas were at pains to communicate. The epidemiologist's attempt to gender the mosquito was thus ecologically informed. It *is* the female *Ae. aegypti* who feeds on blood in order to reproduce. Males do not bite us. The joke also referenced a gendered knowledge about life in the barrios of Ciudad Sandino.

"Males," the epidemiologist explained, "provide the seeds, and then they fly off or die. They don't stick around." Her extension of the conceit drew an uproarious laugh. I was reminded of this two years later at an international dengue conference, when a Cuban entomologist made a similar reference. "You don't want to quibble with her. She is in charge of the children, she has to go find the food, and the man—he's nowhere to be seen!" Mosquito jokes that draw on the trope of the overworked woman almost always get a laugh, even among the stiffest of academic audiences.

Jokes like these anthropomorphize the mosquito. Anthropomorphisms assign familiar human motivations to nonhuman behaviors, but the "humanizing" of animal others actually underscores a sense of distance between human and nonhuman.[68] In anthropomorphism, the strange behavior of the animal "other" becomes recast in the vernacular of the human self.[69] It is possible, however, to identify characteristics common to humans and nonhumans without any reference to humanity or animality. What Kay Milton calls "egomorphism" is a recognition that the nonhuman other is "like me" rather than "humanlike."[70] For the brigadistas, the single mother metaphor fit this description. Their egomorphic gendering of the mosquito emerged from the shared history of failed eradication and expanding epidemics I glossed above. Though not directly referenced, that history "haunted" the discursive space in which the single-mother joke emerged. Much as dog breeds like pit bulls, associated with the bodies of racially marked human "others," "conjure" "spectral . . . histories of racialized power," mosquitoes conjured histories of gendered power.[71] As an ecological aesthetic form, then, the single mother joke was not an expression of distance between human and nonhuman but an expression of attachment.

The single mother joke was funny because it reflected how brigadistas understood their work. Mosquito hunting was public service, but it was also "home" work. As Cecilia put it, "This kind of work is better for women; men go to work in Managua, in construction, in offices. This is work inside the home. Women are more comfortable with that." Yamileth added, "Men are just too direct; you have to make people understand, and women are more suited to that." Doña Josefina put it this way: women possessed "more intelligence for time management." They were better at adjusting to the vicissitudes of urban life. Men didn't know their way around the market, how to find food and clothing; they didn't know how to cook and clean; and most wouldn't be able to balance all of this with a job working "in the streets." Women were also *más dinámicas para el trabajo* (more dynamic, flexible in their work). They had the social skills to communicate and to understand the struggles of *moradores* like them. In other words, their qualifications were based upon negotiation, persuasion, and empathy—the very sociality to which don Francisco appealed.

Still, choosing to do brigadista work was not easy, as Cecilia and Morena explained:

CECILIA: I like to work but my husband doesn't like it . . . in the street, he doesn't like it.

MORENA: We have that in common. *My* husband doesn't like me going out in the streets either or that I work, just like her husband . . .

ALEX: But you two, you two like [brigadista] work?

CECILIA: Yes.

MORENA: Yes, of course.

CECILIA: And now . . . that I am not in the campaign, it's been difficult to find work. I go out washing other people's clothes.

ALEX: They bring the clothes here?

CECILIA: No. I go to their houses . . .

ALEX: But apart from working as a brigadista, selling things on the street, washing, working in the zona franca . . .

CECILIA: As a domestic servant also . . .

This dialogue offers a sense of the variety of strategies these women used to contribute to the reproduction of their families. Mosquito inspections took place in the context of households in which, as Cecilia said, "the man is the head of the family, and you know he needs to earn more money . . . and we the women, what we earn is to cover some of it."

Women brigadistas saw their adaptability and intimate knowledge of the household—rather than their suitability for careers "in the streets"—as their contribution to the dengue prevention process. More than any other reason, when I asked female brigadistas why they predominated, the answer was simple: "Women are smarter." The special knowledge and experiences that women possessed—especially young, single women—gave them an unprecedented level of responsibility for health. Although a reading of mosquito control as a process of *human* self-governance is tempting, it does not fully account for the way in which brigadistas understood their work. They recognized the insufficiency of models, worksheets, and diagrams for understanding the household habitat. The single-mother metaphor was a way of articulating the tangled presence of *moradores, zancudas,* viruses, and things. Both were implicated in *public* health through ostensibly *domestic* activity. If, as Susan Leigh Star once wrote, "power is about whose metaphor brings worlds together, and keeps them there," then the single-mother metaphor was more than just a successful joke.[72] It was also more accurate than the domestic "pet" analogy. Having become together, neither mosquitoes nor single mothers would abide simply being the "controlled" "objects" of a health intervention. The joke recognized both a similarity *and* a difference between women and mosquitoes. They were not just casually alike; rather, each comprised part of a whole, a *living* environment.

In her work on entanglement, Donna Haraway calls attention to the "contact zone," the semiotic and material space in which species work out two contradictory needs: to conserve a relational order, and to improvise new ways of relating.[73] Her identification in "play"—and in late capitalist life—of an oscillation between the empowerment of individuals and the conservation of desired social formations draws explicitly on Bateson's work on the ethics of ecological connectivity.[74] Play is a limited form of communication. *Denial* cannot be mimicked, but aggression and even the act of killing can. Play itself cannot be ordered. We cannot force our children or our pets to play, and we cannot force one another to voluntarily *participate*.[75] Acting, as Haraway puts it, is always "*reacting*." Once we forget that, we risk overselling our own imagination and our own dominance. Ethical behavior in this schema comes from recognizing the "pattern which connects" humans and other beings, living and nonliving.[76]

The ecological pattern that made *Ae. aegypti* both a "domestic" creature and a "public" threat was fittingly overlaid onto patterns of remixed gender roles in postrevolutionary Nicaragua, where women highlighted the *domestic* character of *public* health work. Nicaragua's 1979 revolution celebrated gender equity, women's political involvement, and economic independence, and it was through the Sandinistas that gender-based movements for labor, reproductive, and legal rights emerged. Starting in the 1970s, women enjoyed an unprecedented level of involvement in civil society, notably in community health committees.[77] After the 1990 defeat, however, even militant Sandinista women began to feel drawn back into domesticity: power would come from moral and informal economic guardianship of the household. Florence Babb, commenting on life in Managua a decade before I arrived, noted that "the frequent invocation of women as 'mothers,' whether by Sandinistas seeking their solidarity or by governments desiring to reinstate traditional family values (and often enough, by women themselves), [was] understood by many to place additional responsibility on women to underwrite the social costs of development and nation building."[78] Most of the brigadistas I met came of age in this period, when state investments in public health and urban infrastructure declined, precipitating a momentous ecological coincidence. It was precisely when structural adjustment began to replace social solidarity as the guiding principal of Nicaraguan political life that *Ae. aegypti* found her "domestic" niche.[79] Ironically, it was amid a revived discourse of domesticity that zonas francas, garbage scavenging, and the pursuit of microloans for small businesses replaced state employment and collective production as standards for women's employment. It was not until the 1990s that dengue fever became a widespread public health problem in Nicaragua. The reemergence of the virus and *Ae. aegypti* in Latin America coincided with the demise of the nascent socialist state and the implementation of promarket measures.[80]

The single-mother metaphor made sense in a habitat that women and mosquitoes shared, even if they shared it as antagonists. Brigadistas understood that, more than likely, it would be *women* who would have to take out trash, look for impromptu focos, and clean out water receptacles. Any "failure" to control the insect was a gendered one. Killing mosquitoes was possible and even desirable, but to be satisfying, such killing had to occur—paradoxically—in an "inclusive" fashion.[81] Don Francisco was right—the "biological war" was social. The search for mosquitoes was an opening up, rather than a closing, of brigadistas' worlds. It thus should not be too surprising that at the end of a day of mosquito inspection, I would hear groups of brigadistas describing the strange new places in which they had found evidence of mosquitoes, all while showing one another what they had collected on the day's route: a few spare mangoes or limes, or perhaps some aluminum cans to sell to the recycling broker near the market. Like mosquitoes, the brigadistas had visited briefly, flitted into the most intimate spaces of their neighbors' homes, and come back a bit heavier and a bit more able to feed and clothe their own households. There would always be new focos to find, new natures in houses.

AESTHETICS AT PLAY

The recognition of a homology between insects' and women's lives problematizes public health strategies that paint the insect as an enemy and those who harbor them as unsanitary citizens.[82] Joking and storytelling about the search for mosquitoes afford a rereading of MINSA's technocratic public health intervention. The recognition of an entanglement between women and mosquitoes points not to a conventional scientific moment of "surprise," in which new knowledge reaffirms that the world "can be held to account" by rational ordering, but rather to a moment of "unsurprised astonishment," a fascination that admits of vulnerability but also affirms a caring engagement.[83] In the case of insect-borne and zoonotic diseases, the "politics of life" involves a population of entangled beings and things, including insects, houses, water, blood cells, dogs, and fruits.

What, then, makes the people who live in such worlds *care* about them? Classical aesthetics—which, in part, involves the separation of clean from dirty spaces—certainly gives a meaningful, ethical thrust to the governance of health, if health is narrowly construed as the vitality of human populations. Ecological aesthetics helps us understand what becomes of health when we recognize "life" as more than human: as a collective, generative, "multitude of livelihoods."[84] Experiences that permit people to perceive the "shared ontologies" between themselves and nonhuman others—the ways in which they become (and die) together—might be what make them caring subjects.[85]

The philosopher Michel Foucault saw aesthetics and politics intersecting in two ways. In a rational, technical sense, aesthetics are about *discovery* of a truth about health through a "hermeneutics of suspicion," centered on the body and its surroundings.[86] "Knowledge of the self" becomes a rational *duty* rather than an individual *choice*.[87] It is tempting to interpret dengue programs in this sense. House-to-house inspections and the Plan Chatarra were designed instill a suspicion of the home environment: a search for objects—and people and insects—"out of place."[88] A "dirty house," namely, one that contained mosquitoes, signifies the presence of an ethically questionable—albeit bounded and knowable—human subject within. This form of aesthetics is environmental. It entails "ordering things."[89] In another sense, however, aesthetics might be about *caring for* selves and environments. Foucault envisioned an alternative aesthetics: one of what he called "self-fashioning." The aesthetics of self-fashioning operates not on suspicion but on discovery, entanglement, and even pleasure. Those who recognize themselves as subjects of an ordering knowledge system or biomedical technology can, in an aesthetic "transformation," free themselves of its disciplining constraints.[90] This requires that persons be able to recognize themselves as regulated and disciplined by "regimes of truth."[91] This recognition opens up a space of "care."

Ecological aesthetics are about not only visualizing ethics—seeing *right* and *wrong*—but also the *how* and *why* and *whom* of relationships.[92] In MINSA's pictures and brochures, the clean home is an expression of the healthy self and her fit into a healthy social order. Applying larvicide, eliminating focos, and breaking households into bureaucratic boxes are techniques for reinforcing *detachment* between people, mosquitoes, and the spaces they occupied. Doing brigadista work well, however, required a passion for learning about and hunting out mosquitoes, along with an admiration for their refusal to be found.[93] Brigadistas were enthralled by the presence of so many significant others (mosquitoes, of course, but also dogs, plants, turtles, and trees) in their urban habitat. Senses of health came not from strict separation of these elements but from engaged participation in their entanglement.

Earlier, I referred to three explanations for the "failure" of participatory dengue control programs: a lack of "scientific" rigor; an overdependence on poor, strained individuals; and the tendency of people to disobey the orders of medical authorities. There is a fourth explanation. I heard it from both international experts and from Nicaraguan brigadistas and hygiene workers. It is, in brief, that the imagined "participant" is the wrong person. The mosquito intervention should be directed at children, not adults. "Children have the ability—the *desire,* to learn new things," a MINSA hygiene worker told me. "Adults are passive, apathetic. So I say, teach the children." At the CDC Dengue Branch in Puerto Rico, I heard numerous anecdotes from scientists about the effectiveness of harnessing children's fascination with nature. Indeed, the SC Johnson company once produced a dengue-related video game for Puerto Rican schoolchildren that allowed them to go on a virtual "hunt" for mosquitoes in a digital backyard (using SC Johnson insecticides, of course). Capitalists and scientists alike intuited that for children, hunting mosquitoes could be *fun:* it could be "play." Play is in this sense an individuated, psychological indulgence of the naïve, but play can be something more. Ecological aesthetics points to ways in which the play of metaphors and jokes, like physical play, is "serious fun," a queer parody of an otherwise troublesome set of gendered and speciated relations.[94] Even in the absence of slick marketing, brigadistas, too, were fascinated by mosquitoes.

PART THREE

Knowledge

If you want to understand how serious the problem is, you have to understand the statistics. Use the *data* to raise the people's consciousness.

CIUDAD SANDINO HOSPITAL DIRECTOR, *November 2008*

FIVE

Stories of Surveillance and Participation

DOÑA GUILLERMINA spoke with a thick "Nica" accent, a kind of cockney Spanish in which hard *t*'s and *s*'s were often dropped. Born in León, she had lived at various points in her life on Nicaragua's Atlantic coast and in Americas Dos, los Pescadores, Manchester, Ruben Darío, and Acagualinca, Managua barrios that were inundated during Hurricane Mitch, when hundreds of families, including doña Guillermina's, lost their homes. After fifteen days in a hastily arranged emergency refuge located in a local school, doña Guillermina was told that she could be resettled in Nueva Vida. She had two children at the time, and her husband had taken up with another woman while they were camped in the school.

On a rainy night, doña Guillermina and her children, a boy of two and a girl of five, arrived by cattle truck to a recently plowed wheat field. For weeks, the three of them huddled under donated plastic sheets, living off of food and water provided by the Army, nongovernmental aid groups, and municipal leaders from Ciudad Sandino. Doña Guillermina described how a network of mutual support grew among those early refugees. "We began to organize ourselves," she told me. At that time, "nobody had anything, so if I needed to go off and get water, my neighbor would watch the children and our things until I got back. Everyone helped one another." In her telling, the trauma of relocation was a galvanizing force. As she told me, "Ever since then, people have known me as a leader in my community. Now . . . when they come looking for volunteers or brigadistas, everyone says, 'Go ask doña Guillermina.'"

Doña Guillermina was a both an optimist and a shrewd student of politics. In 2008, she became a founding member of Nueva Vida's local branch of the Council of Citizen Power (Consejos del Poder Ciudadano, or CPC), a neighborhood-level political-cum-social networking group established by the new Ortega administration. Each CPC's membership was divided into interest areas, from child and elder care to public health to voter registration. CPCs were given charge of government-subsidized food aid—mostly milk, rice, and beans—as well as of distributing children's toys at Christmas. The government expected its ministries and all local administrations to consult the CPC on public projects and to involve them closely in educational, health, and economic initiatives. These included dengue prevention, which was doña Guillermina's particular interest. CPC members were generally loyal to the regime, but doña Guillermina and her compatriots complained that the new government was not paying enough attention to what they called the "social" side of community organizing.

In this, the new FSLN administration seemed, at least to some, more similar to its center-right predecessors than to the Sandinista regime that ran the country in the early 1980s. The liberal governments that defeated the Sandinistas in the 1990 elections had slashed medical budgets and imposed user fees for health services.[1] Over the decade after Hurricane Mitch—a decade in which such governments also had power—the sense of trust and reciprocity that marked doña Guillermina's early days in Nueva Vida had broken down. Even as some parts of Managua saw the construction of modern highways, housing developments, and shopping malls, sewage and water in Ciudad Sandino remained inadequate.[2] Schools were still crumbling, and crime and drug use were rife. Ortega promised to change this and to reverse the austerity imposed by his predecessors, but the CPC, at least in its early manifestation, seemed even to some of its members more like a party vanguard than a social service organization. Doña Guillermina and other CPC members in Nueva Vida complained that, far from solving social ills, the CPC's more callous political operatives were compounding them. Churequeros, it was rumored, had been hired by Ortega loyalists in the CPC to carry out attacks on political opponents and to stage "protests" in and around the capital during municipal elections. On a more mundane level, CPCs started to behave like another stratum of obstructive bureaucracy. By the end of 2008, a letter of introduction from a CPC member became a necessity for individuals seeking jobs (state or private), access to social services, and stalls in the market, among other things.

Doña Guillermina saw herself as an advocate for better government services, but when it came to dengue, she told me that the people in her neighborhood—not the government—were the main obstacle to success.

"They don't want to understand," she said. "They don't want to participate." I asked doña Guillermina and two other local CPC activists if they felt that more active political organizing might encourage such participation.

Don José answered quickly. "The problem isn't the party. It isn't the president. It's that the *people* are willing to let this [dengue] happen."

Doña Guillermina's neighbor doña Thomasina was more direct: "If we're going to go out into the streets, it should only be to overthrow the government. Otherwise, people need to take responsibility."[3] Like the MINSA celestes—and the MINSA brigadistas themselves—doña Guillermina and her CPC allies routinely described their dengue prevention work as profoundly frustrating. Although dengue was a growing epidemiological problem in Ciudad Sandino, the threat of dengue did not always elicit the kind of openness and curiosity about the urban environment that they hoped it would. They feared that they were failing.

Not surprisingly, MINSA's central authorities didn't like to talk about failures, or obstruction, or a lack of popular will. In early 2009, the ministry released an official declaration that its dengue strategy, featuring the CPCs, had "succeeded." The headline of a January 21, 2009, article in the newspaper *El Nuevo Diario* declared, simply, "MINSA Controls Dengue." The article trumpeted a ministry report that claimed that the number of new cases had been slashed by 50 percent from 2007 to 2008.[4] The very next day, however, MINSA declared a new "war on mosquitoes," in which the CPCs would be key soldiers. MINSA officials would give CPC leaders information about *Ae. aegypti,* and the CPCs would carry out the campaign. The head of MINSA's vector-borne disease unit described this "war" as "[consolidating] citizen participation . . . because MINSA doesn't have a lot of human resources."[5] The people, in this rhetoric, were coming to the aid of the health ministry, just as they had in the 1980s.

When they spoke of "responsibility," then, doña Guillermina and her fellow CPC members were not talking about the kind of "personal responsibility" that has become shorthand among many development and dengue control experts for a jettisoning of dependence on government.[6] Instead, they were talking about a more collective engagement. They were referring to the kind of mutual care they had seen in action in the early days of Nueva Vida and that older CPC members had seen in the days of Ciudad Sandino's founding. Politicians and policy makers took an interest in counting mosquitoes and infected people, but it was the job of local-level doctors, nurses, and brigadistas to make dengue matter in the lives of their neighbors. Workers at that level wanted knowledge about dengue—the kind of aesthetic sensibility that excited them so much—to translate into meaningful action. Yet CPC operatives, brigadistas, and other local-level MINSA workers remained ambivalent about the entanglement of public health science with politics. The increased imperative to search for hard data about dengue and mosquitoes seemed to promote the concentration of power away from the community and into the hands of politicians, technocrats, and international scientists.[7]

As far back as the 1970s, public health planners in Nicaragua have been aware of the potential of community-based work to be a vehicle for political discipline and even repression. To counter this, MINSA's earliest protocols for community-based dengue control came to emphasize shared responsibility and feedback between brigadistas and the health ministry.[8] These inclusive programs diminished during the 1990s, but in the mid-2000s international dengue scientists began using places like Ciudad Sandino as laboratories for testing the idea that local people could be effective collectors and disseminators of epidemiological and entomological information. When they returned to power in 2008, around the same time, Ortega and the FSLN began working to make Managua's barrios what they had been during Nicaragua's revolutionary period: laboratories for a proactive, grassroots, "participatory" politics. Through the CPCs, the party attempted to marry social compassion to political revitalization, while scientists attempted to make dengue control a common interest. Community health workers like doña Guillermina were placed in a "double bind," acting as both agents and targets of the state's most visible (and invasive) health project.[9] As Erin Koch has argued, stories about people in such a position "show how global health standards are refashioned as local techniques."[10] Brigadistas and CPC activists like doña Guillermina were state-sponsored observers of dengue and scientific witnesses to the interactions between mosquitoes and people, but they were also local residents, steeped in the memories of revolution, earthquakes, floods, and hurricanes.[11]

POLITICAL ENTANGLEMENTS

Contemporary dengue control operates through a combination of what experts call "surveillance" (the systematic monitoring of human illness, human habitats, and mosquitoes through data collection by trained scientists and technicians) and "participation" (the enrollment of householders in the management of those habitats, illnesses, and insects). Participation, then, often appears as a means to an end: an intervention that, properly executed, should result in a desired change in surveillance data (i.e., fewer illnesses, fewer mosquitoes). Self-consciously participatory strategies for dengue control have proliferated since the 1990s. These strategies seek to build sustained changes in what public health scholars sometimes call "knowledge," "attitudes," and "practices" regarding mosquitoes and dengue.[12] When these strategies have failed to achieve long-term reductions in the number of dengue cases or the number of mosquitoes in a given area—and many experts believe they have—explanations have varied: lack of sufficient knowledge inputs, thin social networks, government apathy, or simply a dwindling enthusiasm.[13]

Above all, public health planners have complained that accounts of what is actually going on—how people do or do not participate—remain narrative rather than systematic. Planners lament that while there are plenty of "stories" about what kinds of participation work, there exist precious few "hard data" about which behaviors, and which rates of behavior change, lead to decreased incidences of dengue. If an earlier phase of disease control saw scientists focusing intensely on mosquito habitats, to the exclusion of human living conditions (a process that reached its apex with WHO's DDT-based malaria and yellow fever eradication programs in the 1960s), then a successive phase has seen them turn their gaze back onto people. This new strategy aims to convert what people do and think about stopping mosquitoes from anecdotal stories into measurable information, not unlike the records of larval and pupal prevalence that brigadistas were asked to collect. Tasked with protecting populations from harm, public health institutions, by insisting on converting stories into data, create what Didier Fassin has termed "a relationship of otherness" to the publics they claim to serve. They do this even as they claim to privilege attention to everyday local "beliefs" about health over acute experiences of illness.[14]

Community health workers like doña Guillermina were not entirely comfortable with the implications of converting stories into data. In Ciudad Sandino, doctors, epidemiologists, brigadistas, and entomologists, all of whom called themselves "fieldworkers" *(trabajadores de campo)*, produced reams of entomological and epidemiological data about dengue, but they did this by creatively operationalizing the concepts of surveillance *(vigilancia)* and participation *(participación)*. These concepts were as freighted with meaning in Nicaraguan political and historical discourse as they were neutral, mobile, and sanitized in epidemiological discourse. Ciudad Sandino's health workers occupied a paradoxical position, acting as exponents of both a data-gathering health complex and an increasingly self-conscious party-state. Making dengue matter, both as a biomedical problem and as a political issue, required deft manipulation of this subject-position. To careful students of politics, it is perhaps unremarkable that knowledge generated by epidemiologists (statistics, graphics, case counts) became integrated into the deployment of political power. What is more intriguing is the way in which the reverse was also the case. In Nicaragua, local-level fieldworkers, from brigadistas to epidemiologists, routinely manipulated *political* discourses and practices to carry out the *technical* work of dengue control. Dengue had meaning as a threat to the individual lives of the people who lived in Ciudad Sandino, but dengue also brought doctors, nurses, and brigadistas into the volatile project of deciding who would belong in the community and how the state would enter their lives.

GLOBAL HEALTH COMES TO NUEVA VIDA

Starting just before the return of the Sandinistas and the advent of the CPC, MINSA saw major improvements in its capacity to track dengue epidemics. These improvements came thanks in large part to initiatives by the WHO and to the work of nongovernmental scientists and foundations, most prominent among them Dr. Eva Harris, a University of California–Berkeley microbiologist whose connections to Nicaragua dated back to her days as an *internacionalista* in the late 1980s. Harris began researching dengue in Nicaragua in the 1990s, winning a prestigious MacArthur Fellowship for pioneering a low-cost method of identifying dengue, leptospirosis, and other pathogens by polymerase chain reaction (PCR).[15] In the mid-2000s, Harris, who cofounded the nonprofit Sustainable Sciences Institute to bring technologies like PCR to the low-income countries where diseases like dengue struck most often, joined MINSA scientists to launch the Pediatric Dengue Cohort Study. The cohort study was a three-year survey of dengue incidence among children in district 2 of Managua, a middle- to low-income section of the city on the shores of Lake Managua, not far from Ciudad Sandino.

In the study, each child's hospital visits were monitored with bar-code identification cards, and cases of fever presenting in district 2's Socrates Flores Health Center were given extra attention and testing, in order to identify dengue infections as accurately and quickly as possible. The cohort study pioneered new methods for doing this, including saliva tests for antibodies, faster viral isolation, and tracking of cases using Geographic Information System science.[16] In the process, Harris became something of a celebrity in Nicaraguan public health circles, lauded for including Nicaraguan scientists in the research process. Most of the cohort study staff were Nicaraguan, and the Sustainable Sciences Institute made it a priority to train and place Nicaraguan scientists in the lead at every level of its project. During the time of my research, the cohort study helped MINSA acquire a state-of-the-art diagnostic laboratory, giving Nicaragua's dengue surveillance system the potential to be among the most sophisticated in the Americas.

The cohort study was an example of what epidemiologists call "enhanced surveillance."[17] Enhanced surveillance requires not only close attention to clinical cases of fever but also precise geographical mapping of those cases. Ideally, enhanced surveillance links fever counts to counts of mosquitoes in the target community. The goal is to shorten the time it takes to learn the locations of dengue fever clusters, in order to avoid widespread, unwieldy— and politically charged—declarations of "emergency."

But the cohort study did not just aim to bring Nicaraguan scientists into enhanced surveillance; it made unprecedented efforts at outreach to Nicaraguan communities.[18] In 2004, in conjunction with the cohort study, a program known by the acronym SEPA (Socializing Evidence for Participatory Action) began piloting a new method for training nonscientists around Managua to collect data about dengue and *Ae. aegypti* and to devise locally appropriate methods of controlling both human cases and insect populations.[19] SEPA's planners saw a need to speed up the flow of information about disease incidence from Nicaragua's neighborhood clinics to its regional epidemiologists and its sophisticated new national lab. Their "evidence-based methodologies" sought to close what planners thought of as a "motivational gap" between laypeople's knowledge about dengue transmission and their decisions to take preventative action.[20]

In SEPA, community leaders assembled their own groups of brigadistas, who went from house to house in their respective barrios, teaching people how to manage dengue by mosquito source reduction. SEPA's designers, who were mostly epidemiologists from the NGO Community Information and Epidemiological Technologies International (CIET), wanted to test the hypothesis that source reduction could be done more effectively without costly chemical larvicides. CIET called its pesticide-free method the

Camino Verde, or "Green Path."[21] SEPA distinguished itself from conventional approaches not only in its rejection of chemicals but also in that it was active year-round, convening brigadistas each week for house-to-house visits that also included time to discuss other problems in the barrio, such as gang violence, hunger, and the deterioration of streets. As a reward, the brigadistas—often teenagers and children—would receive practical scientific training, a small snack each week, a sense of investment in the research process, and a chance to forge intracommunity bonds. (Unlike MINSA, which paid brigadistas like Morena, Yamileth, and Xochitl, SEPA offered no individual monetary remuneration to its brigadistas.)

From 2004 to 2007, CIET piloted SEPA in several barrios of Managua, including the Bello Amanecer section of Ciudad Sandino. In 2008, to the delight of the epidemiologists in charge, the neighborhood leaders who participated expressed a desire to expand the project. Nueva Vida would be one of the neighborhoods included in that expansion. With backing from the community leaders, CIET epidemiologists convinced MINSA to provide the funding—about $50 per month, per barrio—to continue the program. This expansion coincided with Ortega's return to the presidency and the founding of the CPCs.

THE OPTICS OF SURVEILLANCE

SEPA's barrio leaders were, like the regular MINSA brigadistas, a largely female group. Some were shopkeepers, others were unemployed, and some of the younger ones were students. Several of the older members had been involved with the CDS in the 1980s. The CIET epidemiologists, some of whom had supported the revolution as internacionalistas or political activists, were aware of this, and they spoke of the CPCs as an opportunity. With more government support, SEPA might prove that the Camino Verde was a more effective preventative method than, as one CIET scientist put it, the "fetishism" of using mosquito-killing chemicals.

SEPA's leaders wagered that the community mobilization that Ortega's government was attempting could be integrated into its participatory dengue reduction program. For enhanced surveillance to work, it had to take a population-wide hold. The will to be a political participant—and to be politically observed—had to be fused with a will to be an epidemiological, scientific participant. This will had to take hold in what one CIET epidemiologist called the "soul of the barrio," the household. The blending of scientific and political rhetoric was slowly written into the program. At a retreat for SEPA participants marking the start of the program's fourth year, CIET leaders handed out certificates of recognition to "Distinguished Brigadistas" from each SEPA barrio. Each certificate bore not only the words "Camino Verde" but also "Poder Ciudadano."

Despite SEPA's scientific bona fides, suspicion pervaded barrio-level practice, as I learned when I joined a SEPA brigade led by doña Guillermina.[22] Doña Guillermina lived in stage 3 of Nueva Vida, just a block away from the neighborhood's only bus line and two blocks more from the empty lot that passed for a park. Her house was built of concrete, with a large patio surrounded by sheet metal. The front door, made of wrought iron, was, like the front doors of most houses, almost always padlocked shut. Her brigadistas would arrive through a door she had cut into the sheet metal. There they would gather, and after the day of house visits, she would serve them cola, crackers, or cookies provided by MINSA. On the wall of her patio, she kept a handmade display of the *Ae. aegypti* life cycle.

Every Monday afternoon at three o'clock, doña Guillermina would summon her brigadistas, who included a few children from the neighborhood, her own three teenage children, and the occasional adult helper. While many other SEPA leaders counted teenagers and university-age men and women among the ranks of their brigadistas, most of doña Guillermina's were far younger, some as young as eleven years old. The children worked in teams, canvassing the barrio armed with diagrams of the *Ae. aegypti* life cycle and a rehearsed speech about techniques for cleaning barrels and sinks to control mosquito breeding. They also carried nets and plastic bottles, with which they would collect samples of the mosquito larvae they found. On good days, the brigadistas could cover five or six blocks, and they quickly learned which houses were likely to be "positive" for larvae and which would be "negative." On my first trip through the barrio with these brigadistas, I returned to doña Guillermina's patio to see the children tapping the sides of their bottles, watching the larvae and pupae in various stages of development swim up and down in the brownish water. The CIET organizers did not see their age as a problem. For them, curiosity among youth was a true democratization of public health: barrio children should be the front line of "enhanced surveillance." Inspired, I resolved to return for each week's inspections.

As the following excerpt from my field notes for October 20, 2008, shows, the line between epidemiological and other kinds of surveillance was not always clear:

"Sir, we're here to talk to you about dengue," doña Guillermina explained to a shirtless man, about thirty years old, who was standing in the doorway of his concrete and metal house. Josué, a quiet, thin, curly-haired twelve-year-old brigadista, stretched his head around the doorway into the man's mostly empty room, catching a glimpse of the telenovela that flickered on his TV screen.

"Dengue, yes. Very bad," the man sniffled.

"Well, you know there's dengue in Nueva Vida right now. We've had several cases, and we know that dengue is spread by a mosquito, *Aedes aegypti*."

"Yes, yes. Of course," replied the man gruffly, with the hum of the melodramatic novela soundtrack, violins and vaguely operatic singing, filtering out behind him.

"We're here from the SEPA program to do a little inspection of your house to see if there are mosquitoes living here."

The man hesitated and looked at doña Guillermina with suspicion. "Are you with the rojinegro [red and black] brigades?" [The rojinegro brigades were Sandinista community cleaning and sanitation groups organized by the CDS in the 1980s.]

"No, sir," Guillermina replied. "This work is not red and black. This work is white and blue." Guillermina was referencing the colors of the Nicaraguan national flag, pointedly juxtaposing them with those of the FSLN party flag. The man let us in and turned down the television, but he watched us closely as we examined the water barrels, sinks, and dog dishes around his house. He looked puzzled as Josué drew a vial of water out of one of his sinks and showed him the *Aedes* larvae inside. Then he asked us for *abate,* mosquito larvicide. We had none to give out. Instead, Guillermina showed him a diagram of the life cycle of *Ae. aegypti,* demonstrating how it would develop in just over a week from egg to biting adult if he did not clean his water receptacles [figure 10]. She then reminded him of the symptoms of dengue: fever, vomiting, eye pain, sore joints and muscles. The man was not impressed.

"Why do you come? Just to look at the water? Brigadistas always bring *abate.*" He didn't protest beyond that, but he continued to stare as we moved on to the next house.

"That's the problem," Guillermina told me as we left. "They all think this is political work, and people are sick of politics. This is social work. Those are two different things, political and social work. . . . People need to understand this, but they don't."

As in all the houses she visited, doña Guillermina attempted to explain to the man that he needed to take responsibility for any mosquitoes that

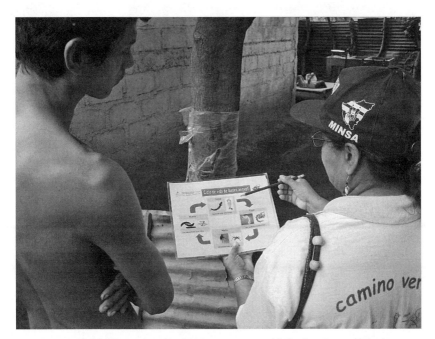

FIGURE 10. Brigadista explaining that mosquitoes could develop from eggs to larvae to pupae to adults in just over one week. (Photo by the author, 2008)

might live there. The mission of SEPA was to educate householders rather than to kill the mosquito larvae on their behalf. The distinction doña Guillermina was making, between the social and the political, resonated with one made by the dozens of other brigadistas with whom I carried out home visits. "I'm part of the CPC," she told me. "This is true. But I am a *community* worker. I work for my barrio, not for the party. I'm a Sandinista, not an Ortegista." SEPA's connection to the CPCs was understandable from a practical point of view, since many of the SEPA neighborhood coordinators were older people with long-standing ties to their communities. In Nueva Vida, however, where social ties were much younger and much more tenuous, this wasn't necessarily an advantage.

Doña Guillermina's misgivings notwithstanding, by the middle of 2008 word of SEPA's work had leaked into the mainstream of MINSA. Ciudad Sandino's health center director became especially keen to translate the lessons of SEPA to the rest of the city's brigadistas. As he told a group at a 2008 training meeting, "We have data that say that dengue is getting worse. If you want to understand how serious the problem is, you have to understand the statistics. Use the *data* to raise the people's consciousness *[concientizar]*. The people have to be conscientious, because dengue costs money. It costs them money when they get sick; it costs the hospital money when they come for consultation; and it costs us money to buy *abate*." Adapting a term he had borrowed from SEPA's organizers (and one that is well known in the development industry), he called this work "Participatory Action Research" *(investigación de acción participativa).* In trying to foment participatory action, the director drew on SEPA's data-oriented message. Statistically, dengue was serious enough to merit attention. The population was at medical risk. Economically, dengue was costing MINSA money. The population was at financial risk. His appeals to statistics and risk were scientific, but he also drew on a deeper history of participation, one peculiar to Nicaragua.

He pointedly mentioned *consciencia,* a sense of civic duty. Brigadistas began as volunteers, working outside the revolutionary government but active in its literacy, antihunger, and health projects in the brief period between the triumph of the revolution and the boiling point of the contra war. Drawn from secondary schools, factories, and neighborhood associations, brigadistas had served as the faces of the early FSLN's commitment to grassroots social service. It was thus no mistake that SEPA's volunteers bore the name *brigadista* as well. Planners were hoping to foment what scholars working with grassroots community groups during the revolutionary period termed *revolutionary praxis.*[23] As a "community"-minded CPC member, doña Guillermina was caught between her sense of obligation to use science to solve practical problems in the community and a parallel sense that the discourse of data-driven responsibility and surveillance might undermine such solidarity. In Spanish, *sepa* is the imperative form of the verb "to know." SEPA's model linked the democratization of science to the political surveillance and the scientific description of communities.

"LOCAL KNOWLEDGE" MEETS "GLOBAL HEALTH"

SEPA was a variant of a new form of participatory epidemiology that began developing in the 1990s. Its closest ancestor is a strategic public health marketing plan that the WHO calls Communication for Behavioral Impact (COMBI). Like SEPA, COMBI emerged out of a widely held concern among public health experts that although knowledge about the basics of dengue transmission (mosquito bites person; person gets sick) was high in most endemic areas, there was no reliable metric for human behavioral changes that might result from such knowledge.[24] The leaders of national-level dengue prevention programs needed to have a mechanism for finding out what kinds of actions people were taking, how those actions correlated to dengue prevalence, and how those actions might be sustained over the long term. Simply counting mosquitoes was not enough. In fact, those who favored the adaptation of participatory methods for dengue control found the use of entomological indices as proxies for human behavior largely unhelpful.[25] Community participation programs, they argued, should include something more than vector control. In their opinion, "best practices" should create "monitoring and feedback" among fieldworkers, scientists, and community members.[26] The goal of COMBI, like that of SEPA, was to create a *standard* procedure for capturing the *local* dynamics of epidemics.

The WHO's COMBI guidebook explicitly states that its goal is to "move beyond identification of risk behavior . . . to understanding the reasons that people do what they do." Its method for doing this is "situational market analysis," or the application of "anthropological methods" to marketing.[27] The idea is to use consultation with communities to identify what information is necessary and what "barriers" prevent individuals from "choosing" to apply that information.[28] Community health workers should be able to deliver to their supervisors nuanced, firsthand knowledge about people's experiences with the dengue prevention program. Supervisors can then adjust their interventions with a view to overcoming "situational" barriers.

The protocol for SEPA, the variant that CIET tested in Nicaragua, avoided COMBI's "market" language, favoring a seemingly less economic and more technical and scientific ethic, what CIET called the "participatory search, open circulation, lay interpretation and collective discussion of local evidence." CIET's summary of SEPA's goals, however, joins COMBI in trumpeting the power of "hard" data:

> When citizens are involved in research and evidence is openly and collectively discussed in focus groups, workshops, households, community meetings, and the media, communities are in a better position to tackle their development problems. The results of the fact-finding process should provide information for households and individuals to make decisions; they should inform service delivery to ensure that services are more responsive to the people; and they should ultimately be able to influence social policy. . . . SEPA's reliance on scientifically valid evidence is . . . a defining trait. . . . SEPA is evidence-based rather than expert-based.[29]

Though one favors market-oriented promotion and the other emphasizes collective decision making based on supposedly objective science, SEPA and COMBI are linked by a strict separation of evidence from experience, and of experts from laypeople. Whether couched as marketing or mobilization, the notion in these programs is that *data,* properly collected and disseminated, can lead to better decisions about health.

Within the WHO, PAHO, and MINSA, proponents of COMBI and related strategies like to compare dengue with noninfectious problems such as auto accident injury or hypertension. Seatbelt use, diet, and smoking cessation programs succeed, the argument goes, when public health experts find a way to sell them to the public. Good marketing overcomes concerns about comfort, taste, and fashion. WHO's COMBI manual emphasizes the need to document what it calls "qualitative" behavioral indicators, including "the existence of circulating rumors . . . that promote non-participation" and whether or not "target populations" perceive a given intervention as "relevant" and "effective." Notably, all of the qualitative questions in the COMBI model—including the existence of rumors—can be answered in a simple binary way: either there are rumors or there are not rumors; either there is a perception of relevance or there is not; either people see smoking as connected to high blood pressure or they do not.[30] In this way, "local knowledge" becomes legible as "evidence." SEPA's method simply reverses this, turning epidemiological and entomological "evidence" into local knowledge without changing its positivistic, quantitative character. Importantly, both strategies maintain the essential transferability of evidence and scientific validity, and the separation of these from a kind of immutable "local" experience.

While some within MINSA expressed enthusiasm about SEPA and COMBI, others wondered whether strategies like the Camino Verde could work at a national scale. The director of PAHO's dengue program in Nicaragua, looking back on her experience trying to adapt COMBI for a Nicaraguan audience, told me not only that mosquitoes and numbers were mobile, but also that ideas about dengue were steeped in history. "In the past, I thought that pesticides, that insecticides, should be eliminated, full stop." Now, she was not sure. "I think you have to start with the vectors," she told me. "When you inform the people more, they demand more." Once people knew that they were being watched—and being asked to watch mosquitoes—they could watch back. What if, in the weekly prevention visits, they saw not a group of expert technicians helping them factually document behavior but a government looking in on their private lives? This possibility made successive administrations wary of implementing COMBI, and indeed, she and others within MINSA were uncertain about its potential. No amount of public outreach, it seemed, could overcome deep-seated suspicions about the health ministry's relationship to the party and the state.

As the PAHO official explained, people in Nicaragua, including the staff of the national vector-borne disease program, placed a high value on pesticides like the *abate* that brigadistas carried on their home visits. They weren't dependent on such pesticides per se, but they did see them as material evidence of the government's investment in health. While SEPA's planners doubted the long-term effectiveness of pesticides, in Ciudad Sandino the health center's head epidemiologist and several vector-borne disease technicians expressed doubts about the benefits of the Camino Verde. Some even worried that SEPA's condemnation of chemicals would make householders more reticent than they already were about allowing paid MINSA brigadistas—brigadistas like Morena, Cecilia, and Xochitl—into their homes.

For those brigadistas, the job required a delicate set of exchanges: of *abate* for cooperation, and of privacy for safety. The ability to effect such exchanges was integral to the ability to gather and share data. They relied on a combination of empathy and routinized authority, a mix that set up brigadistas and householders as similarly participating and observing. In one MINSA training session I attended, experienced brigadistas were asked to tell newcomers how they convinced reluctant homeowners to let them inside. One group put together a short play, a *sociodrama*, about the difficulty of doing this. With an accuracy that had the other brigadistas laughing out loud, they acted out a typical encounter with a householder. The imaginary brigadista came to the imaginary door and greeted the occupant, played as female. But the homeowner was resistant. "We're all clean here," she said.

"Oh, I'm sure, *doña*," replied the brigadista melodramatically. "But we have to visit all the houses and inspect them. It's my job, you understand. They supervise us."

"Yes, but we're all clean here," the homeowner repeated. "Maybe you can just pass me a little bit of *abate*. For the ants, *amor*. You understand. We've got no mosquitoes here."

"I'm sorry, I can't do that, doña. It's prohibited. And you see, there are lots of cases of dengue in the barrio right now, including *dengue hemorrhágico,* which I'm sure you know is deadly."

"Dengue," the doña replied curiously. "What's *dengue?*" (Laughter erupted from the audience.) "All I know is that here it's all clean. And you know the mosquitoes and the flies, they come from all the mud puddles, and from the neighbors over there. You should see the mess she's got in her house. What a dirty woman. She's a *churequera* [garbage scavenger], you know. From there, there's where all the sickness comes from, not here. Now, can you give me a little *abate?* For the ants, you understand, *mi amor.*"

In the end, the imaginary brigadista succeeded by explaining what dengue was and that the woman's children were susceptible. "You have to scare them," said the doctor who was leading the training session. The appeal was to the individual's responsibility for her family's health but also to her obligation as a citizen to be vigilant. Brigadistas couldn't just "give out" *abate.* The sociodrama illustrated the delicate dance required to foment a "will" for this public and private vigilance, and it is noteworthy that the brigadista herself, in referring to "supervision," also drew on the trope of surveillance. In this instance, the brigadista acted as both agent of MINSA and cosubject, in order to draw the reluctant, "clean" homeowner into compliance.

The resistance of homeowners to inclusion in larval surveys stemmed in part from a suspicion that the brigadistas, as data collectors, might possibly single them out as "high risk," but it was clear to all of the brigadistas with whom I spoke, including those who performed the sociodrama, that being a part-time, underpaid state official, and doing so in *someone else's home,* was far from easy. A common refrain from the more than 10 percent of householders who refused to allow brigadistas inside was *¡Ustedes mandan en la calle, pero yo mando en mi casa!* (You're in charge on the street, but I'm in charge in my house!).[31] In the campaigns, I also witnessed and heard of householders threatening to set dogs loose, sexually harassing female brigadistas, threatening to call the police, and coming to their doors with machetes. As in other countries, many of the poorest in Nicaragua felt alienated from and mistrustful of the state (left-wing or right-wing), and as the sociodrama and my own survey data indicated, most considered the principal foco for mosquitoes to be in the streets.[32]

By pointing to the streets, homeowners were questioning the house-to-house prevention model, looking to public space rather than private space for blame and responsibility. There is limited scientific merit to this. *Ae. aegypti* is highly adapted to home habitats and to small bodies of water with low amounts of organic material. Ecological accuracy notwithstanding, questions about MINSA's neglect of public space were acknowledgments of the antidengue campaigns' stigmatizing tendency. Householders who met brigadistas' visits with angry complaints about the sanitation of streets and parks saw a punitive socialization of the private environment and a malign neglect of the public environment. In other words, they saw in state observation an overdetermination of the problem. As residents not only of houses but also of the streets, they reasonably saw their conditions as entangled.

The association of dengue prevention with the exercise of state power, then, was too frequent to avoid. As a PAHO official put it, referencing the 2008 change in Nicaragua's government from the liberal regime of Enrique Bolaños to the FSLN government of Ortega, "When the liberals were in power, they thought COMBI was socialist; now some Sandinistas say it is 'neoliberal.'"[33] From one perspective, data-driven "monitoring and feedback" played into the worst excesses of "big government," and from another, it permitted the state to put the responsibility for mosquito and dengue control disproportionately on the shoulders of citizens ill-equipped to bear such a burden. With COMBI and SEPA, government functionaries found themselves having to relocalize "local" knowledge. Though these processes were designed to render Nicaraguan experiences of dengue legible to global health experts, those who implemented them still had to do the work of making them look homegrown in the eyes of Nicaraguans themselves. Exchanges of *abate* for participation and the stories that lubricated those exchanges were helpful in this work.

DATA VERSUS STORIES

The routines of science and politics were certainly not in lockstep. Science was supposed to be detached and dispassionate, while politics was moored—perhaps too firmly—in place, history, and experience. One was concerned with gathering data: discrete points of information about the worlds of people and mosquitoes. The other was concerned with manipulating well-known stories. Keywords like *conciencia, socialismo,* and *neoliberalismo* evoked the emotionally charged experiences of the revolution and its aftermath. Yet for health workers, particularly at the most intimate levels of MINSA's organization, success in public health depended upon an entanglement of scientific and political practices, a blending of data collection with storytelling.

The tension between data and stories was a recurring topic at a COMBI-inspired course for public health workers at Cuba's Pedro Kourí Tropical Medicine Institute, which I attended in August of 2009. There, course leaders challenged a room full of community health workers from around Latin

America to ask themselves how they knew when they had achieved "participation," "empowerment," or "mobilization." Ideas shot across the room. For the Cuban delegates, "mobilization" had a decidedly political meaning, bound up with revolutionary and party activities.[34] You didn't necessarily "mobilize" against dengue. "Participation," however, made sense, and Cuban households were participating. (It was the law.) Cuba's dengue numbers were, by far, the lowest of any country in the hemisphere. A group of Costa Ricans, representing a small city that claimed some success the previous year in dengue reduction, explained that it had achieved "empowerment" by calling town meetings, gathering community groups together, and pressuring them to do something about mosquitoes, dengue, and household hygiene. Empowerment, for them, was little more than the application of political will. After the Costa Ricans made their pitch, a confident young Colombian doctor took the floor, slid a memory stick into the seminar room's computer, and began to explain—in exhaustive detail, with PowerPoint slides—how she had achieved "real participation" by educating children and youth.

At some point, a seminar leader reminded the group that their goal was to create systematic models for participation. "Otherwise," she said, "these are just stories." The seminar leader told students to privilege communication based on data over communication based on narrative.[35] "Stories," as the experts at the Cuba meeting explained, were impossible to measure or to replicate.

Experts and policy makers like to say that the field of dengue prevention has moved beyond the hubristic notion that human beings can dominate and manipulate nonhuman populations of insects and viruses. Today, bugs of all sizes are recognized as so adaptable and flexible that eradication plans that depend solely on technological measures such as swamp drainage, fumigation, DDT, or pharmaceuticals will likely fail to stop disease. Despite this humility in the face of dengue's nonhuman elements, the prevention discourse exemplified by COMBI and SEPA retains problematic assumptions about the ability of public health experts to measure the behaviors of *human* populations. If the unruliness of insects and viruses is now a given, the comprehensibility of people has remained somewhat unquestioned.[36]

This is not to say that concepts of local culture, local knowledge, and even local behavior are not important to those who advocate increasing community participation in dengue surveillance. Indeed, such concepts are deployed throughout the WHO's COMBI guides and SEPA's dengue prevention materials. The problem is that these aspects of human life have become targets for standardized data collection, even that which is purportedly "qualitative." SEPA's promotional materials include a collection of personal reflections by community participants, many of which include sentiments reflecting those I documented in the last chapter among Ciudad Sandino's brigadistas—sentiments about social connection and the joy of learning about the environment.[37] Yet even these stories appear in the modality of before and after. They are either preliminary or post hoc local "testimonies" about the power of data.

A look at Nicaragua's more routine forms of dengue control, like the ones represented in the sociodrama, shows how the geographically and historically particular stories, told not just by community members but by doctors, entomological technicians, and epidemiologists, continue to matter, in all their softness and complexity, despite an increasingly standardized, data-driven discourse of participation. Stories—charged with politics, rumor, and racial and ethnic undertones—are far from epiphenomenal to the progression of epidemics. Statistics produced by scientists do not erase them—quite the opposite. As Charles Briggs found in a study of cholera in Venezuela, stories about disease often reinforce the primacy of purportedly scientific and objective, data-driven knowledge and suppress other kinds of knowledge. Working in Cuba, Sean Brotherton notes that rumors about what the health ministry does *not* say about the extent of the dengue problem—unconfirmed statistical data—may actually promote collective action against mosquitoes.[38] While planners often see themselves as confronting memory, rumor, politics, and other aspects of "local culture" as obstacles to be overcome, on-the-ground practitioners in Ciudad Sandino discovered that those factors were not obstacles at all. In fact, the ability to dramatize dengue and to make participation tantamount to a role in that drama was what enabled them to collect data in the first place.

In his observations of experimental mahogany forests in Brazil, Hugh Raffles notes that the production of knowledge about forests—what he calls the "hunt for natural processes"—presumes the existence of facts (and trees) external to politics. The stories of those trees, which include the actions of humans, disappear. The same seems to happen in the process of public health data collection. A human decision to discard garbage or empty a water container is not just a point of data, any more than a mahogany tree in a Brazilian forest is just a tree, devoid of history.[39] Rather, the tree, the mosquito, and the human action are ongoing processes, steeped in history and identifiable "not by their intrinsic attributes but by the memories they call up."[40]

Conventional models for dengue control, then, elide a tension between the organization of the external world into data, which we experience as fact, and the "confluence of action and responses," which we experience as stories.[41] Doña Guillermina and her friends were frustrated because they found themselves turning complex processes into points of data whose status as "medical" and thus external to politics was necessary to the success of the participatory prevention project.

STORIED ROUTINES

Even though some MINSA officials like Ciudad Sandino's health center director were enthusiastic about SEPA and COMBI, these strategies were never adopted region- or country-wide. Yet even in routine prevention work, health workers like Ciudad Sandino's head epidemiologist mixed data with political dramatization to make dengue matter, symbolically and materially. The epidemiologist knew the code words of Sandinista politics. At various points in the meetings she held with CPC representatives, she described dengue as "our enemy," an "atomic bomb," and a "desperate" situation. At one meeting, with CPC representatives from zona 7, she mentioned a recent case of dengue hemorrhagic fever, but before she finished recounting the facts of the case, a representative spoke up and blamed it on the *llanteros* (tire changers) who threw old tires out into the gutters near the León highway, which ran through the neighborhood. Everyone knew that tires attracted mosquitoes, the representative reasoned, so MINSA, the city, the police, or someone needed to stop the dumping. The epidemiologist quickly turned the conversation around, though, to community involvement, asking the group, "If we have cases of dengue in our barrios, whose fault is it?"

"*De nosotros mismos* [It's our fault]" was the response from the assembled leaders, almost in unison.

The epidemiologist seized the moment of silence she had created and warned her audience that it was impossible for her small staff—herself, a nurse, and a secretary—to control dengue problems unless citizens reported them. Raising her voice, she told them, "*Hay que denunciarlos.* You have to denounce the people who are putting you at risk."

"Yes. The doctor's right. It's our fault," one CPC leader repeated. He and his compatriots seemed to get the message, and they began strategizing over how to approach the offending residents.[42]

By giving the epidemic a political valence, appealing to the responsibility of CPC leaders to mitigate it, the epidemiologist was attempting to personalize a population-wide problem. Importantly, *she* was not assigning blame. In MIN-SA's *lucha popular* model, that was the job of the CPCs. If a particular *llantero* was not facing his responsibilities, the CPC leaders were uniquely positioned to rectify his behavior. In Nicaragua's health system, such political dramatization has long been a principal strategy for turning public health problems into facts. Epidemiologists in outposts like Ciudad Sandino could collect data from their clinics, but they had few ways to effectively track behaviors, like tire dumping, that put the population at risk. Even before the return of the FSLN in 2007, they counted on a kind of citizen report known as a *denuncia* to decide which behaviors merited attention and resources. With the advent of the CPCs, however, rules about whose denuncia would be answered became more circumscribed. Despite the epidemiologists' willingness to go along with the government's new plans for mobilization, their appeals to the CPCs showed diminishing returns. In Ciudad Sandino, the CPCs submitted a fair number of denuncias, but they consistently failed to organize local brigades. As in the 1980s, social and medical problems kept coming, but unlike in those heady days, mass mobilizations did not.

Most denuncias concerned the actions of individuals, not public institutions. Complaints included the selling of spoiled meat at the market, the improper dumping of garbage, and other actions with environmental and health consequences. These documents combined geographical, emotional, biomedical, and political ways of framing suffering. One poignant example, written by a young mother from Nueva Vida to the Ciudad Sandino department of hygiene and epidemiology regarding a clandestine aluminum recycling plant, illustrates this blending:

Tuesday, November 28, 2007

To whom it may concern:

Esteemed *licenciadas* of hygiene and epidemiology, this is to make you aware of the situation my family and the residents of blocks "P" and "O" have been enduring for the last five years. We have been affected by an aluminum workshop that is located behind my house in block "P," which we have not denounced before because I lived for a time in Managua because I had a child hospitalized in *La Mascota* who later died. But now I am back in my house and my three children and I are experiencing skin and bronchial illness, and every day we're more affected, to the point that the fruit trees in my house have dried up. Everyone on the block is hoping that whatever is necessary will be done. The workshop operates all night and keeps everyone who needs to work in the daytime from sleeping.[43]

In general, denuncias appeared in this way. In almost all cases, the names and addresses of plaintiffs and accused were included, as well as the precise locations and times of significant events. Importantly, testaments of emotional *as well as* biological harm were included.

To ensure a prompt reading, denuncias had to come in writing, and they had to include a stamp and accompanying letter of approval from a CPC secretary. By invoking the denuncia to manage the dengue emergency, epidemiologists could tap a punitive political authority they did not themselves possess. They needed the aid of local volunteers to turn dengue into a solvable medical problem.[44] Epidemiologists could put dengue into the technical language of case counts and mosquito indices, but they needed individuals to feel responsible for the epidemic. Health centers could only give out the "facts" about the relationships between tires, mosquitoes, and dengue. Through the denuncia, those facts hit individual targets.

GOOD EPIDEMIOLOGISTS, GOOD TALKERS

One afternoon, sitting in the Ciudad Sandino epidemiology office, I began to reminisce with my coworkers about my initial 2006 field visit to Ciudad Sandino, when Dr. Arnoldo Muñoz was the head epidemiologist. This was before the CPCs came into existence, but the Ciudad Sandino health center had an active dengue program, focused on prevention efforts through meticulous surveillance, or *vigilancia*. I recalled that, back then, *vigilancia* involved not just health center staff and brigadistas but city employees, garbage men, and schoolchildren. Since 2007, I had seen few such prevention efforts.

Dr. Muñoz left Ciudad Sandino to become the head epidemiologist at the health center in another Managua barrio, but he and I remained in close contact. (This move was not unusual. Ciudad Sandino's health center cycled through several lead epidemiologists over the years of my fieldwork.) Muñoz had a master's degree in epidemiology and was studying for a separate master's in public health. We met on a regular basis to discuss my research and his own. During 2008, his barrio recorded many fewer dengue outbreaks than Ciudad Sandino did, and I wanted to find out how epidemiological workers in Ciudad Sandino might explain that difference. As one of the public health nurses recalled Muñoz's preventative activism, I asked her why she thought the two locations were so different epidemiologically.

"Dr. Muñoz works in [a place]," she answered, "[where] the houses are nicer. . . . The people have more money. Plus, it's very hilly there, so maybe the water runs down and carries off the mosquitoes!" We laughed.

"But really, you know, Dr. Muñoz is a militant Sandinista, like his whole family." (Muñoz's mother was especially active. She was a high school and university economics teacher and a party leader). "And that gives him good connections in MINSA, in his health center. Muñoz is a good talker."

Muñoz himself told a slightly different story. The more he learned about epidemiology, he used to tell me, the more he became disillusioned with politics. The distinction he made between the technical work of epidemiology and the spectacle of politics was not unlike those I heard from dengue specialists in other contexts, but in the end, he agreed with his former colleague in Ciudad Sandino that, for better or for worse, politicians ruled MINSA. After 2008, MINSA's top brass were almost all Ortega loyalists, and so were the majority of health center directors. Privately, Muñoz worried that despite his master's degrees, he would never be promoted, given his tepid enthusiasm for the direction in which Ortega and his cronies were leading the party. Publicly, however, Muñoz was indeed a "good talker." He had managed to organize preventative campaigns with the CPCs that were sometimes effective but always visible.

Sitting in his office one August afternoon, Muñoz showed me the results of a one-day campaign in which CPCs and health center staff visited about two thousand homes, giving educational talks about mosquitoes and distributing oral rehydration salts, bleach, and *abate*. (The bleach was for killing the mosquito eggs lodged on the rims of the concrete sinks and plastic fifty-five-gallon drums people used to store water.) I asked him how he was able to marshal the resources to do all this. He told me that he had "several advantages." The first? "I'm stubborn!" Without agitating, by sending letters and evidence of need to his local health center director and to MINSA leaders, he would never be able to carry out MINSA's dengue control policy. Second? He communicated daily with his counterparts in the hospital's vector-borne disease unit, figuring out which areas needed larvicide and fumigation. His main weapon in dealing with MINSA was statistics. He always backed up his claims of need with quantitative evidence of a problem: a pair of confirmed cases here, a mosquito "hot spot" there.

The third element was his work with CPCs. His preferred way of attaching himself to them was material: gifts of larvicide, bleach, oral rehydration salts. Muñoz kept a file in his desk that contained contact information for all the local party block leaders, and he called on them nearly every weekend to organize community brigades. How, then, did he guarantee that the CPCs did quality work? Here, he said, he took advantage of the political situation. The CPCs wanted to be seen as active and conscientious, since this paid political dividends. The health center director that supervised Dr. Muñoz wanted to be seen mobilizing the CPCs. Muñoz insisted that the CPC leaders themselves be out in the streets and that their "conscientious" mobilization be passed on to the brigadistas they chose. Muñoz personally made sure that the CPCs were visible. The packets of pesticide, bleach, and oral rehydration salts he gave them were good social tools because they were both immediately effective *and* effective in the long-term. Bleach killed mosquito eggs but it also cut down on bacterial growth. The pesticides kept mosquito larvae at bay and people also saw them as effective against household pests like ants and flies. Oral rehydration salts were still the quickest method for dealing with sick infants and children.

When I visited one of his weekend prevention programs, I watched as he wrangled his own staff and the CPC leaders in a barrio that sat above the highway leading into central Managua. I arrived in the barrio in the back of a pickup, along with two celestes, and Muñoz pulled in behind us in an ambulance. He had donned a white lab coat. (I remembered the coat from his days in Ciudad Sandino; it was embroidered with the words "Cleveland Clinic.") He grabbed a megaphone and gave the standard speech about dengue, house cleaning, and water containers, peppering it with political keywords: *consciencia, lucha popular,* and *Poder Ciudadano.* He was an entomologist, epidemiologist, and geographer, but he was also an entrepreneur and a storyteller. If the CPCs wanted the party to be looked upon favorably, he reasoned, they should help him produce good, cheap, and, most of all, visible epidemiological results.

Muñoz was deploying two kinds of *vigilancia:* the traditional epidemiological kind, using case counts, maps, and entomological surveys to quantify the dengue problem, and the political kind, using well-placed technological "gifts" to make the problem matter materially and symbolically. *Vigilancia* was chronic work. The point was to create a sense of generalized alertness to the ever-present danger of dengue. As Muñoz liked to tell me, echoing the consensus of most epidemiologists and health professionals in Nicaragua,

"You can't eradicate dengue. Dengue came to Nicaragua for good." Dengue could only be controlled, contained, and managed. His success hinged on the understanding that the FSLN was watching him from above via the MINSA administration and from below via the CPCs. To be sure, the Ortega administration's reason for making the CPCs the center of epidemic response was not only its interest in stopping dengue. (Muñoz had already trained his own brigadistas to do just this, and MINSA still paid them a small stipend to carry out routine mosquito surveillance and control.) The political motives behind the insertion of CPCs as gatekeepers to public services and sanitary chemicals were plain, but as political functionaries with special access to state resources, CPC leaders were useful allies for epidemiologists like Muñoz. Of course, epidemiologists still had some work to do. To show results to a party-state eager to declare "victory" over dengue, it was essential to craft a good story about epidemic response.

MANAGEMENT AND POLITICS

Even before the end of Sandinista rule in 1990, community organizers and brigadistas began to change the way they positioned themselves in relation to the state. When the CDS was at its most powerful, in the early 1980s, it was successful because its leaders appealed to a transpolitical sense of belonging. People had "rights" to read, write, eat, and receive health care not because they were party members but because they were Nicaraguan. In the distinction doña Guillermina made, a "Sandinista" was someone who organized the community for a practical purpose, with political dividends secondary. An "Ortegista" wanted political rewards to precede social ones.

This distinction betrays some nostalgia for the 1980s, something that certainly was palpable among the older generation of barrio leaders. Others, like Dr. Muñoz, told slightly more nuanced tales of the days of the CDS and of the 1980s. Dr. Muñoz recalled a woman who lived on his girlfriend's block when he was a teenager:

> Her name was doña Gregoria, but everyone called her by her nickname, doña Joya. She was a popular woman, coordinator of the CDS. She was popular because she ran all the government programs for health, for education. She was a leader with lots of followers, but not everyone liked her, even if they were enthusiastic about her programs. My girlfriend's parents told me that doña Joya kept a list of the names of all the boys in the barrio. She knew when

they were going to turn sixteen, and she would make sure that their families knew that there would be no more benefits if they didn't report for military service.

I guessed aloud that this must have made people resent doña Joya. "Eventually, yes, when the war became unpopular," he replied. "But when people believed in what she was doing, she was a good leader. The problem today is that there are lots of leaders but not so many followers."

The production of willing and effective participants in the "fight against dengue" was, like the production of effective surveillance, a work of political artifice.[45] Dr. Muñoz's recollections of the past indicate a sense that participants were not simply out there in communities, waiting to be identified. They, too, had to be produced, by "good leaders." In other words, they came into being along with the technological and material apparatuses designed to find and "mobilize" them. When it was most effective in the 1980s, participation felt as politically rewarding as it was socially rewarding. Some of my informants remembered those days with fondness, but they also remembered how quickly the urban masses lost heart, when the government turned social challenges into "wars," with "struggles," "victories," and "marches," and especially when claims to victory didn't come with material evidence thereof. Dengue was getting worse, not better, and everyone knew it. Even in the best of times, *el pueblo* could quickly become a hollow term. *Mejor solo que mal acompañado.* Searching for a reason that participation did not seem to be arising in their city, people in Ciudad Sandino seemed to be substituting the classic epidemiological questions, "How and why did this happen here?" with the questions, "How and why does this *matter* here?"

Despite the misgivings of Dr. Muñoz, doña Guillermina, and others like them, dengue and Nicaraguan politics, mosquitoes and Nicaraguan epidemiology, statistics and sicknesses, remain inextricably entangled. Indeed, dengue, as "social nature," has thrived *within* processes of political upheaval and technological change, from slavery to world wars to the reorganization of the global economy that resulted in a proliferation of zonas francas and chatarreras in Ciudad Sandino.[46] The trail of the mosquito traverses an unruly mélange of life-inscribing, knowledge-making apparatuses, including the epidemiological record, the mosquito surveillance worksheet, and the community map. Dengue prevention of all kinds—self-consciously "participatory" or not—requires citizens to join biomedical authorities in creating narratives about epidemics, mosquitoes, and the environment in which they relate to one another. Throughout the term of my fieldwork, doctors and scientists in MINSA were anecdotally skeptical of the official epidemic numbers, fearing that the government may have been manipulating them. Without capacity on my own to confirm or deny MINSA's claims, I remain agnostic on this point. It is easy to imagine, of course, that epidemiologists, brigadistas, and others *would* make up stories about dengue for political gain. This possibility is likely why many public health experts consider politics to be a barrier to quality care. But seen from another point of view—seen as the context in which disease *and* disease narratives emerge—politics might be something more than a barrier. Narrative production, as historian Gabrielle Hecht suggests, "both open[s] and close[s] political possibilities."[47] For doctors, CPC leaders, and brigadistas, to make a "declaration" about dengue and mosquitoes was to make a statement of authority. This authority issued from a mastery of both the scientific production of data and the political practice of storytelling.

SIX

Dengue Season in the City of Emergencies

YAMILETH'S SON ESTEBAN became ill in 2005. Yamileth, whom I introduced in chapter 3, was a brigadista, and her house was a *casa base,* a place where neighbors could come for basic medical advice. As a *casa base* volunteer, Yamileth knew when Esteban got sick that he needed more skilled attention than she could give. It was the height of the rainy season—the peak period for dengue infection, as well as respiratory and gastrointestinal illnesses.

"I took him to the health center," Yamileth told me in an interview three years later, "but they found nothing in his [blood tests]. Then I went to a paid laboratory [a private diagnostic facility], and there was a contradiction in the exams."

Esteban was sick and getting sicker, and no one could figure out why. On three separate occasions, he was sent by doctors at the Ciudad Sandino health center to a hospital in Managua, only to be sent home with inconclusive diagnoses. On her last trip to the hospital, Yamileth said to the doctor, "Doctor, look, my son is going to die . . . he doesn't want to eat. He's so thin!" Yamileth kept returning with more blood test results and consultation records *(constancias),* scribbled on scraps of lab paper, but still the doctors could find nothing specifically wrong with Esteban.

Then, after two days of testing and retesting (at one point, Esteban even underwent an ultrasound to rule out appendicitis), a doctor in the Velez Pais Hospital found something. He asked Yamileth to accompany him into the hospital laboratory. Yamileth remembered looking into a microscope at her son's blood sample, and she recalled the conversation with the doctor, who explained: "Your son has mixed malaria." According to the doctor, Esteban was stricken with two forms of malaria parasite: both the one that typically circulated in Managua and the one usually seen only on Nicaragua's Atlantic coast.

Following normal malaria protocol, the doctor asked if Yamileth or any-one else in her family had been traveling lately. Yamileth thought about it. The neighbors traveled, but they only went to León, less than two hours north of Ciudad Sandino. The unusual strain of malaria was not endemic there either. Unable to trace Esteban's parasite back to its supposed origin, the doctor seemed to doubt his own analysis. Though the disease still struck rural areas of the Department of Managua, malaria of any kind was rare in urban Nicaragua. His next diagnostic *constancia* for Esteban listed three ill-nesses: malaria, pneumonia, *and dengue.* Esteban was now staying overnight in the hospital for observation.

"This was so hard for me. From one illness to another, then another, with nothing that could be done," Yamileth recollected. "Then, one morning the doctor returned and told me, 'Look,' he told me, 'you have to go get another exam for the boy.'"

"Why?" Yamileth asked him with exasperation.

"Because it's possible that this boy is diabetic," the doctor answered.

Yamileth was distraught, but she managed to find ten U.S. dollars to pay for another blood test, which came back negative. After a few more days in the hospital—still with no clear diagnosis—Esteban began to improve, re-gaining his appetite. He was sent home, but Yamileth, mindful of the sug-gestion that dengue might have been what made Esteban sick, remained apprehensive.

"All I could think was that [my two other young boys] were going to get sick . . . but only he was sick," she remembered. "That was in 2005. . . . But then a year later, when it *was* dengue, we all got sick. Everyone but my hus-band and my daughter."

DENGUE AND TEMPORAL INCONGRUITIES

When relatives got sick, Nicaraguans like Yamileth entered a public health system that was, by any reasonable standard, vastly underresourced. Still, they were beset with a barrage of devices and forms of explanation: micros-copy, ultrasound, blood sugar assays, geographies of malaria parasites, and suspicions of bacterial-pulmonary infection. This medical and technical lit-any underscored something that doctors and nurses and parents all knew well. Children die in Managua too often, and too often the causes of their deaths are multifactorial, or indeterminate. Still, in Managua, biomedical cures—promised by MINSA doctors and advertised by private clinicians—*appear possible*. Mary-Jo DelVecchio Good has articulated a key aspect of global health, a "biotechnical embrace," whereby "multiple regimes of truth," including patient histories, clinical narratives, and political economic histories, muddle the distinction between local and global knowledge. "Local meanings and social arrangements," Good writes, "are overlaid by global standards and technologies in nearly all aspects of local biomedicine."[1] In Esteban's case, the truth claims of the hospital diagnoses were technical, based upon an assumed scientific authority, yet they were entangled with material and social circumstances particular to Nicaragua—and even to Ciudad Sandino.

Yamileth trusted doctors' orders, but more specifically, she worked to reconcile *her* story about Esteban's illness with those of doctors. Note the importance of time in Good's "regimes of truth:" the "histories" and "narratives" that seem sometimes to overlap with and sometimes to diverge from "local knowledge." Medical anthropologists have long been interested in the disjuncture between linear, historical clinical narrative and the phenomenological experience of disease.[2] In Michael Taussig's classic essay "Reification and the Consciousness of the Patient," he describes how patients surrender their understanding of time and even self as a series of social relationships to a medical understanding that sees bodies and illnesses as objects. Biomedicine suspends the time of experience and relationality in favor of a time of homogeneous empty sequence.[3] In fitting particular experiences to a standardized clinical history, medicine seems to flatten time out, putting it into an abstract narrative of cause and effect in which past, present, and future are clearly delineated. Patients surrender their understanding of time—and hence of their own bodies—to that of the clinician.[4] Likewise, epidemiological narratives about risk rely upon discernable reckonings of events-in-sequence. Biopolitical analyses of global health approaches to diseases like dengue, avian influenza, and other kinds of what experts call "emerging infectious diseases" emphasize how systems of surveillance and preparation link individual subjective experiences of disease-to-come with models of population dynamics. As a governmental apparatus, global health instills a kind of temporal discipline that, as in Taussig's analysis of the clinical encounter, serves particular power interests. In contemporary global health, concerned with the rapid spread of diseases like dengue, biomedical attempts to standardize temporality have, by some accounts, led to a moral, technical, and political posture of "anticipation," of orientation to a future occurrence of epidemics.[5] This involves the reconciliation of local experience with both "global" (in the standardizing sense of the word) clinical temporalities and "global" (in the geographical sense of the word) concerns about future catastrophe.

Accounts of global health centered on a discourse of anticipation say much about how those in the global north understand emerging disease but they tell us less about the places where epidemics have already emerged. This is where Lock's concept of "local biologies" and Good's notion of an "embrace" become useful.[6] Examinations of local biologies in global health from anthropology highlight the temporal demands that technologies like anti-retroviral HIV therapy or tuberculosis therapies make on bodies. Drug regimens demand particular sequences of drugs and rigid routines of self-management. Such standardized biomedical technologies tend to meet uncomfortably with local routines of bodily care, colonial and postcolonial histories, and culturally specific senses of personhood.[7] To date, however, most work on local biology tends to look at temporal politics as situated only in bodies. Animal-borne diseases like dengue involve extra-bodily temporalities.

In Nicaragua, dengue is a seasonal emergency. Epidemics swell in the rainy season, usually from August to November, when conditions for mosquito propagation are optimal. The embodied experience of dengue blends seasonality, with its connotations of regularity and reliability, and emergency, with seemingly opposite connotations of the unexpected and chaotic. Seasonal emergencies are full of what the economic anthropologist Hirokazu Miyazaki calls "temporal incongruities."[8] Biomedical technologies, human socialities, and nonhuman ecologies demand different, and not always reconcilable, forms of temporal attentiveness. Concern about dengue emerges somewhere in the overlaps among the biweekly cycles of insect growth, the hidden flaws of an immunological memory that spans years, and the everyday tasks of householding. Nicaraguan health workers construct a notion of health by, as Miyazaki puts it, "making use of" the disjointed temporalities of the objects and processes they want to understand. They do this as parties to a biotechnical embrace, taking up technologies that are built not for local biologies but for standardized bodies and uniform spaces.

Yamileth's brief story demonstrates the power of biomedical technologies and their attendant promises to shape bodies and subjects but it also shows how biomedical temporalities clash—ideologically, materially, and politically— with other temporalities. Esteban's case drew together ideas about clinical and epidemiological time with other senses of time. His case was about cycles of dengue transmission, but also about the life histories of parasites and the life cycles of mosquitoes. These were connected in turn to patterns of rainfall, heat, and climate. Temporal reckonings of health from biomedicine and epidemiology were refracted through reckonings from ecology and meteorology. Disparate time scales paralleled disparate geographical ones: both Yamileth and Esteban's doctors tried to reconcile the suspected occupation of blood cells by parasites with the seemingly improbable travels of those same parasites across the rugged Nicaraguan landscape and through the entangled spaces of the clinic, the *casa base,* and the family home.

Political ecology and environmental anthropology, informed by science and technology studies, have leveled a critique of nature similar to that of medical anthropology's critique of the body, namely, that what science and policy present to us as objective facts about the supposedly natural world are in fact sets of social relationships.[9] What we know as "nature" has the ability to hide the historical conditions of its own production. Landscapes change—sometimes with human help, and sometimes without—but because those changes occur at speeds and scales that do not match human embodied experience, their deep sociality is difficult to comprehend.[10] Even human bodies contain temporal incongruities. Consider the phenomenon of "antibody dependent enhancement," which likely causes many hemorrhagic dengue infections. A body exposed to a single dengue serotype (for example, to Dengue 1) develops immunological "memory" of that particular serotype, but problems arise when the same body confronts another serotype. The antigens that are dominant in Dengue 1 are recessive in the others. This means that antibodies produced to neutralize Dengue 1 bind to the antigens of the new serotype, but instead of neutralizing it, those antibodies actually help enhance the infection, helping the virus replicate *more* quickly than before. Because of this shortcoming in immunological memory, second infections can lead to more severe infections. Community health workers like Yamileth knew, in general, that past infection might matter for present and future ones, yet they often were not privy to the particular histories of their own immune systems' encounters with the pathogens.

Measurements of dengue's prevalence in the landscape, from immunoglobulin assays that traced antibodies to case counts to mosquito assays, marked time, but the making of those measurements—an embodied activity that implicated experts and "local participants" alike—left its own traces on the landscape. Mosquitos, viruses, and habitats are frequently reified as hazards that can be overcome through proper education, training, and hygienic discipline. Emerging disease in this view looks like nature's war on us, when in fact the stories of dengue, influenza, and HIV-AIDS—even though all these diseases have major nonhuman components—show them to be not ones of conflict but rather of a series of temporally incongruous entanglements.

In this variegated temporal and spatial field, Nicaraguans' trust in biomedical authority remained fairly strong. Even when diagnoses clearly conflicted with one another, *constancias* and prescriptions were normally quite closely guarded. Diagnostic confusion is part of the dengue season in Nicaragua. Increasingly, so is death.

One such death, that of Maria Luisa Gutiérrez, a thirteen-year-old girl from Managua who died in the La Mascota hospital in 2009, briefly captivated the attention of journalists and the public. A hospital death, even the tragic passing of a child, was not always public news, but *El Nuevo Diario* chose to put Maria Luisa's story on its front page. That year, the dengue season coincided with the onset of what the WHO called "pandemic influenza A-H1N1" and what most people in the United States knew as the swine flu. *El Nuevo Diario*'s story's title presented Maria Luisa's case as a medical mystery: "Did She Die of H1N1, Tonsillitis, Dengue, or Medical Negligence?"[11] Like several other children that year, Maria Luisa presented with symptoms of more than one disease. Though talk of H1N1/dengue "coinfection" was commonplace among doctors, nurses, and epidemiologists, Maria Luisa's case highlights the temporal incongruities that framed the practice of care in Managua's hospitals and health centers during each dengue season.

At a clinical level, cases like those of Esteban and Maria Luisa point to the possibility that the mingling of two pathogens in a single body could cause severe and unforeseen complications.[12] At an epidemiological level, the appearance of an inordinately large number of sick children in Managua's health centers indicated that the mingling of viruses was overloading an already strapped public health service.[13] As Maria Luisa's doctors told reporters, the particular strain of dengue that was eventually found in the girl's body (a serotype-3 variant) tended to cause an "unusual" sequence of symptoms.[14] Pediatric patients like Maria Luisa were deteriorating from severe fever to abdominal aches to life-threatening capillary leak syndrome at a faster rate than with other serotypes—even faster than with serotype 3 strains known to have circulated in Nicaragua in previous dengue seasons. As in Esteban's case, disparate disease temporalities were meeting in Maria

Luisa's body: the progression of viral-immune system reactions became entangled with the seasonal progression of epidemics and the close, painful, collectively embodied "progress" of a particular person's illness.[15]

When she first got sick, Maria Luisa's parents took her to their neighborhood clinic. The Socrates Flores Health Center does not look remarkably different from the health center in Managua where Dr. Muñoz worked, or from the Ciudad Sandino Health Center where Yamileth sometimes worked as a brigadista and where she first took Esteban. But Socrates Flores was actually unique among Nicaragua's public medical facilities. Since 2004, a team of scientists based there had been involved in the Pediatric Dengue Cohort Study, the longitudinal study of dengue in urban children organized by the Sustainable Sciences Institute, which I introduced in chapter 5.[16] The study isolates viral strains and traces them via a worldwide genomic database as they spread to and from Nicaragua. Funding for the study came from the Bill and Melinda Gates Foundation, via the Pediatric Dengue Vaccine Initiative, a global partnership among national health ministries, pharmaceutical corporations, and academic scientists.[17] Thanks in part to the success of the cohort study, Nicaragua's National Diagnostic and Reference Center (CNDR) is now one of the most sophisticated molecular epidemiology laboratories in the Americas. Equipped with state-of-the-art viral detection equipment, CNDR is now a key node in the global tracking of dengue. By 2009, CNDR was making dengue more visible in Managua, and making Managua more visible to global health practitioners and policy makers.

But Maria Luisa was not part of the cohort study. Socrates Flores still received the majority of its patients in the same way Ciudad Sandino's health center did: through a public, walk-in "emergency" ward and several overcrowded consulting rooms. Eventually, laboratory tests might turn dengue cases like hers from "suspected" to "confirmed," but the seasonal procedures undertaken by brigadistas, epidemiologists, doctors, and others before and after it made the dengue problem matter, in a material and symbolic sense, long before her death made it into the newspaper. In 2009, as in every other dengue season, most suspected cases of dengue would never receive laboratory confirmation. The cost of the tests and the difficulty of transporting samples from around the country to CNDR made that impossible. As I explain later in this chapter, "suspected" cases mattered to local confrontations with dengue as much—and probably more—than "confirmed" ones. In both suspected and confirmed cases, mosquitoes died, ambulances were mobilized, and neighbors were put on alert.

Dengue underscores the recursive relationship between climatic and ento-mological cycles and economic, political, and technological routines. As Tim Ingold suggests, the resonances between human activities and the tem-porally disparate cycles of geology, climate, and ecology "are *embodied,* in the sense that they are not only historically incorporated into the enduring features of the landscape but also developmentally incorporated into our very constitution as biological organisms."[18] In places like Managua and Ci-udad Sandino, people, insects, rainfall, and viruses meet along the uneven pathways formed by local urban infrastructure and global health programs. These trails, each with their own temporalities, connect health centers to dif-ferent forms of life. Those cycles that seem mostly human (the economic, political, and technological) do not just constitute reactions to nonhuman cycles of climatic, viral, or insect development. Instead, temporal patterns of nonhuman behavior disrupt, reconstitute, and recalibrate human ones, and vice versa. Dengue entangles a multiplicity of temporal ontologies—or ways of apprehending and perceiving the passage of time.[19] These include the em-bodied yet strangely "other" workings of the immune system, seasonal cli-mate patterns, mosquito life cycles, health ministry budget allocations, epi-demiological patterns, political cycles, and the abiding expectations of future disaster (bound up with memories of past ones), including epidemics but also earthquakes and floods, that shape urban Nicaraguan experiences.

Maria Luisa's death and Esteban's illness can be understood as part of a seasonal cycle of rising suspicion, confirmation, and containment. This cycle played out not just in clinics but across Nicaragua's urban landscape. Nearly every aspect of the dengue complex, from prevention to clinical encounters to emergency response, operates in a seasonally patterned way. The cycle starts in the dry season. From January to June, brigadistas spread knowledge about the cyclical patterns of insect growth and how those patterns mesh with the cycles of household management. As the rains begin in July and August, doctors contemplate the patterns by which human immune systems respond to novel viral serotypes, sometimes producing unexpected reac-tions. Epidemics themselves swell at the height of the rainy season, which begins in late August and lasts into December.

In my ethnographic notes and interviews, the term *emergency* appears in reference to everything from the 1972 Managua earthquake, to Hurricane Mitch in 1998, to a taxi drivers' strike, to the 2008 financial collapse, to the botched municipal elections of that year, to the blockades of Ciudad Sandino's dump. Like *surveillance* and *participation, emergency* was an infectious political trope. The words *epidemia* (epidemic), *brote* (outbreak), and *crisis* (crisis) were just as likely to appear in discourses of violence and moral breakdown among community and church leaders as among epidemiologists. Indeed, as I have argued, the area's history was steeped in emergency. In many ways, then, the discourse of emergency was effective at making dengue matter in urban Nicaragua. The reliable breakdown of routine surveillance and the fracture of delicate infrastructures prompted reflection about the entanglement of care and politics.

Ethnographies of catastrophe underscore the importance of scientific and political economic processes in making meaning out of supposedly "natural" disasters. Often, weather or seismic events become ways to reinforce a divide between people and a capricious and unpredictable "nature," but in Nicaragua's dengue epidemics, such a divide was rendered impossible maintain by the seasonally timed, concomitant spikes in rainfall, mosquito populations, and illness.[20] The reliability of emergency prompts a new question. As Erica James asks regarding the politics of trauma in Haiti, "Where is the line between drawing attention to the suffering of others in order to assist them and appropriating the suffering of others for institutional or personal gain?"[21] On the one hand, to "assist" others in a coordinated fashion requires reliable metrics for declaring when and where "suffering" has occurred. Global health metrics such as confirmed case counts aggregate suffering across populations and turn it into a solvable problem. On the other hand, once quantitative thresholds (of rainfall, of morbidity, of mosquito prevalence) have been breached, as James suggests in her question, the "suffering other" ceases to be an undifferentiated member of a population and becomes a political subject.[22] A dengue emergency, as a seasonal disruption of the normal relationship between people and nature and between people and systems of power, is not just an opportunity for the consolidation of state or technical power. In an emergency, the making of political subjects, the making of scientific facts, and the opening of spaces for ethical reflection (spaces both environmental and bodily) all happen at once. In a seasonal emergency, that intersection of activity and debate happens at a particular, reliable time of year, marked by weather and epidemiological patterns. Attention to such seasonal frictions, between rainfall, mosquitoes, viruses, and human biology, shows how politics and history "channel" regionally and globally oscillating cycles of epidemics and weather and render them meaningful.[23] Thus, the emergency constitutes not a singular event but a confluence of several ways of reckoning time: phenomenological, clinical, social, historical, climatic, and epidemiological.

Nicaragua's seasonal responses to dengue were moments in which people recalibrated their relationships to the nonhuman environment and to the systems of social order in which they found themselves.[24] According to the Intergovernmental Panel on Climate Change, changes in long-term temperature and humidity induced by intensified human activity are likely to produce more intense dengue epidemic seasons.[25] Even absent drastic climate change, political and economic upheavals, from financial crises to regime changes, have already intersected, both to enable the rapid spread of people, viruses, and mosquitoes and to produce a high-tech global health complex that is reframing how scientists and local people understand dengue. This final chapter is an attempt to track the ways in which people in Ciudad Sandino and neighboring Managua, those "cities of emergency," engaged the seasonal rise and fall of dengue epidemics amid other temporal concerns.

Effective public health requires linking personal experience to population concerns through plausible and actionable connections between time and space. Changes in the urban landscape occur in discernable patterns, and in dengue epidemiology these changes gain significance when they cause disturbances to bodies. Studies of human exposure to chemicals, nuclear fallout, and pharmaceutical regimes—to name a few notable examples—have demonstrated how bodily chemistry and the time scales of half-lives, retroviral efficacy patterns, and pesticide drift become woven into human senses of disease temporality.[26] The environments of health, then, undermine our attempts to reify the consciousness of patients, as well as of nonpatients who are also enveloped in seasonal emergencies. Both care and politics emerge in the attempts by an agglomeration of actors to stuff an unruly and thoroughly social body-nature back into sets of discrete events that take place in discrete places. As a practice of care and politics, public health, at least in the context of vector-borne diseases like dengue and other clearly "environmental" health problems, emerges in contests over ways to align temporality and geography, yet in dengue, a multiplicity of temporalities obtain—those of the body, the mosquito, the rain, the immune system, chemicals, and political history. This makes dengue difficult to render politically or morally legible, yet it also makes dengue emergencies a form of what Hugh Raffles calls "effective geography": moments that reveal that what undergirds social and natural action is not a neat sequence of occurrences spread in linear fashion across a uniform space but "a profusion of entangled events."[27]

As Esteban's and Maria Luisa's cases demonstrate, uncertainty and chaos are central features of dengue and other seasonal epidemics. Through formal and informal bouts of testing, questioning, pleading, and intervening, seasonal states of emergency engendered what Lauren Berlant calls "modes of attachment that [made] persons public and collective and . . . collective scenes intimate spaces."[28] Taking dengue as a seasonal occurrence, we can understand it as a more-than-human mode of attachment, in which not only chaos and uncertainty but also identifiable, patterned dynamics of ecology and politics are at play. It is important to note that the seasonal cycles of dengue I describe here were somewhat new in Nicaraguan medical experience. Until the 1990s, dengue was simply not on most people's lists of major health concerns, even if the rains did bring about spikes in diarrhea and respiratory illness. Given the uneven, overlapping ways in which health technologies, mosquito populations, and the built environment changed from year to year, each iteration of the dengue season slightly reframed the ways in which people dealt with the paradox of intimacy.

AUGUST: PAYDAYS AND EMERGENCIES

The director of Ciudad Sandino's health center was facing a crisis. The entomological reports from the first week of the latest house-to-house source reduction campaign were not good. Worse, funds had run short. Today was Friday. It should have been payday for the brigadistas, who, after a day's work tracking mosquitoes in Nueva Vida, would be lining up outside the administration building to collect envelopes containing their cash stipends. But there did not appear to be any money available. Not unless something else—perhaps gasoline for the ambulances, or funds for the monthly meeting of the diabetics' club—gave way. To make matters worse, don Francisco, the head celeste, had recently been transferred to another district. Don Luis, his replacement, was having trouble keeping morale high among the brigadistas. Don Luis was younger and was completing a master's degree in entomology at the National University of Nicaragua. He was thus a rising star within MINSA, but he was a poor communicator.

The job of delivering the news about the missed payday fell to don Nacho, the oldest and most experienced of the remaining celestes. Don Nacho lived in

Ciudad Sandino and was a neighbor to many of the brigadistas. Perhaps they would trust his word. After the brigadistas gathered at the Nueva Vida health post that day, don Nacho performed the *revista*, checking that all the brigadistas were present with their equipment in good order. He then addressed them, starting off, as don Francisco often had, by scolding them about the entomology reports. "I was out there yesterday, supervising your work," he said, "and I found *too many* eggshells, coconuts, bottles, and cans being missed. Here in Nueva Vida—especially in Nueva Vida—that is not acceptable, *muchachos*." Don Nacho then lowered his voice. "*Oígame.* I have a piece of bad news." The brigadistas appeared to step half a foot closer as he told them that there would not be any payment at the end of the day. The brigadistas were first incredulous, then angry. They threw down their clipboards and bags, demanding that don Nacho explain himself. Perhaps, he guessed timidly, their national ID numbers had not been processed correctly. Morena, who had dealt with dishonest managers at her previous jobs in zonas francas and in the local market, knew what to do. She wrote down the ID numbers of each brigadista and enlisted a volunteer representative from each of the four work groups.

Morena and her appointed cohorts led don Nacho on the twenty-minute walk back to the health center to confront the director. The health center was officially titled the Hospital Nilda Patricia Velasco de Zedillo, after the wealthy Mexican donor who helped finance its construction in the 1990s. Nobody called it by its commemorative name, however, partly because the name was so lengthy, and partly because the staff had heard that Mexicans considered it rude—and possibly bad luck—to repeat the names of the dead. They more commonly referred to the small collection of buildings as the "little hospital" *(hospitalito)*. On the north side of the complex was the first of the hospitalito's four main buildings, an emergency ward that was open twenty-four hours a day. In early 2007, the emergency ward also became home to an eye care clinic, part of a joint Cuban-Venezuelan mission called Operación Milagro (Operation Miracle). Thanks to the popularity of the eye clinic, the large metal gate that led to the emergency room was usually swarmed with buses, cars, and cabs carrying Nicaraguans from all over the country seeking free care for cataracts, glaucoma, and other ocular ailments. Morena strode into the hospitalito through these gates, where patients found themselves hounded by opportunistic vendors selling coffee and buttered bread in the morning and *comidas rápidas*—tacos, *gallo pinto,* sodas, and the homemade, sugar-sweetened fruit drinks known as *frescos*—in the afternoons. A guard manned the gate, but with the daily influx of eye patients, vehicles, and vendors, he could provide little security.

Once inside the gates, Morena and her fellow brigadistas followed a small concrete path bisecting the administration building on the right and the pharmacy and general consulting clinics on the left. The director's office was located inside the administration building. Its small windows looked into the courtyard where the ambulances parked. The director was protected from the cacophony of cars, motorcycle taxis, touts, and vendors but still in sight of the weary old *campesinos,* stumbling out of surgery just as blind and unsteady as they had entered, rambling about their pain, and fiddling with their gauzy eye patches.

The brigadistas, followed by a sheepish don Nacho, escorted themselves past a weary secretary and put their case to the director. There would be no *abatización,* Morena declared, without a paycheck. The director saw this coming, but he was visibly frustrated that don Nacho was not able to control the brigadistas. Morena and her cohorts threatened to strike. They threatened to denounce the director to his supervisors in Managua. The director quickly relented, averting at least one crisis. But as he told Morena and the others on that day, and would tell them again and again, "A brigadista has to be ready to serve the community in any kind of emergency."

The brief battle over paychecks was a battle of triage: whose interests would prevail when not all interests could be served? The brigadistas were addressing one looming emergency—the dengue one—but their lives, too, were precarious. "We raise families, too. We have to feed them, too," Morena said afterward. "What if they stopped paying the full-time staff? Would *they* keep showing up to work?" Morena's personal bodily concerns—about the basics of getting enough to eat—became public concerns, just as the workings of dengue in the bodies of patients became public. The temporal incongruity at play here was between two kinds of calendrical events, one economic (the payday) and one epidemiological (the looming dengue outbreak). Dengue took its moral and political form in the space between these.[29] Concerns about the incongruity between economic and biological time only intensified as August turned to September.

When a suspected case of dengue was reported to the epidemiology office in Ciudad Sandino, the health center's staff did not wait for a laboratory-confirmed diagnosis of dengue to spring into action. Standard procedure in suspected cases was, first, to kill mosquitoes. Responsibility for short-notice fumigation visits fell to the celestes. In Ciudad Sandino, the celestes who did most of this rapid extermination were don Nacho and his younger male colleague, don Noë. Once a suspected case came to the attention of the epidemiology office, arrangements would be made for either don Nacho or don Noë to be transported by pickup truck or ambulance to the house of the patient. This involved the signing of forms and the approval of the hospitalito's head epidemiologist, verbal arrangements with one of the two resident ambulance drivers, a signature from the head celeste, and the approval of gasoline expenditure by the director. The commissioning of a gasoline-powered vehicle was particularly important, and particularly disruptive. In the course of my fieldwork, the call for don Nacho or don Noë to "attend a case of dengue" led to the suspension of several other vehicle-dependent activities, such as routine water quality testing, quarterly rabies vaccination campaigns for dogs, or the transportation of brigadistas to an outlying zona for mosquito control visits.

You could tell when don Nacho or don Noë had come to your neighborhood by the distinctive sound of their main piece of equipment, the *motomochila*. The *motomochila* looked like a heavy-duty leaf blower. It was essentially a small two-stroke engine mounted to a backpack frame. The engine powered a fogging machine that released a vaporized, diluted solution of an aerial insecticide, most often a variant of malathion, cypermethrin, or other organophosphate, through a long, wide plastic tube. The machine made a terrific moan that echoed off of the concrete walls and metal roofs, and don Nacho and don Noë showed no small amount of enthusiasm when they got the chance to use it. Arriving at the patient's house, they would order all inhabitants and neighbors outside and then saturate the already dense, hot air inside with the chemical fog, a neurotoxin that was calibrated at MINSA's central vector-borne disease headquarters to kill adult mosquitoes on contact.

Malathion and its organophosphate relatives are powerful agents, but as with other pesticides, mosquito populations can develop resistance to them. Not all mosquitoes will die in a given fogging. Some will survive the poison, and eventually their offspring will dominate the population. Thus, levels of insecticide in the *motomochila's* dilution had to be high enough to kill a significant number of mosquitoes but low enough to make the evolutionary march to mosquito population resistance as slow as possible. A massive dose of high-powered insecticide would be effective in the short-term but render the chemical useless in the long term.

MINSA's head entomologist for the Department of Managua called achieving this dilution level a process of "experimentation." He and his staff maintained their own *insectario,* a mosquito nursery where they bred control colonies of *Ae. aegypti* and other species. Each season, they tested various insecticides at various strengths on both the control colonies and on "wild" mosquitoes harvested from traps placed throughout the city. The head entomologist showed me the graphs he produced from these tests, reflecting mosquito death rates from various mixtures. He delivered this information to his superior in the vector-borne disease unit, who helped him determine an official yearly dilution level for the district. Since the resources for poison were limited, the decision about an acceptable death rate was part biology and part economics. Even if the number of suspected dengue cases fluctuated over the course of the year, MINSA's budget for poison was constant, set just once a year.

During our interview, the entomologist drew me a graph of *Ae. aegypti* prevalence from the 1990s to the 2000s. The graph showed that, when the government stopped investing in mosquito control measures (aerial poisons and the *abate* given to brigadistas), the numbers climbed. Since the 1990s, the staff of the vector-borne disease program had been slashed. The entomologist faulted nonexperts in the political class for paying too little attention to the science of surveillance. During outbreaks, he said, MINSA would bring out the *motomochilas* and target neighborhoods with dramatic hygienic measures, but in their treatment of the mosquito, they always took the "cheapest" route. "Mosquitoes," he said, "are animals of custom like us." "Wild" populations adapted to chemical control regimes (as well as higher altitudes and higher average yearly temperatures), so it was up to "fieldworkers" like himself to adapt to them through seasonal experimentation. Trying to tackle the problem at the last minute was scientifically pointless, if politically savvy. Since the end of the revolution, MINSA had lost "respect" for its entomological fieldworkers, for their understanding of the complexity of mosquito life cycles and their tuning to variations in climate. They had been turned from "specialists," valued for their expertise, into "technicians," valued for their ability to make do with the resources given, to follow orders, and to produce clouds of questionably effective smoke.

That those who encountered dengue on a daily basis called themselves "fieldworkers" seems significant. Like anthropologists, community health workers in Nicaragua were both learning *about* the world around them and learning *in* the world around them. Their skills were incorporated, both in the sense that they emerged from a bodily interaction with mosquitoes and in the sense that they became essential to MINSA's ability to monitor human and insect bodies.[30] The frustration that the head entomologist described had to do with a temporal incongruity. His attempts to contemplate and comprehend evolution—time in the longue durée—were tripped up by allocation—both the annual distribution of budgets and the designation of spaces and techniques for addressing disease. The entomologist's claims about the disjuncture between mosquito evolution and political allocation drew as much on worries about future mosquito ecologies as on nostalgic ideas about how the making of local dengue biologies proceeded back in the revolutionary period. He was thinking in evolutionary cycles but was constrained by the vagaries of political ones. For him, the sound of the *motomochilas* was a declaration not of knowledge but of alarm.

OCTOBER: CLINICAL NARRATIVE
AND HISTORICAL MEMORY

Maria Luisa got sick in October. October is the high point of Nicaragua's rainy season. By that time in the year, the humidity permits virus-carrying mosquitoes to thrive, and in poorly ventilated houses and inadequately serviced neighborhoods, it leads to yearly spikes in dengue, as well as diarrhea and respiratory infection. Simultaneous epidemics of multiple diseases were thus not unusual for the season. The fact that influenza—H1N1 or otherwise—was among these epidemics in 2009, however, *was* unusual. While the normal influenza season (May to July) did not overlap with the August to November dengue season, H1N1 was a latecomer to Nicaragua, arriving in full force just as dengue began to reach its epidemiological peak. This unfortunate timing was overloading Nicaragua's already strapped public health service. Dengue and H1N1 had other things in common. They were both viruses that mutated as they moved through and with animals, humans, and inanimate elements of the landscape. In bodies like Maria Luisa's, these viruses—and biomedical and political stories about them—became "knotted up" together. Ecologically, dengue and influenza thrive in partiality, and in uncertainty.[31]

In the news story about Maria Luisa's death, MINSA officials assured the reporters that all such incidents were subject to investigation, but one day later, Maria Luisa's parents registered a denuncia against the Socrates Flores Health Center, where their daughter was initially treated. The denuncia recounts how she was diagnosed—without any blood tests—with H1N1 and was prescribed Tamiflu. During the H1N1 epidemic, this was more or less standard practice. The Socrates Flores Health Center served thousands of patients, and MINSA and the Ortega government were clearly interested in being seen to have influenza under control. Less than twenty-four hours later, however, Maria Luisa returned to Socrates Flores. Here, her parents' narrative starts to resemble the one Yamileth told about Esteban. On the second visit, Maria Luisa was diagnosed with tonsillitis, and someone prescribed antibiotics. In the denuncia, the family describes how "trusting the doctors' word, we waited for the drugs to take effect." The drugs did not work, and after her third trip to the health center, Maria Luisa was rushed to the La Mascota Hospital in Managua, a children's hospital that also happens to be a work site of the transnational Pediatric Dengue Cohort Study. It was there that she received a blood test that confirmed dengue, but it was too late to save her. She died hours later.

As I explained in chapter 1, Nicaragua's health ministry was built by the revolutionary Sandinista government in the 1980s, and its funding and staff were severely cut in the 1990s and 2000s as part of the post-Sandinista austerity measures undertaken by center-right governments. When Daniel Ortega and the Sandinistas returned to power in 2007, an institutional self-consciousness about public service became prevalent again in MINSA documents, staff meetings, and outreach. In Ciudad Sandino, as I showed in chapter 5, epidemiologists actually spent a great deal of time fielding and even soliciting citizen denuncias. Properly presented (complete with stamps and signatures from a local CPC member) to the health ministry, denuncias allowed individuals to steer the state's attention in particular directions, usually toward individuals whose actions were causing others harm—for example, polluters, reckless drivers, and owners of aggressive dogs. Food poisonings, dog attacks, gun violence, and auto accidents, followed by dramatic public denuncias, are a near-nightly feature of most newscasts in the country. The new government's proactive approach to denuncias might have been an attempt to make such stories less frequent.

Despite the relative frequency with which health centers received them after Ortega's election, denuncias began in Nicaragua as a more indirect method for transcending the geographical confinements of urban poverty: for naming and shaming *government* institutions and officials. The denuncia has its roots in Nicaragua's proud tradition of adversarial journalism. Public complaints, masked as straight news reporting, appeared in the newspaper *La Prensa* during the 1970s, exposing the corrupt bureaucratic practices of the Somoza dictatorship. These included the embezzlement of humanitarian funds intended to rebuild Managua after the 1972 earthquake that destroyed 90 percent of the city. Among the most famous denunicias of this type detailed a scheme whereby Somoza colluded with international plasma dealers to bilk the poor and indigent into selling their blood at exploitative rates.[32] Maria Luisa's family's denuncia fits this older model. Again, children become sick and die frequently in Nicaragua for many reasons, and deaths that occur in the hospital are probably less likely to make the papers than fatalities or injuries that occur on the streets from causes like gun violence or automobile accident. Maria Luisa's family was neither particularly wealthy nor particularly well connected. They named individual doctors in their denuncia, but their complaint was directed at the entire Socrates Flores Health Center.

This is what makes it so instructive. As MINSA officials understood the situation, Nicaragua's postrevolutionary health system was designed and built "for the people." As public trusts, neither Socrates Flores nor MINSA was an appropriate target for a denuncia. A health care provider could be *negligent,* but the public ministry, by definition, could never be unjustly harmful. Doctors at Socrates Flores had not failed to act; they had just acted incorrectly. Besides, as directors at Socrates Flores told me, Maria's family had also been negligent. According to their counternarrative, had the parents administered fluids and drugs in the right manner, they might have saved her. Yamileth had heard a similar admonition when she first brought Esteban to the hospital: "Look after this child well," Yamileth remembers the doctors saying, "because whatever happens to him will be your responsibility." For the staff at Socrates Flores, Maria Luisa's multiple diagnoses were tragic, but they were also excusable in the context of a multiepidemic environment in which nervous patients were overrunning overworked doctors. MINSA officials reasoned that Maria's family had expected too much of the health system and too little of themselves. The denuncia has embedded within it a memory of politics otherwise, with other purposes. As narratives about local biology, both the denuncia and the health center's counternarrative integrated the positivism of the clinical case-history with the moral valence of Nicaraguan social justice discourse. A temporal incongruity—an unpredictable encounter between one girl's immune system, a virus (one or many), drugs, mosquitoes, and forms of illness narrative, led to a conflict over who had cared properly and who had not.

NOVEMBER: TRENDS AND EVENTS

While funds for routine dengue prevention in the dry months of the spring and summer were chronically short, when the *motomochilas* started firing things changed. Soon after the sight of don Nacho and don Noë careening through neighborhoods in the back of a pickup truck became frequent, the smell of the MINSA fogging vehicle, a giant version of the *motomochila* that slowly plodded down the street and blanketed front porches in smoke, would become prominent. By the end of November, the director would declare a dengue emergency, mobilizing Ciudad Sandino's brigadistas and hospital staff for a series of weekend-long, house-to-house campaigns in which they would inform neighbors about the epidemic and hand out brochures about dengue. The staff had been prepared to expect to "lose weekends" to the yearly outbreak. In November, emergency mobilizations were routine.

Even if they expected these disruptions, health center staff were still frustrated by them. In narrative terms, if the "declaration" of an outbreak or epidemic represented a crux, a plot twist, governments too often mobilized people and resources *after* the twist. A CDC entomologist who had thirty years of experience fighting dengue put it to me a way that roughly reflected what the MINSA entomologist told me in our interview about how he calibrated insect poisons:

> The fact is that a dengue epidemic goes away as fast as it comes. It has a reliable upward tendency, which gets to a peak, and then trends negatively. And the epidemic recedes almost as fast as it comes simply because . . . everyone who can be infected has been infected. . . . So, *Whoo!* It's gone! But . . . people begin to take actions against the epidemic, and . . . show you some graphs of when the epidemic starts, put some little arrows indicating that "this is where we began to apply insecticide, or we began to organize

the community, and look how it dropped! The epidemic dropped! It disappeared!" But this is a lie. What's going on is that there are some people . . . either they're ignorant and really think that what they did worked, or they manipulate the information to make it seem like what they did worked. But this doesn't change things; nothing has changed. Nobody can control dengue epidemics. But the show, the farce, continues. The spectacle continues, year after year.

Dengue specialists continue to be concerned that states might hijack dengue epidemics for their own narrow purposes, using them as excuses to consolidate power. The misgiving here is not just about the ways in which politics seems to infiltrate the production and deployment of scientific knowledge. Dengue epidemiology and mosquito ecology are prisms through which people articulate their responsibilities to one another (forms of care) just as they are ways for state and global health organizations to articulate their relationships to their subjects (forms of political subjectivity).[33] Much of that articulation happens through the production of a document that looks rather straightforwardly technical: what epidemiologists call an "endemic channel."

The hospitalito's epidemiology office was cramped, but in a good way. The office was important enough to contain a functioning personal computer, along with more filing cabinets, desks, and other equipment than most of the primary care clinics in the center. Its air conditioner would lure a steady stream of employees from other areas of the complex whose business, like mine, was often just a thin pretense for stealing a few moments of gossip and relaxation in the artificial cool and dry. Each week, Licenciada Eufrasia Lewites, an epidemiology nurse in her mid-fifties, translated clinical disease data from paper sheets to a Microsoft Excel database on the computer, updating the city's endemic channels.[34] The endemic channels were part of MINSA's official record of the incidence of infectious disease in each of its local health centers. Lic. Lewites's Excel database was the centerpiece of the weekly report the epidemiologist would send to her superiors in MINSA.[35] The report documented the prevalence of malaria, HIV, acute respiratory illness, tuberculosis, diarrhea, and dengue.

Endemic channels consist of three lines. In figure 11, reproduced from MINSA's 2008 records for Ciudad Sandino, the dotted line represents the historical average of dengue cases over the previous five years. The dashed line represents the "epidemic threshold," which is two standard deviations above the historical average. The solid line tracks the cases of the ongoing

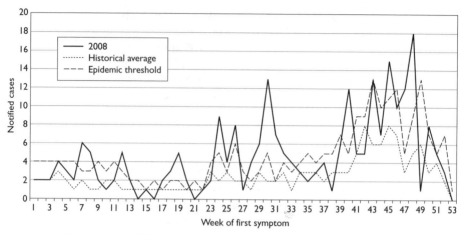

FIGURE II. Reproduction of a dengue "endemic channel" for Ciudad Sandino, 2008.

year. When the solid line stayed below the epidemic threshold, an epidemiologist could declare the city to be in a "normal zone" of prevention. When the line dipped two standard deviations below the historical average, the staff celebrated being in a "zone of success." When the line broke outside the epidemic threshold, a "zone of alert" was noted, and if the breakout remained consistent, hospital officials *might* declare an emergency.[36] Importantly, the process of declaration was iterative. Its structure was similar from year to year, yet its precise operation and the thresholds that put it into action varied.[37]

Ostensibly, Lic. Lewites's job was to put the numbers into the system and nothing more. The epidemiologist would then report those numbers to the director and to her superiors in MINSA, who would decide if an emergency had begun. MINSA staff referred to the pronouncement of an emergency as a "declaration" (*declaración*), a combination of considered decision and objective fact. A dengue "emergency" meant that hospital resources, human and monetary, would be diverted to fumigation for mosquitoes, house-to-house larvicide treatment, and public awareness. Regular clinical hours would be curbed. Scheduled vacations would be suspended. Lic. Lewites's endemic channel and the emergency *declaraciones* it enabled served two seemingly opposite purposes: to establish a trend and to mark the occurrence of an event.

The stability of the trends as scientific and mobile, and of events as idiosyncratic and local, was far from assured. In order to enter the global record and to travel on to national and international viral monitoring databases, a suspected case had to be confirmed by laboratory analysis—far from a guarantee. At the same time, the event—the local stories, rumors, and suspicions that would be launched anew by the blast of the *motomochilas* (Who had failed to control their mosquitoes? Who brought the virus into the zona?)— could easily produce new data. Alerts about dengue were designed to make residents vigilant about dengue symptoms. The seasonal emergency campaigns featured not only the distribution of *abate* and talks about the life cycle of the mosquito but also reeducation about the patterned symptoms of dengue fever: the chills, the rashes, the muscle and bone aches, the eye pain. The sound of the *motomochilas* might plausibly drum up more suspected cases.

Knowledge about dengue would make its way into the public one way or another. MINSA's central authorities could ignore the endemic channels for a time, but they certainly couldn't afford to ignore an *emergencia,* especially if the *declaración* hit the papers or television news before it reached their desks. In fact, MINSA's Office of Health Publicity devoted many of its resources not to alerting the public about epidemics but to monitoring the print and news media. The MINSA publicity office for the Department of Managua contained no less than three radios, two television sets, and one computer. The publicity officer there was trained as a journalist, not an epidemiologist. He explained to me that his job was to "stay ahead" of the public health stories that appeared in print, radio, or television. MINSA leaders frequently heard about what was going on in its various health centers through the media before they received communiqués from directors. Instead of "staying ahead" of the pathogen, then, MINSA wanted to be ahead of the public narrative about emergency.

This process mirrors one that is now routine for contemporary global disease monitors from the WHO and other global health organizations, which often use media reports in addition to epidemiology reports to identify emerging outbreaks and to make predictions about future ones. Geographic databases such as DengueWatch can now sift through a variety of sources, including local news reports—compiled event-narratives known in some corners of the Internet as "trends"—to formulate what some consider to be a more accurate dengue monitoring system than those that rely upon epidemiological trends alone. Tellingly, DengueWatch and the HealthMap technology on which it is based actually use a meteorological metaphor, the "heat index," to gauge the significance of the different kinds of (scientific, journal-istic, impressionistic) reports they collect.[38] Systems like these locate not just hard data but information from the press, social networking sites, and other kinds of discussions—sources not unlike the denuncia registered by Maria Luisa's parents and printed in *El Nuevo Diario*.

Maria Luisa's parents wanted to use the denuncia to connect their daugh-ter's death meaningfully to the dynamics of the wider population and its environment. The denuncia reads more or less like a clinical case file, only with the raw emotions, uncertainties, and frustrations of the grieving left in. In Maria Luisa's case, the global authority of the national diagnostic center, CNDR, blended with the more localized authority of physicians and epide-miologists. The truth claims of the denuncia were multiple. They integrated both the positivism of the biomedical case history and the moral certitude of a Nicaraguan social justice discourse that can be traced from the revolution-ary medical system, through the years of austerity in the 1990s, to the Ortega government's recent attempts to reestablish a MINSA "for the people." The denuncia, like Maria Luisa's three diagnoses, was an attempt to answer the question, "What is going on here?" (in Maria's body, in Managua more gen-erally). At least two of her diagnoses (H1N1 and dengue) came thanks to the material and intellectual connections forged through the Socrates Flores Health Center and the La Mascota Hospital's entanglement in a global viral tracking complex for dengue and influenza. At the same time, the denuncia and the public response of the health ministry were rooted in a particular, territorial history of explanation, a history in which biomedicine was one of several factors.[39]

DECEMBER: EMBODIED PASTS AND SEASONAL ANXIETIES

Just before Christmas, I sat down with Marianna, a Ciudad Sandino Health Center hygienic technician who had served in several emergency health campaigns over the course of her twenty-seven years in MINSA. "What is interesting," I suggested, "is that emergency is a way to raise participation."

MARIANNA: Yes ... they see that when they talk about emergency, everyone gets mobilized. The community worker there, the midwives there, the brigadistas there. Everyone gets involved.

ALEX: Yeah, in the name of citizen participation.

MARIANNA: That's right . . . and some people benefit from this, because they know that more money is coming, although they won't use it in the emergency, they use it in—

ALEX: What do you mean more money comes?

MARIANNA: I mean, when there's an emergency like that, they send money . . . an example [is] a dengue emergency, when there are lots of people to mobilize. Then they [MINSA] send down a lot of money for food, gasoline, transportation, who knows what, and there they go, and the more emergencies there are . . . more money keeps coming.

ALEX: But you really believe that they promote emergencies to get more . . . ?

MARIANNA: You know, lots of people think so . . . because for everyone it's an emergency, including the government itself. "No, we're in an emergency!" [mockingly assuming the "voice of the government"]. And maybe things aren't totally calm and peaceful [*tranquilo*], but they know that if an emergency comes, they'll get money from somewhere.

As Marianna pointed out, an emergency *declaración* was to a large extent a pragmatic move. The procedures of crisis mobilization were familiar to people in Ciudad Sandino and to Marianna in particular. On her right arm, Marianna had a jagged patch of scar tissue, a painful bodily memory of the night when, as a teenager, she was struck by a Somoza National Guardsman's bullet. She grew up in León, the northern city that has traditionally been a hub of intellectual and leftist activity. Marianna came from a poor family, but her mother was politically active, running a safe house for clandestine militants passing through León during the protracted struggle to topple Somoza. Her memories of the revolution were quite lucid, and often very positive. Marianna helped host and care for most of the major players in the resistance, Sergio Ramirez, Herty Lewites, and Eden Pastora among them. In 1979, recovered from her gunshot wound, she followed her boyfriend to Managua to celebrate the triumph of the Sandinistas. Later, she found work in MINSA. Her relationship with the boyfriend eventually ended, though not before she gave birth to two children.

The two results of the seasonal emergency declaration, the trend and the event, ramified out from Ciudad Sandino's tiny epidemiology office in decidedly different ways. For people like Marianna, the event was connected through embodied memory to other related experiences.[40] For Lic. Lewites and her superiors in the office of epidemiology, the identification of an epidemic trend would connect Ciudad Sandino to national and even global systems of epidemic surveillance and research. For the online DengueWatch system, that trend would be a data point, much like the story about Maria Luisa Gutiérrez. In Ciudad Sandino, epidemics had to become emergencies if those at the upper reaches of MINSA were to take notice. Local administrators could more easily steer the resources of a cash-strapped and overextended ministry in their direction by declaring a crisis and promising mass mobilization.[41]

This mobilization was part of a set of seasonal worries. In December, it was not just mosquitoes that were dying. Families around Ciudad Sandino raised pigs and chickens throughout the rainy season, and around Christmas slaughters were common. Some families consumed this homegrown meat themselves, but a sizable informal trade also sprang up. Facing suspicions about a tainted supply, frequently reported in denuncias, MINSA would crack down on formal and informal meat markets at the start of each holiday season. Marianna and the other hygienists would spend their weekdays tracking down unlicensed home abattoirs, warning them about the dangers of food-borne pathogens, and their weekends visiting some of those same households to talk about dengue.

All of this took extra money, time, and material. An emergency declaration initiated a set of exchanges between the central authorities in MINSA and its outlying hospitals. Prompt attention to emergencies was good politics, but institutional negotiations between small health centers and the upper levels of MINSA were only one part of an emergency. What Paul Robbins has called the "practical politics" of knowledge, pragmatic negotiations between the state, scientific authorities, and local people—who may be one in the same individual—marked the interactions between local hospital functionaries like epidemiologists, MINSA authorities, and people whose claims to citizenship seemed to rest on their vulnerability to outbreaks.[42]

Experts have struggled for decades to partition epidemiology from politics and to make "epidemic" a globally applicable, technical term, one that references a specific set of statistical circumstances. Indeed, the use of endemic channels is part of the WHO's standard manual for dengue prevention and control.[43] Despite these efforts, the process of declaring epidemics remains highly local, subjective, and politically charged.[44] Emergency declarations call the population to account for an ecological and medical situation that has become unruly. In an inverse of this process, Maria Luisa's family used the denunica to call the doctors at Socrates Flores to account, not only for their daughter's death but also for the loss of control that it represented.

JANUARY: ARID REFLECTIONS

After the rains began to subside, doña Eugenia and I drank sweetened instant coffee on her patio and munched on buttered club crackers. She recalled the mass mobilizations of the 1980s, when she and other members the Sandinista Youth were called to participate in projects ranging from bringing in coffee harvests to repairing potholed streets. By the time of our afternoon coffee, another dengue season was at an end, and I asked doña Eugenia to compare the Sandinista Youth work with the house-to-house dengue emergency work we had been doing over the past few weekends. Social and political knowledge production had been blended in Ciudad Sandino since the days of OPEN III, when base communities helped organize resistance to the Somoza dictatorship. Sixteen years of center-right rule had certainly diminished the power of grassroots organizations, but for doña Eugenia, the difference was that, in the case of dengue, the whole thing was avoidable. In earlier days, CDS leaders and other activists *planned* their mobilizations. She found a parallel in the hospitalito's method of carrying out yearly vaccination campaigns.

"Now in the vaccination campaigns," she explained, "the entire hospital staff goes out ... leaving no one behind for regular consultation." Yet vaccination, like dealing with dengue or with the December surge in the pork and chicken trade, was an expected yearly responsibility of the hospital. Where was the planning? When the vaccination campaigns began in the 1980s, she and other community activists would spend a few days in advance announcing the coming of medical staff to the neighborhood. Doña Eugenia recalled this method. "'Listen up!' we'd say, 'we're going to be vaccinating for measles, mumps, et cetera, in the house of doña Fulana on this and this day!' And on that day, everyone would line up and get their injections. We could do a whole barrio in two days."

Remembering my conversation with Marianna, I suggested that perhaps treating problems like dengue as "emergencies" was good for ministry and hospital leaders, since successfully managing an emergency made them look responsible and occluded the "chronic" nature of the problems they faced, namely, shortages of vaccines and medicine or a seasonal need to monitor markets. Doña Eugenia was doubtful. "Maybe that's what they think," she countered, but she felt the hospital directors were less calculating than that. They were just "bad managers." Maybe they deserved to be denounced.

Emergency could thus be read as both a political and a moral condition. If the denuncia seems like a peculiarly Nicaraguan form of communication, the biomedical diagnosis and the epidemic declaration seem rather nonterritorial. Whereas the denuncia called attention to the physical and structural vulnerability of children like Esteban and like Maria Luisa Gutiérrez within the national health system, the multiple diagnoses—especially these *particular* diagnoses in this *particular* part of Managua—enrolled them in a standardized (if multisited and multiscalar) process of knowledge production. Diagnoses and epidemic declarations rely on both rigid data collection and compelling, place-specific narration. They are devices that link health to place, interchanging scientific and social categories, seemingly "local" emotional vocabularies with seemingly more dispersed scientific, economic, and political forms of representation. Disease geographies combine local struggles to temporalize health with seemingly standard and nonterritorial scientific ones. They involve weighing the "technical" aspects of health against its "meaningful," "moral" aspects.[45] To construct public health as a seasonal emergency, people had to make use of the incongruity between biological and social time, and between the regularity of the trend and the multiplicity of entangled events.

HEALTH IN SEASONS

In Ciudad Sandino, in each dengue season, brigadistas, epidemiologists, and entomologists, along with global health scientists, tracked changes— subtle and staggering—in climatic, virological, and entomological cycles. These changes occurred recursively with changes in economic, political, and technological routines. Even when one is not directly made sick, an epidemic can make a person feel a stranger in her own world. In the context of infectious insect-borne disease, this sense of alienation can be particularly acute, since the mobilization of diagnostics, mosquito fumigation, and other technological and scientific tools militate against the entanglement of bodies with their surroundings.

In seasonal dengue emergencies, conceptions of health emerged in the process of confronting temporal incongruities; of attempting but never quite managing to reconcile the cyclical behavior of mosquitoes with that of people and weather. As cases got reported, and the *motomochilas* started firing, the longer-term considerations of mosquito population adaptation (a concern of entomologists) clashed with the poison's ability to effect instant (and politically valuable) mosquito death. When seasonal emergencies happened, the vagaries of immunological memory made past infections painfully relevant in the present. Even though a global health complex that now reaches Nicaragua can identify viruses in people's blood and keep records in sophisticated genomic databases, that complex has yet to resolve the imperfect memory of the immune system. There is still no vaccine or drug against dengue. Likewise, those whose job it is to sequentially organize facts about disease—turning them into trends—increasingly rely on the narration of seasonal emergencies as events.

Global health problems—routine and extraordinary—reveal the deep attachments that attend even the most seemingly standard of objects and tools, from the case file to the epidemiological chart, and the multiple kinds of authority and meaning these can take on.[46] The perspective of entanglement further complicates this. In the case of dengue prevention in Nicaragua, human technologies weren't the only devices for making meaning. Such power also resided (among other places) in insects, in multiple circulating viruses and microbes, in rainfall, and in the human-built world that connected them.

In his essays on colonial development and science in Egypt, Timothy Mitchell discusses the ways in which Egyptian institutions of public health and infrastructure worked to tame the Nile and stop the *Anopheles gambiae* mosquitoes that carried malaria. Mitchell introduces the concept of "technopolitics" to describe the rise of institutions of economic development, public health, and public works. Technopolitics involves the manufacture of an illusion, namely, "that the human, the intellectual, the realm of intention and ideas seem to come first and to control and organize the nonhuman."[47] Technopolitical power coalesces when the illusion of a divide between human intention and nonhuman "resistance" can be maintained, but as Mitchell argues, the Nile and the *Anopheles* mosquito were anything but static. They came into being, as material forces and as objects of knowledge, along with the technologies and policies designed to contain them. At every turn, hydrological cycles and mosquito growth cycles adapted to and infiltrated human systems of control. Similarly, the divide between human and nonhuman force in Nicaragua's dengue epidemics remains anything but clear. It was made and broken through contests over how things and people in the landscape (and their temporalities) created and recreated attachments.[48]

Eventually, the dengue events I witnessed during my research would enter global health databases as epidemiological data, and those databases would shape the process by which Nicaraguan epidemiologists "declared" future outbreaks. (Each year, the endemic channel is revised to reflect new trends, so a year like 2009, for example, in which incidence increased fourfold, raised the thresholds of "alert" and "success" in the channel for 2010.) As a social phenomenon, dengue was thus the offspring of two different activities: detached observation of populations and negotiations among individuals within those populations. The real work of care and politics happens somewhere in-between, in the spaces occupied by brigadistas like Morena and Yamileth, by epidemiological technicians like Lic. Lewites, and by individuals like Maria Luisa Gutiérrez.

Maria Luisa's family registered their denuncia because they did not have access to rigid, scientific knowledge about their daughter's illness. Socrates Flores presumably did, and, in interviews with me, officials confirmed this assumption by blaming Maria Luisa's family for failing to adequately respond to the "truth" of her condition. There is a parallel between a health center's limited access to "true" information and the partial knowledge evident in the denuncia. The story, it appears, goes down multiple potential trails, all of them alive with meaning.

To navigate those trails, it is useful to think about how Maria Luisa's case fits into anthropological ideas about "disease emergence," another category of temporal analysis that is both material and symbolic. The age of "emerging infectious diseases" (EIDs) has indeed brought on a new system of surveillance and tracking mechanisms that appear to take epidemiology from the local to the global scale. EIDs seem to have unique abilities to subvert borders and upset bureaucratic and social orders. Biosecurity concerns have thus created space for the exercise and proliferation of surveillance technologies: a "globality" that, paradoxically, takes root at the most microscopic of scales—that of the mosquito, the virus, and the blood that connects them to humans.[49] Diagnostic technologies such as those that were partially available at Socrates Flores are key to this. At the same time, the age of EIDs is also an age of unprecedented humanitarian attention to health.[50] The dengue cohort study based at Socrates Flores was a humanitarian project, one designed to bring the tools of diagnosis and treatment to those who needed them most. Whereas biosecurity promotes the management of bodies across environments and spaces, humanitarianism operates through the geographic *location* of suffering. The seasonal embodiment of dengue emergency, however, shows how place is more than location. It is, rather, the articulation of several incongruous temporalities at once through technology and experience.[51] As a practice of care and politics, public health requires the elaboration and dissemination of effective temporal models that link individuals to populations. It is in their dissemination, however, that people are invited into engagement with the world.

Conclusion

ALONGSIDE MOST EVERY ROAD in Ciudad Sandino there is a footpath. Occasionally this path takes the form of a concrete sidewalk, but more often it is a well-worn trail, a hard-packed, sometimes even shiny, line of dirt. Such trails contain a wealth of stories, and in this book I have tried to tell a few of them. The work of telling such stories is never complete. I see this book and most any other work of anthropology as something akin to a trail guide: the kind of document a backpacker might buy or borrow before setting off on a trek. Such documents, like trails themselves, need constant care and maintenance. The stories they tell are momentary distillations of the host of actions, some human, some climatic, some animal, some even chemical, that have put the trail in its present condition. The trail guide is not about a mountaintop or a valley or a waterfall or any other particular feature. Rather, it is, very literally, about what happens along the way to and from those features. Thus, it needs constant updating, constant care.

The focus of this book has not been a particular epidemic or a particular case of dengue. By calling attention to the connective pathways between people, viruses, habitats, and, of course, mosquitoes, I have tried to faithfully reflect the ideas that Ciudad Sandino's residents expressed about health—in particular, that it was a search for "good company." As I have reconsidered the adage to which I referred in the introduction, *Mejor solo que mal acompañado* (It's better to be alone than in bad company), I have come to view it as an argument for humility in the face not only of political or economic barriers but also of a vast, sometimes frightening, but at all times fascinating nonhuman world. As global health institutions, philanthropists, and scientists begin to confront humankind's relationship to the nonhuman environment, critical medical anthropology is as relevant as ever. The contribution of this book has been to show how, in the weedy spaces where global health hopes to have its biggest impact, a sense of place as something that is constructed in "good company" may provide a valuable ethical roadmap or, perhaps, a collaboratively constructed, if partial and momentary, trail guide. The silent moral of that idiomatic expression—at least in Ciudad Sandino— was that one was never alone, so making good company was an unavoidable responsibility.

For my colleagues and students in medical anthropology, the purpose of this book has been to suggest that the stories of single mothers-turned- brigadistas, of scavengers and chatarreros scapegoated by their government and exploited by their patrons, of endemic channels, of weather patterns, of mosquito life cycles are, together, constitutive of health. That is why Ciudad Sandino's landscape has been as much a part of the preceding discussion as the bodies that make up the city's population. By focusing on both bodies and the urban landscapes they inhabit, I have used the particularities of den- gue in Ciudad Sandino to understand how the regulation of human *and* nonhuman life produces specific forms of belonging and exclusion.

As the medical historians Gregg Mitman, Michelle Murphy, and Chris- topher Sellers put it: "[Health] is the product of a network of material, so- cial, and symbolic relations between and among human and non-human ac- tors. In cutting across the categories of human and non-human, health offers a useful means for rethinking nature and how we come to know the natural world."[1] Speaking of both animal-borne infectious diseases and novel envi- ronmental health threats such as industrial pollution, they use the term "landscapes of exposure" to identify the physical and cultural networks through which historically and politically situated interactions between people and nonhumans of all kinds emerge. Landscapes are products of human-environment interaction, but they also are politically contested. At- tention to health landscapes helps to dismantle a conceptual divide between human bodies and the environment.

The goal of *Mosquito Trails* has been to suggest a reinterpretation of global health along similar lines. I have tried to use the story of Ciudad Sandino to show how health landscapes are inhabited by humans, microbes, and the vec- tors that carry them. The landscape is the physical expression of place: neither a timeless environmental ideal nor the endpoint of a single historical trajec- tory. The habits of the *Ae. aegypti* mosquito fit the economic and social trends of the times: the "flexibility" and mobility of people and things, a prolifera- tion of disposable consumer products, trends toward market-based health, an emphasis on rights to entrepreneurship over rights to collective action, and the submission of public spaces to private accumulation.

A central message of this book is that people, pathogens, vectors, and their shared surroundings are always in the process of becoming, together. Environments do not just cause health problems; rather humans and non-humans *incorporate* one another's actions. And those actions—even when they occur in times and places seemingly distant from one another—have a bearing on the kinds of beings they become.[2] Even though I have chosen to speak of entanglement in lieu of exposure, there is no denying that human beings make an inordinate impact on their nonhuman surroundings and must answer for the health outcomes (for people and nonpeople) of those impacts. Thus, I suggest that the politics of life in infectious disease complexes is as much about ecologically imagined, multispecies communities— about landscapes that include people *and* mosquitoes *and* garbage *and* viruses—as it is about biomedically imagined human bodies. Again, *entanglement* references the ongoing coconstitution of people and (living and nonliving) things. As Ciudad Sandino's experience with earthquakes, floods, hurricanes, and dengue epidemics shows, politics has long been inflected by nonhuman activity. Nicaragua's history of imperial privation, dictatorship, and popular revolution is also marked by a series of spectacular "natural" catastrophes. These events left their marks in bodies and in the landscape. While much of contemporary global health orients itself to the future, seeking ways to anticipate or head off pandemics, I believe that anthropology's role should be a bit different.[3] In order to critically examine global health, we cannot be futurists. Rather, for anthropologists, understanding dengue and diseases like it entails *trailing,* working from behind, or even along with, pathogens and vectors and people, gathering knowledge from the traces they—and we—leave. These traces, I argue, play a significant role in how we think of health.

I therefore see this book as both an academic and a pragmatic exercise. Dengue is in part a manifestation of structural inequalities, but like other ecological systems, dengue and human reactions to it must be understood dialectically. In other words, it is too simple to say that inequality produces dengue epidemics, or that environmental factors "affect" health. Dengue epidemics can and do happen in wealthy and middle-class places. Nevertheless, it is safe to say that the majority of dengue patients live in poor, urban areas, which means that inequality informs the production of knowledge about dengue epidemics perhaps more than any other single factor. An "apolitical ecology" of dengue would couch disease as a product of a series of rational *choices* by people like those whose stories I have tried to relate in the preceding pages. It would presume also that the harboring of water containers and garbage (again, key breeding grounds for mosquitoes) was somehow driven by an insulated *cultural* impulse. Finally, it would presume that human actions vis-à-vis mosquitoes and viruses and environments are somehow *sovereign,* free or at least above the influence of the insects and microbes themselves.[4] Harboring mosquitoes is not always a choice, even if it is theoretically avoidable as a health hazard. Inadequate water supplies and the potential to make money from the collection of recyclables make such avoidance exceedingly difficult. Insofar as the households of Ciudad Sandino are cultural forms, they are forms that are produced by particular—and particularly unequal—political and economic arrangements. Finally, as I hope to signal through my use of the concept of entanglement, there is ample evidence to suggest that human-mosquito interactions in particular are multivalent. Mosquitoes enroll humans in certain ways of thinking about the urban landscape, and these ways are not always necessarily unhealthy.

Entanglement is an enacted condition. People in Ciudad Sandino enacted entanglement by participating in the motion of garbage across streets and across borders, of political paradigms across generations, and of mosquitoes, fruits, vegetables, and *perros bravos* across patio walls. The meanings and material forms of these things, like the meanings and material forms of epidemiological and ecological models of dengue, are contingent upon environmental contexts and environmental history. While it is satisfying to declare that dengue is a "global" disease, such a declaration presumes that it matters, materially and semiotically, in the same way from place to place.

That dengue, like H1N1, malaria, and other vector-borne and zoonotic diseases, is "ecological" is not news to scientists. To examine health both ecologically and anthropologically—to extend "local biology" to the nonhuman *bios* of insects, rainfall, and viruses—requires attention to the landscapes in which disease appears.[5] Dengue is not Nicaragua's disease, but Nicaraguan dengue has some unique characteristics. Nicaraguans' experiences of war, revolution, structural adjustment, and globalization have been inflected physically into the makeup of their cities and culturally into their understandings of health. An anthropology of dengue and other such diseases has to recognize their "multispecies" aspects: to attend to the ways in which multiple life forms gain meaning at different times and amid different forms of life.[6] The mosquito and the agglomeration of four distinct viruses scientists call "dengue" are constantly in the process of becoming. The "single mother" example in chapter 4 was a dramatic one, but it illustrated how people, who embody health not only as "victims" but also as those who *inhabit* places as healthy or unhealthy, may reflect upon the conditions of a disease's production and possibly change those conditions.

Like other "emerging infectious diseases" (e.g., influenza, AIDS), dengue is being treated more and more in the popular and scholarly literature—scientific and social-scientific alike—as a security threat: as nature's war on the (often implicitly Northern, middle-class) human body. Critics of biosecurity discourse have been properly concerned with the way in which such discourse alters the making of human subjects.[7] I want readers to question this notion of "emergence" and the lure of biosecurity as both an explanatory and a critical discourse. The classification of certain diseases as "emerging" references their multiple origins and the complex interactions of people, things, and animals that produce them, but the label threatens to mislead us into thinking that the unpredictability of such diseases means that local biologies and local ecologies no longer matter. Worse still, it can force us to believe that some places matter more than others. Worse even still, it can lull us into thinking that these diseases, in their very unpredictability, happen out of historical time or political economic context. The concept of emergence as deployed in global health discourse lures us into the idea that humans will embody those diseases in the same—that is, predictable, ahistorical—way and that the human body, though under attack, is still the sole, *whole* site and subject of medical knowledge and power.

In short, I worry about the implications of viewing diseases as "global," for it presumes a level playing field—a "standardizable body"—that simply does not exist.[8] I also worry about the way in which a discourse of emergence turns diseases into security issues. One way to allay those worries is by making "global health" a universal moral humanitarian discourse, using biomedicine to solve health problems wherever they occur. The growth of medical humanitarianism certainly complicates our view of power, but humanitarian action has more to do with the state-like territorial sovereignty and state-led epidemiological action of biosecurity that it first might seem.

While I recognize that "securing" health is a major part of contemporary discourse about infectious disease, talk of security, or its absence, misses the much more subtle issue of entanglement. Entanglement *does* account for place and history, and not just in "global" settings such as laboratories or major cities. Entanglements predate the era of biosecurity. Indeed, in nonbiomedical theories of emergence and self-organization, complexity arises out of the progressive interactions of many relatively simple things, in non-linear relationships. Emergent qualities are those that obtain from a multiplicity of things-in-relationships, rather than from one particular set of agents or actors. Neither the mosquito's nor the virus's emergence, on its own, makes dengue the disease that it is. Dengue is an "emerging" disease insofar as it is the outcome of a complex set of entanglements that implicate (among other things) viruses, international trade, mosquitoes, people, their houses, water, public health priorities, and politics. If it is to serve as a critical framework for the study of health, emergence, as a theoretical or empirical trope, demands reflexivity. It demands recognition of what Gregory Bateson calls the "pattern that connects" human life to other forms of life—and to other nonliving things.[9]

The envelopment of places like Nicaragua in global infrastructures of trade and in hegemonic forms of biomedical classification does not obliterate local practice; rather, those infrastructures and forms get integrated back into already existing ways of knowing. Clifford Geertz called "culture" the "webs of significance" that people spin to explain their worlds. Strictly speaking, spiders are not insects, and Geertz was no posthuman scholar, but the metaphor is tantalizing. New webs of significance—new entanglements—emerge when new epidemiological tools go into practice, when garbage becomes globally valuable, when mosquitoes become more than pests but other than pets.[10] Taking the lessons of political ecology, with its probing critique of the concepts of "nature" and its emphasis on local uses thereof in the age of the global environmental movement, I have found it fruitful to give equal attention to the often silenced nonhuman dimensions of health in the age of global infectious disease emergence. Doing this requires attention to knowledge brokers like brigadistas and material brokers like chatarreros. Without reifying the body or place, it is still worthwhile to describe how diseases and people emerge together.

There are a few lessons here for nonanthropologists. The first and most obvious is that politics and poverty cannot be ignored in the formulation of global health projects. Politics, like environmental degradation, should not be treated as an obstacle to accomplishing public health goals. Rather, practitioners of public health need to think about both politics and environments as the very things that frame, even enable, what they do. In Ciudad Sandino, politics was as much a part of the algorithm for creating knowledge about dengue as was clinical medicine or laboratory virology. What remains striking, especially when seen through a long view of Nicaragua's health system, was the way in which the mingling of politics and science was stratified through the system. Whereas upper-level planners such as those who designed the day-to-day, house-to-house mosquito control programs discursively separated science from politics, those who executed policies at the regional and local levels had no such luxury. Politics became a lubricant to epidemiological practice.

At the very lowest level of the system, however, a desire for a separation emerged once again. The brigadistas, unlike those who occupied positions of authority in the local or regional branches of the health center, saw firsthand how the need for facts pulled against the political salience of events. The brigadistas literally embodied the tension between the two: between emotional, storied connection to the epidemic and detached observation of it. They were entangled, like many community health workers, in a set of sometimes compatible, sometimes contradictory knowledge-making practices.

This leads to a second lesson. Community health workers are just that: workers. What they do requires a level of engagement and care that deserves more economic remuneration, benefits, and social recognition than Nicaragua's brigadistas currently receive. The brigadistas in Ciudad Sandino are employees of the government, but their work is not the simple execution of state policy any more than it is the rote application of neutral scientific ideas. As Sandra Harding suggests, "Science has become a kind of governance which ... bypasses democratic politics. Thus 'the scientific' and 'the political'—science and politics—are inexorably intertwined. Science appropriates to itself as merely technical matters and decisions that are actually social and political."[11] This does not mean that science is inherently negative and undemocratic.[12] Rather, discussions of community health work and its place in global health should bridge what Sheila Jasanoff calls the "production end of representing the world" by the powerful and the "reception" and uptake of those representations by the relatively powerless.[13] It seems important to understand how subjects produce knowledge about themselves and about disease and how they come to govern themselves in new ways. Such "epidemic signification" is always situated.[14] The perspectives of scientists, like those of brigadistas, are partial. Each has an intimacy with mosquitoes and viruses and the environment, but that intimacy is of a different kind.

Third, this book is a call for all who are interested in global health to contemplate the relations of people to nonhuman creatures. Given that dengue and so many emerging diseases are multispecies problems—involving mosquitoes, swine, viruses, birds, people, monkeys, and plants—a new understanding, and perhaps a new ethic, seems in order. Viruses, people, and mosquitoes are meeting more frequently and with more deadly results, and scientists are speaking of this meeting with greater frequency. But these meetings continue to be historically and geographically variable. As soon as we treat creatures like *Ae. aegypti* as mere pests or, worse, as "invasive" species, we begin to reaffirm a short-sighted, anthropocentric view of health that simply does not square with the desperate need for the holistic, even radical solutions that climate change and the uneven development of cities demand.

Many popular solutions these days are technological. Vaccines and genetically modified mosquitoes are being developed in laboratories and tested in dengue-endemic areas. Such technological solutions have arisen in response to a purported "failure" of the kind of community-based dengue control projects I have described in this book. That response has been underwritten by major players in global health, particularly the Bill and Melinda Gates Foundation. This "failure" may stem from a refusal by project designers to honestly engage with the locally contingent nature of the prevention encounter. The stories in this book ask us to look at dengue as an opportunity, a shared problem that links households, scientists, and their intermediaries rather than divides them. My hope is that those stories also cause us to look again at the many forms public health can and must take.

In a 2009 survey, two assistants and I asked 259 householders whether they would like to learn more about dengue. About 97 percent said yes, and of these, a surprising 40 percent favored "community meetings" over in-home visits (32 percent), mass media advertising (12 percent), or public signage (16 percent) as the most effective way to learn more. That survey took place in the middle of a widespread epidemic, in which MINSA flooded radio and television with dengue-related advertisements selling the individualized, home-hygiene solution to the disease. The sound of *motomochilas* in nearby houses and of MINSA officials making grave commentary on the situation during radio news reports regularly formed the aural background of our survey interviews. These numbers come also despite the fact that 73 percent found neighborhood relations in their barrios to be "fair" or "weak," and 69 percent said that they discussed health with neighbors "infrequently" or "not at all." Amidst all this, there was desire, on the part of brigadistas as well as householders, to be coproducers of healthy homes, to open up the landscape and health itself to critical scrutiny. Those statistics are rough. They do not close the issue, but they certainly point to a desire among those most affected by dengue for continued experimentation with "low-tech" approaches to health.

One of the axioms of contemporary global health discourse is that "freedom from disease" no longer seems achievable. The question, then, is what should replace that aspiration. The actions surrounding dengue in Nicaragua signal a possibility that instead of either a biosecurity discourse in which emerging infectious diseases, as monstrous harbingers of fear and destabilization, promote a strict regulation of bodies and spaces, or a humanitarian discourse in which biomedical projects are couched as technological salvation for the poor, there may be a third path: a situation in which basic and complex infrastructures, national and transnational belonging, and, above all, a recognition that environments and bodies are entangled, lead to a more relational ethic of health. That the explanations for the dengue epidemics and illnesses in Nicaragua and elsewhere are all partial does more to unsettle assumptions of global biomedical hegemony (of either the humanitarian or biosecurity variety) than to exclude the "local" as a site of meaningful knowledge production.

NOTES

INTRODUCTION

1. Geographers, perhaps more than anthropologists, have theorized the city as a "socionatural" space, though the seminal work in this area is William Cronon's (1990) history of Chicago and the American West. Of particular interest to readers of this book will be Laura Shillington's rich descriptions of human-plant relations in urban Nicaragua, with special attention to fruit trees and medicinal plants (Shillington 2008, 2013). More general theories of urban nature—most with a deep Marxist bent—come from Gandy (2005), Harvey (1996), Heynen, Kaika, and Swyngedouw (2006), and Swyngedouw (2004). Within geography, Robbins (2007) has offered a more subtle approach, influenced as much by environmental history and feminist theory as by Marxism. Recently, anthropologists have begun to engage urban natures ethnographically (e.g., Anand 2011; Zeiderman 2012). The idea of nature and culture coproducing one another is also central to the notion of "entanglement" (Ogden 2011; Raffles 2002), which I develop in this book.

2. Standish et al. (2010).

3. In Nicaraguan Spanish, *cultura* does not refer to what anthropologists normally think of as "culture." Instead, it is more akin to what Bourdieu (1986) calls "cultural capital," embodied know-how about living in the landscape.

4. Among others, the American colonial leader Benjamin Rush described dengue-like illness in Philadelphia in the eighteenth century (Rush 1789). Jose Rigau-Perez (1998) identifies the first known use of the word *dengue* in Spanish in a letter from Queen María Luisa de Parma of Spain, who wrote to her lover, Manuel Godoy, on June 12, 1801, that she had "the cold in fashion, that they call dengue." In the decades after that letter, the term went into wide use across the Hispanic world. Through the *Oxford English Dictionary,* Rigau-Perez traces *dengue* to the Swahili phrase *ka dinga pepo* ("a kind of sudden cramp-like seizure"). The *Oxford English Dictionary* (1989) expands:

On its introduction to the West Indies from Africa in 1827, the name was, in Cuba, popularly identified with the Spanish word *dengue* "fastidiousness, prudery." In this form it was subsequently adopted in the United States, and eventually in general English use. In the British West Indies, called by the Black population *dandy*. Both names appear to be popular adaptations, of the "sparrow-grass" type, of the Swahili name, with a mocking reference to the stiffness of the neck and shoulders, and dread of motion, exhibited by the patients; whence also another name of ridicule, the "Giraffe."

5. As I was completing the writing of this book, scientists reported the discovery of a fifth serotype (Normile 2013).

6. Other species of *Aedes*, particularly *Ae. albopictus*, also known as the Asian tiger mosquito, can be carriers (Sanchez et al. 2006).

7. Guzman et al. (2010: S8). At the time of my study, DHF was an accepted international diagnostic category, recognized in the guidelines of the WHO. Indeed, the specter of *dengue hemorrhágico* had changed public perception of the disease in Nicaragua. After I completed research, however, international specialists agreed on a reclassification of diagnostic categories, and at the time of this writing, DHF is sometimes replaced by "severe dengue."

8. Standish et al. (2010).

9. Hinchliffe et al. (2013), Keck (2008), Kelly (2012), Lakoff (2008), Lowe (2010), and Porter (2012, 2013).

10. In the formulation I have in mind, following political ecologist Arun Agrawal (2005: 165–66), "subjects" are those who are simultaneously subordinated to political and technical authority, empowered by it, and constitutive of its domain of knowledge. Subjects "make themselves" through specific, local practices.

11. The term "local biologies" was coined by Margaret Lock (1993) to call attention to the material effects of social inequality, gender, and geography on bodies. Importantly, local biologies recognize the materiality of human populations, even as they deploy symbolic, linguistic, and historical analyses of health. Attention to local biologies shows how biomedical technologies—from pharmaceuticals to surgical techniques to epidemiology and public health interventions—operate not as neutral tools but, like other technologies, in a complex interaction with the body in its cultural and material context (Lock 2001; Lock and Nguyen 2010; see also Koch 2013; Mol 2002). The literature on political ecology, and anthropology's role within it, is vast. Within anthropological political ecology, the clash of standard and apolitical narratives about the environment with local practice has been a particular point of focus (Brosius 1999; Escobar 1999; Li 2007; Lowe 2006; Nadasdy 2003; West 2006). Though Eric Wolf, an anthropologist, is often credited with coining the term "political ecology," the field has coalesced across disciplines, with human-environment geographers building a particularly impressive variety of theoretical and empirical contributions (Forsyth 2003; Goldman, Nadasdy, and Turner 2011; Robbins 2012; Rocheleau, Thomas-Slayter, and Wangari 1996). The political ecology of health is perhaps the least developed area of the field (but see Mansfield 2008). Importantly, political ecology permits a view of the body itself as an ecosystem. This move links

contemporary scholarship back to early attempts by the likes of Frank Macfarlane Burnet and Rene Dubos to understand infectious disease holistically (Anderson 2004).

12. Dengue produces what Lauren Berlant calls "modes of attachment that make persons public and collective and that make collective scenes intimate spaces" (2002: 288; Raffles 2002: 209). Writing about postrevolutionary Nicaragua, Roger Lancaster (1992: 118) has identified an "intimate knowledge" about class and gender that emerged not from political discourse—or not from that alone—but from more entrenched notions about the relationship between *machismo* and power, between power and bodily practices of labor and dress, while Cymene Howe (2013) has characterized movements for gay and lesbian rights, which were curtailed after the revolution, as a form of "intimate activism."

13. A reassessment of the concept of the site can underscore the false dichotomy between "local" action and the "global" structures that shape it. As Bruno Latour writes,

> Context-building sites [he refers to what sociologists call "global" centers of power] now look like the intersections of many trails of documents traveling back and forth, but local building sites, too, look like the multiple crossroads toward which templates and formats are circulating. . . . the number of traces becomes so great that you would have to be blind not to follow them. Sites no longer differ in shape or size, but in the direction of the movements to and fro as well as in the *nature* . . . of what is being transported: information, traces, goods . . . and so on. (2005: 204–5)

In some ways, such a perspective has been ascendant in anthropology and sociology since scholars began engaging with "practice theory" and the embodiment of power relations (Bourdieu 1977). A critique of scale as a political construct, however, does not deny its power in the world. What it might do, however, is point us to places in which alternative antiscalar social arrangements might emerge (Escobar 2008; Marston, Jones, and Woodward 2005).

14. I am drawing in part on Latour's suggestion that *having*, rather than *being*, is the quintessential social condition. As he states: "Attachments are first, actors are second. . . . the family of 'to have' is much richer than the family of 'to be' because, with the latter, you know neither the boundary nor the direction: to possess is also being possessed; to be attached is to hold and to be held. . . . As to emancipation, it does not mean 'freed from bonds' but *well*-attached" (2005: 217–18, emphasis in original). I combine Latour's emphasis on attachment with Karen Barad's (2007) and Donna Haraway's (2008) concept of "lively" entanglement, in which they suggest that encounters are best understood as "intraactions," that is, actions that occur between distinguishable beings, observers, and things observed. Intraactions are the stuff of becoming, or as Barad (2003: 817) puts it, "an ongoing process of mattering through which 'mattering' itself acquires meaning and form." Entanglement helps us account for the pathways of mosquitoes and other than human things in and out of houses and lives.

15. Haraway (2008). In Haraway's understanding, relationships are "material-semiotic means of becoming" (25–26). She opens up relationships to include "extremely

prosaic, relentlessly mundane" and "knotty" encounters among species, and among objects.

16. I am thankful to Eric Carter (2012) for calling attention to the complexity of the social-ecological dyad as it has played out in the history of global health and mosquito-borne disease more broadly. Carter shows that even when scientists and health policy makers see themselves as hybridizing the social and the ecological (modern terms like "coupled systems" come to mind), they reinforce a fundamental ontological divide between the two. One can make a useful comparison between Carter's largely empirical insights and those of Latour (2005) on the dubious tendency among sociologists to divide "context" from "action." For a longer view of how the social and the ecological have merged amid questions of health, see Mitman, Murphy, and Sellers (2004), Murphy (2006), and Nading (2013a).

17. Thus, dengue prevention constitutes a more-than-human form of biopolitics (Barad 2003; Foucault 2008). The world, as Hugh Raffles says, is marked by a "bewildering instability" (27). Ideas of nature as separate from social life, reinforced in ecological and biomedical science, mask this instability.

18. Nading (2012: 574).

19. Helmreich and Weston (2006: 108).

20. Julie Livingston (2005), discussing changing ideas about public health in Botswana, uses the term *entanglement* in this historical sense.

21. This aspect of dengue is not well understood, and findings from a research group based partially in Nicaragua have shown that prior exposure to one dengue virus may, if only temporarily, sometimes provide protection from the other three (see Zompi et al. 2012).

22. Paul Robbins's web page at the University of Arizona Department of Geography and Regional Development (www.u.arizona.edu/~robbins/) included this phrase.

23. The trope of the rhizome comes originally from Gilles Deleuze and Felix Guattari (1987), but it has been put to productive anthropological use in the work of Ogden (2011) and the Matsutake Worlds Research Group (Choy et al. 2009). Shaw, Robbins, and Jones (2010) deploy the idea to explain the spatial dynamics of human-mosquito relationships in southern Arizona.

24. There are various engagements with the concept and practice of global health across the social sciences. See, for example, King (2002, 2004) and Lakoff and Collier (2008).

25. For more on global health "partnerships," see Adams (2010), Biruk (2012), Brada (2011), and Crane (2013).

26. Lowe (2010) and Nading (2012). By the 1990s, after the success of education campaigns, antibiotic and antiviral medications, and an increase in access to health care across the globe, some experts had declared that they could safely turn their attention to alleviating work-related injuries, cancer, and psychological problems associated with "social suffering" (Kleinman, Das, and Lock 1997). By the end of the decade, however, it became clear that old diseases such as cholera, tuberculosis, and malaria were "reemerging," while new ailments, including AIDS, hantavirus,

and avian influenza, were "emerging" (Wilcox and Colwell 2005). Coming at a time (the 1980s and 1990s) when many public health systems in the third world were being rolled back, privatized, and curbed through structural adjustment, emerging and reemerging infectious diseases threatened to dismantle the progress that international health had made over the course of the twentieth century (Farmer 1999).

27. Haraway (2008: 249) quotes Don Ihde: "In this interconnection of embodied being and environing world, what happens in the interface is what's important." Entanglement and related concepts have been explored recently by scholars working in such diverse contexts as undersea microbial research (Helmreich 2009), human/dog training (Haraway 2008), and mushroom hunting (Tsing 2012). As Laura Ogden suggests, human-being "is constituted through changing relations with other animals, plants, material objects, and the like" (2011: 2).

28. Here I have in mind work on "biosociality," which examines the ways in which genomics has altered conceptions of the sovereign, bounded biomedical subject (Rabinow 2002; Rabinow and Rose 2006), as well as the work of Strathern (1992) on the multiplicity of personhood.

29. See Biehl (2005), Farmer (1992), Lock (1993), and Scheper-Hughes (1992).

30. Put more specifically, they are *biopolitical* endeavors (Foucault 1990, 2008; Rose 2007; Weir and Mykhalovskiy 2010: 22). If people begin to desire to regulate their health, the biopolitical argument goes, they come to see themselves as part of a population that is more or less "at risk" (Hacking 1991). By monitoring biological processes (birth, death, disease), states manage populations at an intimate biological level. Extremely "local" concerns (menstruation, cancer, migraine headaches) become political. By sharing spaces such as streets, parks, and commons, each posing particular dangers to the body, people come to think of themselves as parts of a more or less vulnerable population. Crucially, however, the process by which this happens is contingent. In Michel Foucault's classic formulation of biopolitics, a liberal state and its citizens hold nearly exclusive power to manage this measuring and observing work, but when states, nongovernmental organizations, and businesses *all* take an interest, as in global health, it becomes unclear where such power resides. Noting this, critical medical anthropologists share a concern with the ways in which the body, like nature, is variously experienced as a social metaphor, as a site of phenomenological experiences of pain and pleasure, and as the subject—both focus of interest and site of practice—for state and citizen formation (Scheper-Hughes and Lock 1987). Studies of reproductive technologies (Roberts 2012), therapeutic regimes (Nguyen 2010), genomics (Franklin 2007; Rabinow 2002), medical education (Wendland 2010), and medical humanitarianism itself (Redfield 2013) have begun to ask what becomes of citizens and subjects when what Lock calls "local biologies," the historically, culturally, and materially constructed bodies that contain "disease," meet with universalistic and standardized ideas about wellness and illness (Lock 2001). One clear conclusion is that specific conditions, such as AIDS, malaria, dengue, or even menopause, produce specific "healths" and specific kinds of health-seeking or health-destroying groups of subjects. (The

analogue in political ecology would be the multiple "natures" constructed by conservation regimes and the specific kinds of environmental subjects those natures call into being.)

31. Choy et al. (2009) and Kirksey and Helmreich (2010).

32. Or, perhaps, the "killability" of mosquitoes and microbes (Beisel 2010; Haraway 2008).

33. Freeman (2010: 336).

34. *Zona* is the official name of the neighborhoods in Ciudad Sandino. Although Managua has several large "districts," which encompass multiple neighborhoods (Ciudad Sandino was at one time district 1 of Managua), the neighborhoods themselves are known as barrios. In Nicaragua, the word *barrio* has another connotation: it often means "slum" or "dangerous neighborhood." In Ciudad Sandino, people would most often refer to their home neighborhoods as *zonas* and areas they considered unsavory as *barrios*. A planned subdivision would be an *urbanización*. Newly annexed areas were known as *repartos,* which could be either slums, such as Reparto Rene Schick in Ciudad Sandino, or high-end areas, such as Reparto San Juan, near the Central American University.

35. Ingold (2007).

36. Hutchinson (1996: 44).

37. Casey, quoted in Pink (2008: 178).

38. Ingold (2011).

39. Raffles (2002) and Tsing (2005: 180).

40. The lives of different creatures are thus not simply connected; the connections breed further connections, or what Tim Ingold calls the "meshwork" that connects beings that inhabit the world. For Ingold (2008, 2011), the environment is precisely the zone of entanglement. "It is not," Ingold writes, "that organisms are entangled in relations. Rather, every organism—indeed every thing—is itself an entanglement" (Ingold 2008: 1806; see also Serres 2007 [1982]). Looking for objects, we find relationships.

41. But this is not enough. If shadowing tasks—in this case, labor processes taking place in the gaps between productive life and home life—is the first step to this entangled anthropology, how do we methodologically link houses in motion? Ingold (2007) has suggested that we consider what it means to walk. He contrasts the walked-upon *trail* with the abstract *connector,* the undifferentiated line between points. For Ingold, the walk between points matters as much as the points themselves.

42. If I wanted to understand how a garbage economy confounded dengue prevention and structured the landscape in a way that permitted dengue epidemics to happen, I had to do what George Marcus (1998) called "following the thing." Marcus was advocating a cosmopolitan, multisited ethnography, but such activity is equally appropriate in a contiguous site, because by following things along pathways rather than through abstract classificatory "networks," we are able to disaggregate the environment as something beings "live in" and treat it as an "open" habitat, a fluid space of constant becoming (Bowker and Star 1999; Haraway 2008; Ingold 2011; Lien and Law 2011). Landscapes are always already multisited.

43. Donahue (1986), Garfield and Williams (1992), and Wilson (2010).

44. Andrew Lakoff (2010) has identified "two regimes" of global health, articulating the parallel rise of humanitarianism and biosecurity as dominant discourses (see also Fassin 2005).

45. In many ways, critiques of global health productively follow earlier critiques of development (Escobar 1995; Ferguson 1994; Packard 1997).

46. Farmer (1999).

47. I am sympathetic to this critical argument about disease emergence, but I believe that even such "slippery" concepts retain some analytical potential. Emergence is a particularly apt lens for studying how globalization, urbanization, and environmental change inform conceptions of health and citizenship in nonlinear, unpredictable ways. Despite its prevalence in descriptions of infections, economies, or social movements, emergence is not a property of discrete phenomena. Emergence is a characteristic of fluidity, collectivity, and relationality (see Zhan 2005).

48. For a discussion of this in the context of "clinical tourism," see Brada (2011) and Wendland (2012).

49. The deterioration of revolutionary sentiment and attachments to liberation theology has been well documented across contemporary Latin America. Brotherton's (2012) study of the Cuban health system's postsocialist reconfiguration frames a tension between individualism and collectivity as constitutive of body politics. Reichman's (2011) ethnography of a Honduran coffee-growing village traces these changes more directly to the demise of liberation theology (and Roman Catholicism more broadly) in the face of transmigration, the dissemination of evangelical messages through the internet, and the collapse of the local coffee economy due to neoliberal reform.

CHAPTER ONE

1. *Envío,* September 1981.

2. Gobat (2005) and Walker (1997).

3. For more general Nicaraguan history, with a focus on urban events, see Babb (2001), Mendez (2005), Murray (1994), and Prevost and Vanden (1997).

4. The tale of the "city of emergencies" resonates with the tales of other Latin American cities in the twentieth century, in which the building of infrastructure has been part of the reconfiguration of class, racial, or ethnic politics. Key works include those of Caldeira (2001), Donna Goldstein (2003), and Holston (2008), on modernism, violence, gender, space and class in Brasilia, São Paolo, and Rio de Jainero; Daniel Goldstein (2004) on violence and indigeneity in Bolivia; Scheper-Hughes (1992) on structural violence in northeastern Brazil; and Low (2000) on place and space in Costa Rica.

5. Philippe Bourgois (2002) calls this critical, ecological view of life in urban poverty "street history."

6. Gaonkar and Povinelli (2003: 394). The anthropological study of infrastructure has recently expanded. See, for example, Anand (2011), Appel (2012), Carse (2012), and Zeiderman (2012).

7. The story of Ciudad Sandino is unique, then, in that most of its construction was accomplished thanks to the efforts of people who came from unofficial squatter settlements, popularly imagined in Nicaragua and elsewhere as places marked by an absence of such connections. Ciudad Sandino has come over the past forty years to look less and less like a prototypical "slum," yet it has taken on many of the characteristics—violence, social fracture, and infectious disease—that many scholars and writers commonly associate with slum life. For an example of this pessimistic view of the slum, see Davis (2006).

8. Livingston (2005: 16–17, 21).

9. Other anthropologists have also argued that urban Nicaragua has become socially more fractured in the days since the revolution, just as its infrastructure has led to spatial division and disembeddedness (Babb 2004; Lancaster 1992; Rodgers 2008).

10. I draw this notion of public health from Livingston (2005), as well as from Foucault's classic understanding of the technologies of public health as "governmental," in that they link concern for populations to concerns for individuals. Many such technologies arose with the dawn of the modern city (see Foucault 1984: 282–83).

11. This story is well known in Nicaragua and was retold in a lengthy investigative report by Glenn Garvin, of the *Miami Herald,* in the February 14, 2010, edition of that newspaper.

12. The victorious FSLN was borne out of three disparate and loosely based leftist movements. First was an agrarian guerilla movement in the countryside. This movement spawned in the early 1960s from a second, intellectual antiauthoritarian leftism forged among middle-class students in schools and universities. Third was an urban, union-based revolutionary movement. By the late 1970s, as Anastasio Somoza Debayle's callous and reckless predation of earthquake relief and demolition and construction contracts became overwhelming to the urban underclass, as well as the previously agnostic middle and upper class, the FSLN was able to form a broad-based economic, military, and social movement whose first priority was regime change and second priority was economic reform (Walker 1991, 1997; Wickham-Crowley 1992).

13. The autobiography of poet and novelist Gioconda Belli (2002) captures the preearthquake period—and the revolutionary days—with particular vividness.

14. Walker (1997: 2).

15. Elizabeth Dore (2006) provides the most thorough history of this process. She argues that patron-client relations, particularly between indigenous workers robbed of collective title and large plantation-owning elites, persisted well into the twentieth century.

16. Murray (1994: 25).

17. Walker (1997: 5).

18. Walker (1997: 5).

19. Barreto (2001: 6).

20. Barreto (2001: 14).

21. Pichardo (1993: 13).

22. I take the term "bare life" from the philosopher Giorgio Agamben (1998), who has extended Foucault's philosophy on biopower to suggest that highly regimented spaces, including cities, are sites not for the cultivation of citizenship but for fine-tuned surveillance of populations. I find Agamben's analysis of limited use, however, in understanding Ciudad Sandino's history, not least because discourses of law and property rights have likely always been skewed against the poor (Holston 2008). From a political ecology perspective, life is much more unruly. Water, geology, and insect behavior are difficult to survey into submission.

23. Sarah Besky (2013) and Julie Livingston (2005) have productively theorized the nostalgia of the poor and marginalized. While nostalgia is not equal to oral history, it is far from useless in social analysis. Indeed, much of what concerns contemporary students of Latin American politics is the political deployment of memories, nostalgic or otherwise (Babb 2001; Brotherton 2012).

24. Gobat (2005: 49).

25. Pichardo (1993: 8).

26. Werner (1992).

27. The term *brigadista* is probably most immediately derived from the Cuban model of community health mobilization (Brotherton 2012). Cuban support was crucial in the early years of the Sandinista regime.

28. *Envío,* September 1981.

29. Werner (1992: ix).

30. Werner (1992: ix).

31. Dore (2006), Garfield and Williams (1992), and Lancaster (1988).

32. Walker (1997: 10).

33. Donahue (1986: 66) and Freire (2000).

34. The 1980s were what many political and economic theorists call the "Lost Decade" of Latin American development. For a review, see Remmer (1991).

35. Brunkard et al. (2007) and Gubler (2002).

36. An article in the left-wing Nicaraguan journal *Envío* described the campaign as follows:

Concurrently [to the contra war], another war is being fought at the cost of millions of córdobas and tremendous grassroots mobilization across the country. It is the massive campaign against the dengue virus now at an epidemic level, particularly in populated areas. The campaign involves the disinfecting of all workplaces, schools, private houses, fields, etc., and the fumigation is being carried out with planes, trucks and on foot. Seeking out every small collection of still water, the goal is to eradicate the *Aedes aegypti* mosquito, carrier of dengue. President Ortega said on September 29, considering the rapid spread of the disease and the damage it has caused the population, including a hemorrhagic complication that can be fatal, the possibility could not be ruled out that this epidemic, plus the Xantonoma plague that is threatening thousands of acres of cotton, is a product of bacterial warfare initiated by the United States as part of its unbending aggressive policy toward Nicaragua. (*Envío,* October 1985)

37. *Envío,* September 1981.

38. Donahue (1986).

39. Revolutionary defense committees have also been an important part of Cuban political life, and Nicaragua certainly took inspiration from the Cuban Communist Party's neighborhood political organization and health mobilizations (Andaya 2009; Brotherton 2012). However, the Nicaraguan model also has its roots in the clandestine, barrio-by-barrio organization of the Sandinista movement (Babb 2001; Higgins and Coen 1992; Lancaster 1988; Nading 2013b).

40. *Envío,* September 1989. Had Nicaragua not been paralyzed by the contra war, these programs might have succeeded in the way that similar brigades did in Cuba during the same period (Whiteford 2000).

41. As has been noted by Babb (2001), Montoya (2003), and others, the Sandinista government actually began imposing austerity measures in 1988, as a last-ditch reaction to the costly war with the contras.

42. Birn, Zimmerman, and Garfield (2000) and Tesler (2006: 134).

43. Although the SILAIS system, which remained in place during the time of my fieldwork, has made regional offices responsible for health care provision, the majority of the MINSA budget, as well as control over the ministry's organizational framework and national public health policy, remains housed in central offices in Managua (Birn, Zimmerman, and Garfield 2000; Tesler 2006: 135).

44. Gubler (1989: 574).

45. Gubler (1989: 575, emphasis added).

46. In an era in which Latin American states have devolved many social services, including sanitation and health care, to local governments and civil society organizations, two perhaps contradictory ideas are at play. First, governments recognize that all citizens have the right to clean, "healthy" cities. Second, with this right comes the "responsibility" to contribute to the sanitation of those cities (Allison 2002: 1542; see also Paley 2001). The democratic appeal to "local" control can be offset by continued structural oppression, since "local participants" often make demands the state refuses to answer, and existing social differences may lead participants to exploit one another (Allison 2002: 1542). In this way, participatory approaches to the construction of healthy communities, such as Ciudad Sandino's antidengue campaigns, can shift blame onto the low-income citizens who suffer when urban ecosystems are "out of balance." Those who fail to participate in mitigating risk become depicted as "maladaptive" or inflexible.

47. Gubler (1989: 576–77).

48. That was 1989. By 1996, Gubler was publishing his own assessments, and they were mixed (Gubler and Clark 1996). The Rockefeller programs had not yielded significant reductions in dengue, and they had not realigned the relationships between dengue-affected communities and their governments. Where gov-

ernments were still trying to tackle dengue, they were often repeating activities that were either ineffective (i.e., outdoor low-volume spraying, which does little to contain mosquitoes that reside under roofs) or "vertical" (i.e., household inspection and abatement by state officials, with fines for those who harbored mosquitoes). Gubler came from the CDC, a U.S. government institution, but he and others did not hide their doubts about the capacity or willingness of states to solve health problems. It was not until the early 2000s that PAHO, an intergovernmental organization, would begin to devise "best practices" for dengue prevention (Parks and Lloyd 2004). For medical anthropologists sensitive to the multiscalar dimensions of dengue, simply integrating "local" knowledge with "state" policy would not suffice, given the "health transition" in which, as Carl Kendall noted at the start of the Rockefeller programs, diseases like dengue were linked as much to such macroscopic forces as trade, migration, urbanization, and the breakdown of already tenuous primary health care systems (Kendall et al. 1991: 266). Within the renewed discourse of "personal responsibility," then, was a counterdiscourse about structural forces that limited such responsibility and, ultimately, about the possibility that knowledge about dengue could be linked to awareness of larger problems affecting the urban poor, through "negotiated relevance" (Kendall 1998). By the 2000s, however, the notion that politics should be externalized from dengue control had become dominant.

49. For more on this process, see Nading (2011).

50. NGOs became increasingly important in the provision of social services, and some formerly Sandinista grassroots movements, particularly the women's movement, transitioned into the 1990s intact (Babb 2001; Ewig 1999; Mendez 2005).

51. Babb (2001) and LaRamée and Polakoff (1997: 185–86).

52. Tesler (2006: 455). Tesler describes brigadistas as "unpaid" (2006: 455), but in Ciudad Sandino and other places, brigadistas did receive small stipends in exchange for participation in antidengue campaigns. The demise of liberation theology is also suggestive here (Reichman 2011). Religious demographics have shifted considerably since the 1980s, and by my count Ciudad Sandino now contains more than 150 evangelical Christian congregations. Most estimates posit that evangelicals make up half the city's population. In 2008, citizens there elected their first *evangélico* mayor, Roberto Somoza Romero. Somoza was not the choice of the Ortega-FSLN party elite, and in 2010 he was forced out of office on dubious charges of corruption. The first attempt to force him out was a staged strike by city workers, orchestrated by the party during my September 2009 field visit. Friends reported that Somoza's religion made him suspect, and that evangelical Christianity was, for many hard-line FSLN activists, a "neoliberal" ideology.

53. Nading (2013b).

54. The branches of government were known by their "power" functions: the presidency was formally *Poder Ejecutivo* (Executive Power), joined by *Poder Legislativo* (Legislative Power) and *Poder Judicial* (Judicial Power). *Poder Ciudadano* was, for Ortega's administration, the new name for the electorate, or at least the 38

percent plurality that had put him back in office. The move to "Citizen Power" is one chapter in a longer debate within MINSA about the relative importance of professionals (including physicians and nurses, as well as mosquito control officers) and brigadistas in the primary health system. As far back as the 1980s, a sizable portion of MINSA's leadership had favored a deemphasis of brigadista work. Though it took most of the 1980s, they successfully pushed for the establishment of a system of local health centers, staffed by formally trained doctors and nurses: the system that the Chamorro government eventually formalized as SILAIS (Donahue 1986; Garfield and Williams 1992).

55. Low (1996: 876).

56. Farmer (1992).

57. From EPTISA's website, www.eptisa.com, "Integrated Project on the Outskirts of Managua (PROMAPER)," accessed January 31, 2011.

58. *El Nuevo Diario*, January 25, 2008.

59. The city's engineers explained to me that the choice to install sewage in these barrios was due to the "higher concentration" of the population there. As the director of environmental services told me, census data on the center or on Nueva Vida were difficult to come by. "If they do an accurate census," he told me, "they have to provide services for everybody, and not just some." The now-defunct fair trade organization Esperanza en Acción, which ran a women's apparel cooperative in Nueva Vida, found in 2010 that Ciudad Sandino had the highest population density in Nicaragua (at 4,500 persons per square kilometer) and that the *alcaldía* generates only US$2.30 per resident in yearly revenue (www.esperanzaenaccion.org, accessed February 6, 2011; the site has been discontinued).

60. INSS was shorthand for National Institute of Social Security. INSS gave a small percentage of government employees and formal sector workers subsidized health care, administered after the 1990s by private companies, with separate wards within MINSA hospitals (Tesler 2006: 239).

61. Donahue (1986: 66).

62. The line between rights and privileges is also being redrawn in postsocialist Cuba, particularly with respect to access to drugs (Brotherton 2012).

63. Though unions were not illegal, it was common knowledge among the largely young and predominantly female working population that organizers were often fired and blacklisted. In Nueva Vida, a fair-trade apparel cooperative briefly flourished as an alternative source of employment to the zona francas (Fisher 2013).

64. Paley (2001).

65. Murphy (2004).

CHAPTER TWO

1. Following doña Flor and the *recolectores* along the waste stream convinced me that one contribution of anthropology to understanding dengue epidemics is the anthropologist's position as one who can *move* alongside and among the actors who

live those problems. Privileging mobility hedges against the temptation to reduce the social and cultural elements of environment to the words we hear in interviews (Ingold 2000, 2011; Pink 2008). Movement exposes how environmental politics derives as much from everyday moments of conflict and conciliation, often within households, as it does from punctuated events in more traditionally "public" spaces such as parks, city halls, and streets. This approach affords a view of the urban landscape as a winding string of variegated habitats, rather than as a bounded "field" where political problems are contested or, in the case of dengue, where mosquitoes and garbage meet. Studying entanglement is about following that winding string. Such an approach reveals how the everyday, house-to-house movements of people like garbage men and *chuɾequeros* (garbage scavengers), as well as other living beings like mosquitoes, shaped both the local landscape and the global, ostensibly place-neutral techniques of urban planning and public health designed to make that landscape more livable.

2. This is an approach that dates back to the earliest days of mosquito control (see Carter 2012; Kelly and Beisel 2011; Kinkela 2011; Sutter 2007).

3. See Anderson (2004) and Mitman, Murphy, and Sellers (2004) for a review of how ecological ideas have served biomedicine over the last century or more. See also chapter 8 of the fourth report of the Intergovernmental Panel on Climate Change (Confalonieri et al. 2007; see also Patz et al. 2005). Some leading dengue scientists see a lack of empirical data to support the claims of the panel that climate change is helping dengue to spread. Dengue mosquitoes are certainly adapting to new environments (viz., higher altitudes with measurably lower mean temperatures), but *Ae. aegypti* has lived north and south of the subtropics for decades. One of the first outbreaks of dengue, or "breakbone fever," to enter the Western medical literature was in Philadelphia in 1789 (Rigau-Perez 1998). Opponents of the connection between global warming and mosquito-borne disease have argued their case with particular verve. Dissenters include one scientist, Paul Reiter, who has appeared on the Glenn Beck radio program and in a British documentary accusing those who elaborated the panel's position on climate change and vector-borne disease of intentionally misleading the public (Reiter and Murphy 2007).

4. Following Ulrich Beck (1992), Alan Peterson and Deborah Lupton (1996) contend that people's recognition of the environment as a source of new dangers and a crucible for the resurgence of old ones has produced a new "reflexivity."

5. Briggs suggests in the conclusion to his study of Venezuelan cholera epidemics in the 1990s that the production of sanitary citizens is increasingly seen by international health practitioners as the responsibility of states (2003: 319–20). The imperative to act out and reproduce sanitary citizenship in Venezuela proved more divisive than unifying.

6. Appadurai (1988).

7. Analysis of patron-client relations is nothing new for anthropology (see Mintz 1960), but it has remained an important element of recent studies in the region, including historical studies of Nicaragua (see Dore 2006; Raffles 2002; Scheper-Hughes 1992). This relational analysis of politics resonates with political

ecology, and it is perhaps no surprise that Eric Wolf, himself a student of patron-clientage and its fate under capitalism, coined that term. A close examination of the intersection of garbage, mosquitoes, people, and policy calls attention to the ways in which these things "contain and are constituted by their relations" (Robbins 2012: 94; see also Besky 2013).

8. See Escobar (2002) and Fox (1994). For a classic discussion of how capitalist relations change patron-client relations, see Mintz (1960).

9. *La Prensa,* August 4, 2008.

10. Ashencaen-Crabtree, Wong, and Mas'ud (2001) and Gubler (1989).

11. Robbins (2012).

12. Matthews (2008); see also Seabrook (2008). Scholars are now recognizing the contributions of the world's two million scavengers to this surprisingly lucrative market. By extracting valuable material from dumps, streets, and sewers, scavengers may help both to forestall the ecological degradation of cities and to maintain the sustainability of urban economies. According to development economist Martin Medina (2007), when exploitative intermediaries are eliminated, and when states encourage rather than punish the formation of scavenger cooperatives, informal garbage collection can "improve national industrial competitiveness," "[save] municipalities money", and expand the environmental benefits of recycling (Medina 2008: 3). In Ciudad Sandino, ownership of garbage was fluid, or "open," in the language of resources. Recyclable waste shared two characteristics with other "open" resources, such as fisheries, range, and forests. Excluding user groups from access was impossible (or at least prohibitively expensive), and each new user or user group that gained access subtracted from the success of others (Feeny et al. 1990: 3–4).

13. These data are based on a basic demographic survey I conducted with two assistants while interviewing adult (older than sixteen) churequeros in September and October of 2008. Fifty adults were surveyed. Although more than 120 people could be found in the dump in a given day, interview data and a census taken by churequero leaders suggest that the number of full-time scavengers was closer to eighty. These income statistics are thus a rough guide based on self-reporting by full-time workers.

14. *El Nuevo Diario,* October 14, 2008.

15. Rumors in Ciudad Sandino and Managua persisted that FSLN operatives were hiring churequeros and other underemployed or marginalized people to act as its agents in stirring up unrest. More than a year after the dump protests, this turned out to be true: the party-paid group of churequeros was hired to attack Ciudad Sandino's elected mayor in a staged "protest" against alleged corruption within the *alcaldía.*

16. *El Nuevo Diario,* March 24, 2008.

17. Patron-client relationships are "moral economic" in that they depend upon a careful management of exploitation (Scheper-Hughes 1992; Scott 1976; Thompson 1971). As Sarah Besky (2013) explains in her study of the "tripartite moral economy" that shapes tea plantation life in Darjeeling, India, moral economies are generally

seen as two-way relationships between the powerful and relatively powerless, but care for place and its nonhuman, material elements complicates this view. For Besky, the tea-producing landscape is not a passive element in moral economic relations. Likewise, it seems wise not to see garbage or mosquitoes as passive either.

18. The literature on common property resources distinguishes between resources and property, since property need not necessarily be a tangible thing but may also be a right of exclusion. Private property is that to which an individual owner has rights of exclusion and inclusion; collective property is that to which polity has such rights; open access property is that to which no specific rights obtain, and common property is that to which rights are claimed by a specific user group (see Agrawal 2001; Feeny et al. 1990). In analyzing urban life, it is easy to think of *common* resources—distinguished from "open" ones by the fact that a limited number of users can claim them—as things of the past. Most public spaces, such as roads, dumps, and sewers, are considered *collective* property, built by the state and with rights to inclusion and exclusion arbitrated through jurisprudence. In the case of Ciudad Sandino, however, garbage, erstwhile private property that had been released into collective space, became a kind of open access property, whence it was freely harvested and traded and transferred again to the realm of private property. During the 2006–2008 scrap boom, churequeros were forced to define themselves retroactively as a "community of resource users" and to defend their access (Schlager and Ostrom 1992: 249).

19. An alternative narrative arose, in which the FSLN had actually instigated the protests, but I found no evidence of this.

20. This phrase, borrowed from Carol Rose (1986), is a reversal of Garrett Hardin's (1968) famous dictum of the "tragedy of the commons." Here, it seems, is an example of how generalized access to a public resource—rather than sadly overexploiting that resource—might strengthen otherwise "atomized" poor communities (Ackerman and Mirza 2001). As the case of Ciudad Sandino demonstrates, while it is attractive to view recyclables as resources whose recovery and sale on a market are both socially and environmentally beneficial, such a view does not fully account for the city's integration into fundamentally uneven global production and consumption systems.

21. Robbins (2012: 95).

22. Adams and Kapan (2009).

23. *El Nuevo Diario,* July 24, 2008, and *La Prensa,* August 7, 2008.

24. The contrast between this situation and garbage politics in other parts of Latin America is striking. In work ongoing in Brazil, anthropologist Christopher Alley (2010) has shown that in the context of dengue epidemics, garbage scavengers and informal garbage collectors, who have had strong labor unions for decades, managed to position themselves as stewards of environmental health. There, brokers were nearly never involved in the discussion over the social etiology of dengue; instead, dengue epidemics became an opportunity for the scavengers, rather than the brokers, to assert their legitimacy and claims to citizenship. The erasure of scavengers from the discussion between MINSA and the recycling industry is noteworthy.

25. Purcell (2002).

26. *El Nuevo Diario,* September 29, 2009.

27. Ideas about waste and pollution run deep in anthropology and the social sciences (see Douglas 2002 [1966]). As geographer Sarah Moore puts it, garbage and the people who handle it are "abject" phenomena, in that it they are both reviled by the society that creates them and, paradoxically, necessary components of that society's reproduction (Moore 2008). Michelle Murphy elaborates: "Abjection designates 'unlivable' and 'uninhabitable' zones of social life which are nonetheless densely populated by those who are not enjoying the status of subject, but whose living under the sign of the 'unlivable' is required to circumscribe the domain of the subject. . . . [Abjection] makes and marks a domain of supposed impossibility" (2006: 152). In the case of infectious disease, ideas about pollution and abjection translate into ideas about places as pathological, in what Paul Farmer (1992) calls a "geography of blame."

28. I am grateful to Eric Carter for encouraging me to explore the patron-client idea in this chapter. For the theory of parasitism, I draw on the work of Michel Serres (2007 [1982]), who argues that parasitic relations—relations of disruption and disturbance—are the norm rather than exceptional in social life. This idea resonates with Marx's (1976) ideas about relations between the proletariat and the bourgeoisie, but more important, it links classes of relationships (human-nonhuman, human-human, nonhuman-nonhuman, animate-inanimate) that normally get separated. In other words, the parasite is a device for thinking of the ways in which environments are inhabited—constantly made and unmade—rather than simply occupied. I also draw on the work of Timothy Mitchell (2002), who, though not drawing directly on Serres, uses the term "para-sites of capitalism" to describe active presence of mosquitoes and people in the intersecting spaces of war, hydroelectric development, and global malaria control.

CHAPTER THREE

1. Karen moved to Nueva Vida several years after the hurricane and after the original resettlement of hurricane refugees. The refugees, for their part, told other stories about bill payment. Two of the most prominent were (a) that they had been given their homes with the understanding that water and gas were also "donated" and (b) that they had moved into homes unaware that previous occupants had failed to pay their debts.

2. Heintze, Garrido, and Kroeger (2007).

3. *El Nuevo Diario,* August 22, 2007.

4. The phrase "senses of place" comes from the work of Feld and Basso (1996). Keith Basso (1996), in particular, has examined how attachment to places through narrative forges sense of collective identity. Language—including names and metaphors—helps create entanglement.

5. The social epidemiologist Nancy Krieger (2005; Krieger and Davey-Smith 2004) has developed this idea most forcefully, arguing against the tendency in her

own discipline to ignore the historical conditions that produce class, racial, and gender differences. She argues for an understanding of inequality itself as "embodied" (see also Mitman, Murphy, and Sellers 2004).

6. *El Nuevo Diario,* August 22, 2007.

7. For vivid accounts of evangelical and Pentecostal transformation in Central America, see Kevin O'Neill (2010) and Reichman (2011).

8. I have changed the name of this church to obscure its exact identity. The *pastora's* story of conversion abroad in the United States was typical. Latin American Pentecostal religion, especially in Central America, has largely been a product of South-North transmigration (Reichman 2011).

9. Elizabeth Roberts (2012) shows how Catholics, too, have learned to blend religious and biotechnical embraces.

10. For seminal work on original antigenic sin in dengue, see Halstead, Rojanasuphot, and Sangkawibha (1983).

11. For a full explanation of this process, see nature.com's resource on dengue, www.nature.com/scitable/topicpage/host-response-to-the-dengue-virus-22402106, accessed December 13, 2013.

12. Compare, for example, Kuno, Gubler, and Oliver (1993) and Midgley et al. (2011). Recent studies have suggested that prior infection by future viruses can possibly confer protection—if temporary—from others (Zompi and Harris 2013).

13. Martin (1994); see also Napier (2012).

14. As Nikolas Rose puts it, "Biological senses of identification and affiliation [make] certain kinds of ethical demands possible; demands on oneself, on one's kin, community, society; on those who [exercise] authority" (2007: 133). In discussing how rural Indians "become environmentalists," Arun Agrawal emphasizes how a sense of duty to the environment arises through practice: "Although the politics and analytics of identity consider significant the external signs of belongings, it is the tissue of contingent practices spanning categorical affiliations that is really at stake in influencing interests and outcomes" (2005: 163). In Ciudad Sandino, homemaking and brigadista work were such contingent practices.

15. See Babb (2001). Elsewhere (Nading 2013b), I have described this work as moral economic negotiation, drawing on the trope of "brokerage."

16. Biehler (2007).

17. Harding (2008: 1).

18. Haraway (2008).

19. Carter (2012: 161) traces the history of household standardization and homogenization in mosquito control to the heyday of DDT. Lock and Nguyen (2010) level a similar critique of the "standardizable body" that dominates global and international health discourses.

20. Harris (1984).

21. Koch (2013: 309), describing tuberculosis treatment in post-Soviet Georgia, calls practices that standardize bodies and spaces "responses to disease that emphasize medicine as a moral commitment to society."

22. Koch (2013: 312); see also Koch (2011).

23. In discussing thresholds as "limits," Koch (2013: 313) draws on the work of Claire Wendland (2010) with Malawian medical students. Wendland finds that Malawian doctors developed a moral commitment to care in the absence of standardized medical tools. The meaning of being a doctor was adjusted to political, economic, and historical contingency.

24. Geertz (1973: 93).

25. Reichman (2011).

26. Haraway (2008) and Hinchliffe and Whatmore (2006: 123).

27. Ciudad Sandino had few "homeless" individuals. Even people who spent a great deal of time living off of the streets, such as scavengers, had small dwellings, often semilegal or untitled.

28. Caldeira (2001). Caldeira's "city of walls," in Brazil, was a series of exclusionary spaces, cordoning rich from poor. In Managua, as Rodgers (2004) has argued, the well-to-do have created a more fluid network of "disembedding." Instead of being a series of "fortified enclaves," Managua is now a place where entire layers of the city (highways, shopping malls, *and* exclusive neighborhoods) are effectively off-limits to the poor majority.

29. In some parts of Ciudad Sandino and Managua—including in Nueva Vida—people would pay private, informal collectors to haul trash away. These *carretoneros* would routinely sort through garbage for items of value and dump the refuse in illegal dumps. The installation of formal municipal garbage collection in most of Ciudad Sandino noticeably reduced the number of such dumps in the landscape.

30. Deleuze and Guattari (1987: 311) call such routines of entanglement "refrains": comforting, repeated patterns of expression that forge continuity in an unstable world. "But home does not preexist," they write; "it [is] necessary to draw a circle around that fragile center, to organize a limited space. . . . The interior space protects the germinal forces of a task to fulfill or a deed to do. . . . Finally . . . one launches forth. . . . To improvise is to join with the world or meld with it."

31. Ferguson (2008: 571).

32. Ferguson (2008: 577).

33. Bourdieu (1977), Martin (1994), and Scheper-Hughes and Lock (1987).

34. Shillington (2008).

35. Shaw, Robbins, and Jones (2010).

36. Deleuze and Guattari (1987: 311–12); see also Bateson (1979) and Ingold (2011).

37. Recognition of this pushes a reassessment of the classical opposition between *polis* and *oikos*. A classical understanding of city life has traditionally confined those—women, children, and "others"—who supposedly belong in the *oikos* to subservience and the production of "mere life" *(zoe)*, while "public life" *(bios)* has been seen as the realm of the *polis* (Moore 1994: 87; see also Rabinow and Rose 2006). Theories of biopower call attention to the ways in which political life increasingly revolves around the production and reproduction of "mere life" (Holston

2008: 311–12). The entanglement of humans with nonhuman animals and microbes, however, troubles this argument (Helmreich 2009; Koch 2011; Paxson 2008).

38. Gal (2002).

39. Rochleau, Thomas-Slayter, and Wangari (1996: 298); see also Mansfield (2008) and Shillington (2013).

40. Dwelling happens in an in-between space, neither public nor private, for which Elizabeth Grosz uses the classical term *chora*: "*Chora* . . . is the space in which place is made possible. . . . It is the space that engenders without processing, that nurtures without requirements of its own, that receives without giving, and that gives without receiving. . . . It is no wonder that *chora* resembles the characteristics the Greeks, and all those who follow them, have long attributed to femininity" (1995: 116).

41. Hinchliffe and Whatmore (2006).

42. Kirksey and Helmreich (2010).

43. Subject formation occurred through what Stefan Helmreich (2009: 23–24) calls "symbiopolitics," the politics of the associations *between things* and the implications of those associations.

CHAPTER FOUR

1. Lockwood (2002: 3).

2. Lockwood (2002: 19–20). Raffles (2010) describes a similar kind of fascination in his work with the artist and entomologist Cornelia Hesse-Honegger, whose drawings of insect mutations that resulted from fallout due to the Chernobyl disaster have allowed her to critically approach the relationship between ecology, life, and health in a nuclear age. Raffles later traces this posture back to the work of earlier entomologists Jean-Henri Fabre and Karl von Frisch.

3. Lockwood (1999: 366).

4. Bateson (1979), Foucault (1997), and Harries-Jones (1995).

5. In an interview with Stephen Riggins, Foucault asserts that the "transformation of one's self by one's knowledge is, I think, something rather close to the aesthetic experience" (quoted in Milchman and Rosenberg 2007: 57).

6. Karen Barad (2003) calls this process one of "intra-action," whereby observers, things observed, and instruments of observation make one another. Intra-action is how "matter comes to matter."

7. Ingold (2011: 79).

8. Bourdieu (1977) and Robbins (2007). Combined with the exhortation to kill virus-laden mosquitoes, we might see this ordering work as a rationalization or "medicalization" of household space. Another way to understand these documents might be to see them as what Asher Ghertner (2010) calls forms of "aesthetic governmentality," whereby ideas about the look and feel of spaces reinforce particular behaviors within them.

9. Suarez et al. (2005: 499).

10. Harvey (1996).

11. Bateson (1979) and Neves (2005).

12. Here, I want to use the idea of "ecological aesthetics" to contribute to discussion about the "politics of life" amid a process of "mutual becoming" (Deleuze and Guattari 1987; Haraway 2008; Ingold 2011; Neves 2009: 147).

13. Ingold (2011: 75, 115).

14. As mosquito control pioneer William Gorgas once said, "This system of destroying mosquito larvae is . . . essential. . . . *caring* for the cisterns, water barrels and containers is the essential work" (quoted in Shaw, Robbins, and Jones 2010: 380).

15. Neves (2009: 146); see also Hale et al. (2011: 1854) and Litt et al. (2011).

16. The term "multiplicities on the move" comes from Foucault's late work on security (Foucault 2009: 125). The notion of multiplicity, however, is most often associated with the work of Deleuze and Guattari (1987).

17. See Carter (2012) and Packard (2007) for historical reviews of malaria management, and Anderson (2006) for a broader discussion of how hygiene was linked to health and race in colonial tropical medicine. For discussions of approaches to *Ae. aegypti,* see Dick et al. (2012) and Lowy (1997).

18. Mitchell (2002).

19. As historian Paul Sutter argues, malaria and yellow fever control programs in Panama, based on the premise that by "eradicating" mosquitoes, authorities could stop the virus, contained within them an important counternarrative (Sutter 2007). Sutter's archival data show that entomological technicians working on the American canal project in Panama carried on an internal dialogue about the origins of the malaria problem there. In brief, entomological workers in the Canal Zone believed that environments conducive to malaria were not simply products of untamed tropical nature; rather, malaria was—at least in some instances—a product of colonial landscaping itself (2007: 749). For Sutter, the debate shows "how the dominant U.S. ideology of tropical conquest, manifest here as a landscape aesthetic, came into conflict with the perceived ecological dictates of mosquito control" (750).

20. Reed's work around the turn of the century was actually a confirmation of a theory put forth in 1881 by Cuban physician Carlos Finlay (Cueto 2007: 30–32).

21. Ross, quoted in Chwatt (1977: 1072).

22. The discursive separation of "clean" settlers from "dirty" natives constituted a particular kind of body politics, in which the "closed, ascetic" (white) colonial body was opposed to the "open, grotesque" native one (Anderson 1995: 640). Elsewhere, Warwick Anderson has pointed out that the ecological epidemiology of Frank McFarlane Burnet and Rene Dubos was a kind of precursor to modern ecological health (2004: 40–41). The narrative of insulation of human bodies from a dangerous and germ-ridden environment was paralleled in colonial medicine by a recognition not only of the inherent porosity of human bodies (the circulation of blood, parasites, and viruses via mosquito bites are just one example) but also of the

role of colonialism itself in producing dangerous environments. The emphasis in ecology on host-parasite interactions was not, as Anderson points out, immune to reductive racial thinking or complicity with colonial projects, but it was an important alternative to anthropocentric discourses about "closed bodies."

23. Anderson (2006).

24. Cueto (2007: 33).

25. In fact, Cruz felt so strongly about the undifferentiated vulnerability of the Brazilian population that he pushed for mandatory smallpox vaccination in 1904 (Meade 1986). The move for compulsory vaccination led to mass resistance and rioting, but Cruz ultimately prevailed and by the middle of the next decade was praised for his commitment to generalized health through sanitation.

26. Carter (2008: 280). The construction of such spaces under the guise of "environmental sanitation," or *saneamiento,* is central to Carter's (2012) history of malaria control in twentieth-century Argentina. For Carter, malaria and mosquitoes helped facilitate a convergence of knowledge production and state formation. The Argentine state's claim on malaria prevention as an area of concern (hardly a given in the early 1900s) was one way the state itself came into being. The Argentine state adapted the *saneamiento* approach from approaches developed in Italy, but they did not copy the approach wholesale. Rather, they adapted it to what they saw as the particular conditions of their country's "malarious" zones, particularly the rural northwest.

27. Mitchell (2002: 40–41) tells a similar story as he recounts the confluence of colonialism, capitalism, and entomology that created modern Egypt. Importantly for both Carter (2012) and Mitchell, individuals adapted mosquito control strategies to suit what they saw as particular national or regional economic necessities and ecological contingencies. In 1933, the Tennessee Valley Authority (TVA) in the American South began operating on the assumption that economic development and malaria control should be combined. The building of hydroelectric dams in the valley went along with careful ecological studies of *Anopheles* mosquito breeding patterns. Water levels in newly dammed rivers were dropped and raised in order to control riverine breeding; screens were applied to houses; insecticides were used; and education campaigns were implemented. Malaria, dengue fever, and yellow fever, which had been resurgent in the economic hard times of the early 1930s, were significantly rolled back by the start of World War II. Such large-scale, cross-class, and cross-race interventions were not limited to the United States. Even at the height of the malaria mosquito eradication movement between the 1940s and 1950s, programs tended to be adapted to particular landscapes and political environments (Carter 2014).

28. Carter (2007: 644; 2008: 280). In his study of this disaggregation in the context of colonial and postcolonial Egypt, Mitchell (2002) insists that this process is integral to the consolidation of "technopolitical" power. Another example comes from the American experience. Dengue, malaria, and yellow fever took a considerable toll on the U.S. military during the World War II, yet military experiences also exposed the burden of these diseases on populations in the tropics. In the wake of World War II and the founding of the World Health Organization, and

the consolidation of the U.S. Public Health Service and the Malaria Control in War Areas program into the new Communicable Disease Center (CDC), an effort to eradicate mosquito-borne disease began (CDC 2014). DDT was central to this effort (cf. Brown 1997; Gladwell 2002; Kinkela 2011). The genesis of the chemical is thus bound up in the techno-optimism of the postwar period and the developmentalist rhetoric that characterized international relations in the years after the Marshall Plan (Escobar 1995; Packard 2007).

29. Carter (2012: 122).

30. By 1930, Soper was taking Cruz's early successes with expanded species eradication and testing their limits, again in Brazil (Lowy 1997: 401–2). That Soper did his early work in Brazil is significant. Brazil was not an American possession or theater of military operations, but it was the site of Cruz's sanitation campaigns in the 1900s and 1910s. Soper worked for the Rockefeller Foundation, a private, pre-World War II version of the World Health Organization. Rockefeller promoted mosquito eradication in part because it was technical work. Men like Soper were scientists; statisticians accompanied all projects, and the humanitarian results were made clear through the quantitative results they produced. The focus on malaria *mosquitoes* as drivers of poor health, and hence as causative of poverty, led to apolitical, entomological solutions. Such solutions were attractive to the Rockefeller Foundation, an organization whose name was associated "with the ills of monopoly capitalism" (Stapleton 2004: 208).

31. Despite its initial promise, the DDT-driven approach to mosquito eradication somewhat ignored the local dynamics of mosquito habitat formation (Carter 2012). As Mitchell (2002: 48) suggests, Soper and his superiors at the Rockefeller Foundation, as well as from the Health Office of the League of Nations and the Pan American Sanitary Bureau, which would later morph into the World Health Organization, presumed that they could control *all Anopheles* mosquitoes around the world because they had succeeded in controlling them in Egypt.

32. Crucially, the push to include *Ae. aegypti* in the WHO program came not from Europeans or North Americans but from the Bolivian delegation to a new WHO subsidiary, the Pan American Health Organization (PAHO) (Cueto 2007: 78). The decision to "eradicate" *Ae. aegypti,* as well as the plan for implementing that decision, flowed from South to North (Schleissmann 1967: 604).

33. Randall Packard (1997) has suggested that the infectious disease eradication projects of the 1950s and 1960s were rooted in a new kind of developmentalism that arose after the war's end. The "success" or "failure" of the malaria eradication program cannot be separated from its political economic context, specifically that of the Cold War. In this way, the global malaria eradication program may be tied fruitfully to the technology-driven "discourse of development" that came to dominate international humanitarian, military, and diplomatic practice for the rest of the century (Escobar 1995). The watchword *development* has survived various changes in discursive and practical framings, just as the term *eradication* still peppers global health discourses. Both have been aided by another powerful discursive package that reemerged in the postwar period, *ecology* (Escobar 1999).

34. USDHEW (1965b: 11).

35. USDHEW (1965b: 11).

36. USDHEW (1965a: 21).

37. USDHEW (1965a: 21).

38. Shillington (2008).

39. That binary maps roughly onto the brigadistas' social/technical distinction and resonates with the historical findings of Carter (2012) on Argentinean malaria programs.

40. For further discussion of the quantity/quality discourse, see Nading (2013b).

41. Packard (1997: 279–80) and Schleissmann (1967).

42. One of the earliest and deadliest of these new outbreaks was the 1981 Cuban event, in which over 150 individuals, mostly children, died. Before that epidemic, there had been only sixty reported cases of severe dengue in the Americas (Guzman 2005; Taubes 1997).

43. The mobilization against DDT began soon after it took hold as a global standard in mosquito control. DDT was quickly adopted in the fight against fire ants in the U.S. South and as an agricultural pesticide, and environmental activists—most notably the biologist and author Rachel Carson—led a successful effort to eliminate its use (Buhs 2002; Carson 1962; Kinkela 2011).

44. See Gubler (1997), Halstead (2003), Hammond et al. (2005), Lugo et al. (2005), and Sanchez et al. (2006).

45. Briggs (2003).

46. Gubler (1989).

47. Kendall (1998).

48. Heintze, Garrido, and Kroeger (2007); compare Perez et al. (2007).

49. Duane Gubler, a microbiologist and one of the founding fathers of the "participatory" approach, summed up his feelings in a 2013 interview, when he was asked which "three wishes" he would want fulfilled, given dengue's continued spread. They were, in order, "That tropical cities were much smaller. That there were good reliable water systems in those cities. That the people in those cities would take responsibility for environmental management in and around their homes" ("Partnership for Dengue Control: A Conversation with Dr. Duane Gubler," www .denguevaccines.org/partnership-dengue-control-conversation-dr-duane-gubler, accessed 3/4/14).

50. Ingold (2011: 69) calls this an "inverted" view of the organism. Its opposite would be a view of organisms themselves as entanglements.

51. Douglas (2002 [1966]).

52. The biology and ecology of dengue—and knowledge about them—are what Richard Levins and Richard Lewontin (1985) refer to as "dialectical," that is, emerging in particular historical and political-economic contexts, rather than naturally and objectively.

53. The case for sylvatic transmission has been buttressed thanks to the recent discovery of dengue serotype 5, which is thought to be transmissible to primates (Normile 2013).

54. Arguello (2009).

55. Gubler and Kuno (1997).

56. Endy, Weaver, and Hanley (2010).

57. Slosek (1986).

58. Dengue's history parallels that of transcontinental trade, especially in slaves, sugar, and spices, and the circulation of people and mosquitoes from forest-village zones to the new cities of Southeast Asia, where the virus is thought to have originated (Endy, Weaver, and Hanley 2010). In the Americas, the coming of dengue was probably preceded by that of *Ae. aegypti* and the yellow fever virus (McNeill 2010).

59. Lakoff (2008) and Shukin (2009: 183–84). In his work on biopolitics, Foucault suggested as much: the ordering of the environment reflects a governmental ethic that is productive and conservative of "life," narrowly defined as the vitality of *human populations* (Foucault 2009; Rose 2007).

60. Ingold (2011: 3–4, 210).

61. People, mosquitoes, and viruses were entangled, sometimes literally, in what Deleuze and Guattari (1987: 10, 242), who were thinking in part of viral zoonoses and epidemics, call "lines of flight."

62. Bateson (2000 [1972]) and Kohn (2007).

63. Brigadistas, as both local householders and representatives of a state ministry charged with managing a household disease, acted simultaneously as "perceivers" of disease pattern and participants in its disruption (Bateson 2000 [1972]).

64. Beisel (2010: 47); see also Haraway (2008).

65. Nadasdy (2007) and Neves (2005).

66. As Deleuze and Guattari (1987: 242) suggest, "That is the only way that Nature operates—against itself."

67. Ingold (2011: 210).

68. Candea (2010: 252).

69. Said (1979) and Sawyer and Agrawal (2000).

70. Quoted in Candea (2010: 252).

71. Freccero (2011: 178, 190).

72. Star (1991: 52).

73. Haraway (2008).

74. Bateson (1979).

75. Bateson (1979) and Kohn (2007).

76. Bateson (1979).

77. Garfield and Williams (1992).

78. Babb (2001: 201).

79. Castro, Khawja, and Johnston (2010).

80. We might therefore see the metaphorical joke about single mothers as what Stephen Pfol, following Walter Benjamin, labels a "profane illumination," a kind of "power-reflexive knowledge … attentive to the complex ways in which technoscientific claims are situated within historical knots of power" (2005: 585). A more familiar trope might be Raymond Williams's "structure of feeling," a mode of expression that self-consciously and partially articulates new forms of "presence" (1977: 135).

81. Tsing (2010).

82. Briggs (2003), Peterson and Lupton (1996), and Suarez et al. (2005).

83. Ingold (2011: 75). Embedded in brigadistas' fascination with *Ae. aegypti* lie some lessons for biopolitics. While we can certainly interpret public health as a set of techniques for the management of populations, as Angela Garcia (2010: 31) points out, the pastoral power on which public health depends may also perpetuate "ethical ideas of caring."

84. Ingold (2011) and Kirksey and Helmreich (2010: 544, 555–56).

85. Neves (2009: 146).

86. Milchman and Rosenberg (2007: 56).

87. Foucault (1997: 266, 269).

88. Douglas (2002 [1966]).

89. Rose (2007: 53).

90. Foucault (1997: 131); see also Tobias (2005: 66).

91. Foucault (1997: 292) and Tobias (2005: 82).

92. Harries-Jones (1995).

93. That observation may seem counterintuitive, but as Matei Candea suggests, "detachment," a studied posture of scientists and amateur ecologists alike, coexists with, rather than opposes, relationship. Detachment in this sense is a form of openness. It "[allows] things to appear in their own time and form" (2010: 253). Detachment, seen as a way of relating, is akin to "unsurprised astonishment" (Ingold 2011).

94. Bateson (1979), Haraway (2008), and Neves (2009).

CHAPTER FIVE

1. Birn, Zimmerman, and Garfield (2000) and Tesler (2006).

2. Rodgers (2004).

3. Brotherton (2012: 130) relates the story of a Cuban doctor who expressed much the same sentiment. As the doctor told a group of "apathetic" neighbors, "*La Revolucion . . .* helps those who help themselves."

4. *El Nuevo Diario,* January 21, 2009.

5. *El Nuevo Diario,* January 22, 2009. Throughout 2008 and early 2009, stories about dengue proliferated. Press releases sympathetic to the FSLN lauded the successes of the CPCs in dengue control; however, I found few examples of that success in Ciudad Sandino. Indeed, when I surveyed residents from five different municipal zones in 2009, I found that only 12 percent (32 out of 259) even knew the identity of their local CPC representatives.

6. Such a discourse is prevalent in the world of "participatory" development (Li 2007; Paley 2001). For an example of the use of this discourse with regard to dengue, see Gubler (1989).

7. I came to this insight through comparison with Nadasdy's (2003) analysis of how the search for "traditional ecological knowledge" in biodiversity conservation

projects subjugates indigenous knowledge to science by forcing indigenous people to translate concepts into the narrow, numerical, data-driven parameters of ecology and wildlife management.

8. Campos et al. (2003), Parks and Lloyd (2004), and Toledo-Romani et al. (2007).

9. Even if MINSA wanted their work to include constructive feedback, brigadistas sensed with discomfort that a will to be healthy had to be observed (Bateson 2000 [1972]; cf. Hacking 1991).

10. Koch (2013: 310). Koch's example draws in turn on Margaret Lock's notion of "local biologies," or "how and why claims to the biological and social are leveraged within historical, cultural, embodied, and political-economic relationships" (Koch 2013: 309).

11. To the extent that they were deploying models of the household habitat to generate epidemiological knowledge, their eyes were those of MINSA, yet their gaze, to use Donna Haraway's (1988) phrase, was "situated."

12. See, for example, Rifkin (1996).

13. Heintze, Garrido, and Kroeger (2007); compare Perez et al. (2007).

14. Fassin (2004: 173).

15. Harris (1998).

16. Kuan et al. (2009).

17. Ramos et al. (2008).

18. Kyle and Harris (2008).

19. Kyle and Harris (2008).

20. CIET, Camino Verde, caminoverde.ciet.org, accessed December 15, 2013.

21. CIET, Camino Verde, caminoverde.ciet.org, accessed December 15, 2013.

22. SEPA had been operating in the Bello Amanecer section of Ciudad Sandino (zona 9) since 2004, but activities there had fizzled after the original CIET project ended in December 2007. When the program was revived in Nueva Vida, I was already tracking the activities of regular brigadistas from the hospital. The hospital epidemiologist at the time suggested that I observe the SEPA program. I attended SEPA activities approximately once per week from July to December 2009, and I also was present at three meetings of the barrio leaders with CIET staff in Managua (July and August 2008), the third annual SEPA retreat (August 2008), and several meetings with Ciudad Sandino leaders in Nueva Vida and Bello Amanecer. Experienced SEPA leaders from two barrios in Managua also came to Nueva Vida on five occasions to assist doña Guillermina with her work. I analyzed SEPA's integration with Ciudad Sandino's MINSA health center and its activities, rather than the overall success of the project, and make no claims about its epidemiological effectiveness. CIET has only recently begun assembling its assessments of SEPA's effect on greater Managua's dengue incidence (some results are available at CIET's Camino Verde website, caminoverde.ciet.org, accessed December 15, 2013).

23. Donahue (1986) and Higgins and Coen (1992).

24. Dengue programs are one of several kinds of intervention that inform COMBI (WHO 2012).

25. CIET (2006: 3); see also Elder and Lloyd (2006: 7).

26. Elder and Lloyd (2006: 7–8).

27. WHO (2012: 27).

28. WHO (2012: 4).

29. CIET (2006: 3–4).

30. WHO (2012: 62–63); see also Parks and Lloyd (2004).

31. In Cuba, Brotherton (2012: 130) heard similar kinds of complaints from citizens. In that case, doctors depicted the sanitation of streets as the responsibility of citizen groups akin to the CPC, not of the health ministry.

32. In my 2009 survey, 55 percent of respondents said that the primary breeding ground for mosquitoes (not just dengue mosquitoes) in their community was accumulated water in the streets (*charcos*) (cf. Whiteford 1997).

33. In Nicaragua, COMBI was adapted to become ECACS (Estrategia de Communicación y Accion Comunitaria Para La Salud, or Strategy for Communication and Community Action for Health). Campos et al. (2003) elaborated the dengue-specific version of this strategy.

34. Brotherton (2012) and Whiteford (2000).

35. Their suspicion that community work suffered from a lack of rigorous measurement speaks to what Linda Whiteford and Lenore Manderson (2000) have called the "fallacy of the level playing field," in which poor and marginalized communities lack health because they have not been properly understood by expert practitioners of biomedicine and public health. On the level playing field, the tools of quantitative public health and biomedicine are imagined to enter communities neutrally, filling in "gaps" or "lacks" to create improved conditions.

36. As Margaret Lock and Vinh-Kim Nguyen argue, "The assumption of a standardizable body permits specific material, political, and economic conditions at local sites, and the local biologies that result, to be effectively circumvented, with enormous moral and practical consequences" (2010: 13). This is the logic of modern dengue prevention work. It is based on the idea that viruses can be contained if enough *human* bodies are rendered responsible through surveillance and behavior modification. There is no illusion that mosquitoes or viruses will disappear; rather, there is an assumption that regulation of human activity will render pests and pathogens irrelevant.

37. CIET, Camino Verde, caminoverde.ciet.org, accessed December 15, 2013.

38. Briggs (2003: 6–7) and Brotherton (2012: 131).

39. The project of dengue control was one in which, as Hugh Raffles puts it in his discussion of the creation of experimental forests, "the softness of biological contours becomes bludgeoned into integers" (2002: 169–72; see also Nadasdy 2003).

40. Ingold (2011: 154).

41. Ingold (2011: 154).

42. Anecdotally, epidemiologists agree that when people have experienced dengue fever, either as patients or as caregivers, they become more willing to take action against it. While the trauma of fever is instructive on an individual level, individual

experiences often are difficult to translate into population-wide preventative action. Epidemiologists call this the "prevention paradox." Individuals who are experiencing trauma—or who accept that they are at "high risk" for exposure—are easy to motivate because the benefits of action are clear. When epidemiologists try to organize entire populations to *prevent* trauma, the payoff for individuals is low (Hunt and Emslie 2001). Negotiating the relationship between populations and individuals lies at the heart of both epidemiology and biopolitics (Hacking 1991; Rose and Novas 2005).

43. As part of the recycling economy I described in chapter 2, some people in Ciudad Sandino melted and reshaped aluminum and other metals into pots, pans, and other items for door-to-door sale (see Nading 2011).

44. Public health required not just the identification of outbreaks but the motivation of nonexpert publics to combat those outbreaks. Doing both, as MINSA's underresourced state epidemiologists realized, requires not only answering the general question, "How and why did this happen?" but also the specific question, "How and why did this happen *here?*" (Davison, Smith, and Frankel 1991, quoted in Hunt and Emslie 2001: 442).

45. Brotherton (2012: 129–30).

46. Castree and Braun (2001).

47. Hecht (2010: 214).

CHAPTER SIX

1. Good (2001: 395).

2. Biehl (2005), Good (1994), Kleinman (1988), Lindenbaum and Lock (1993), and Mol (2002).

3. Taussig (1980).

4. Frankenberg (1988) and Lock and Scheper-Hughes (1987).

5. Adams, Murphy, and Clarke (2009), Lakoff (2008), and Lakoff and Collier (2008).

6. Good (2001) and Lock (1993).

7. See, for example, Koch (2013) and Nguyen (2010).

8. Miyazaki (2003: 256). My thanks to Kath Weston for making the connection between Miyazaki's arguments and my own.

9. See, for example, Castree and Braun (2001) and Robbins (2012).

10. See Bender (2002) and Raffles (2002).

11. *El Nuevo Diario,* October 10, 2009.

12. Perez et al. (2010).

13. Perez et al. (2010).

14. *El Nuevo Diario,* October 10, 2009.

15. Good (1994).

16. Kuan et al. (2009).

17. Around 2009, the Pediatric Dengue Vaccine Initiative shortened its name to the Dengue Vaccine Initiative.

18. Ingold (2000: 68).

19. See Bender (2002), Gell (1992), Hodges (2008), and Munn (1992).

20. Oliver-Smith (1996).

21. James (2004: 127).

22. Fassin (2005).

23. Broad and Orlove (2007) and Tsing (2005).

24. While it would be too much to say that these seasonal emergencies were "ritualistic," they were reliably transformational, they did both reaffirm and slightly remake important structuring elements of people's lives, and they certainly were dramatic (Turner 1966; Turner and Bruner 1986). They also arose along with clear ecological changes (Rappaport 1984 [1968]).

25. Confalonieri et al. (2007) and Patz et al. (2005).

26. Murphy (2006), Nash (2006), Nguyen (2010), and Petryna (2004).

27. Raffles (2002: 260n12).

28. Berlant (2002: 288).

29. For more on the moral valences of these kinds of events, see Han (2012). As it becomes tied to particular capital-driven technoscientific projects, global health itself is constructing a new kind of temporality. It both references a distant future—one of universal health—and relies upon an increasingly standardized attentiveness to what Jane Guyer (2007) calls date-events, recurring moments that act as sociopolitical inflection points. In global health, such moments include home health visits, audits, and drug expiration dates, as well as schedules surrounding clinical field trials.

30. Bourdieu (1977) and Ingold (2000).

31. Conscious of the human tragedy of a young girl's death, I nevertheless am struck by the way in which this unruly clash of pathogens and diagnoses, a variant of what medical anthropologist Merrill Singer (2009) calls a "syndemic," rendered bodies both vulnerable and partial. Unruly pandemic entanglements like this are something of a nightmare scenario for global health, yet they are also instructive for understanding the relationship between a seemingly unassailable "health" and an increasingly politicized "life." Throughout this book, I have been concerned with the ways in which human-nonhuman entanglement in the context of disease troubles the theoretical notion of biopolitics: the idea that governance of populations has become coterminous with the management of "life itself." As Fassin (2009) has argued in a reevaluation of the concept, biopolitics is not only about the technologies that regulate and discipline populations but also about the meanings and values societies attach to different forms of life. I want to further suggest, following Stefan Helmreich (2009) and Celia Lowe (2010), that the multiple "forms of life" arranged in biopolitical practice come about in part through our interactions with multiple "life forms" (mosquitoes, pigs, birds) and quasi-life forms (RNA viruses).

32. Morris (2010: 95) and Kate O'Neill (2010).

33. Redfield (2013). The making of "biological" or "medical" citizens depends upon a recognition of the body and the broader vitality, or "life," it represents as a

vulnerable but knowable entity—one that is the *external* object of both political and technical action. Anthropologists have recently turned their attention to the ways in which health has become a locus for the negotiation of the rights and responsibilities of individuals against those of the state. The term *medical citizenship* refers to politically charged negotiations over "who is excluded or sacrificed" when health "resources are . . . restricted" (Nichter 2008: 183).

34. Even in Ciudad Sandino's hospital, where staff had familiar and friendly relationships, doctors were called *doctor* or *doctora,* and licenciados were addressed with their title. Depending on the context, lower-level workers went by their first names or, in the case of formal conversations or with older workers, with their first names preceded by the honorific *don* (male) or *doña* (female). I have followed the "licenciado/a" convention here, mainly because I never called Lic. Lewites by her first name. Lic. Lewites had been a nurse in Ciudad Sandino since the days of OPEN III.

35. Nicaragua places one epidemiologist in each of its health centers.

36. This reflects WHO best practices (WHO 2009: 73).

37. Rappaport (1984 [1968]).

38. See www.denguewatch.org and www.healthmap.org.

39. Well before the article about Maria's death, health workers, nurses, and doctors I knew had begun to suspect that dengue and H1N1 might be causing serious clinical complications. (This made sense, since they already knew that dengue patients who had other illnesses would be more likely to deteriorate.) After the dengue and H1N1 coepidemics subsided, the research group associated with the Sustainable Sciences Institute and Socrates Flores published some of the first studies of dengue/H1N1 coinfection. In one study, three out of four patients had some other underlying predisposition to severe dengue or influenza, including asthma and obesity, conditions that likely were related to poor housing and poor nutrition (Perez et al. 2010). Maria, who was not a subject of that study since she was not part of the pediatric cohort, was an example of this. This study is revelatory because it uses a globally standard technology to call attention to a multiplicity of local problems.

40. Quesada (1998).

41. At worst, as Marianna hinted, emergency declarations were clever ways for hospital administrators to embezzle money. I decided that it would neither be wise nor particularly informative for me to find out whether or not this was true. Suspicions like these grew quite strong during 2008. When Ciudad Sandino's hospital director fired a human resources employee at the hospital, it was rumored that the employee planned to report him for misusing "emergency" funds. The health workers' union placed a public denuncia of the firing and the director on the wall of the general consulting building of the hospital. Among the complaints in the denuncia, two caught my eye. One was a reference to the continued rise in dengue cases, despite the various emergencies. The other was that the hospital had failed to meet its vaccination goals that year, despite the "emergency" mobilization of the staff toward that effort.

42. Robbins (2000).

43. WHO (2009).

44. Briggs (2003: 255–57) examines how the stable transmission of epidemiological data in this way, from the very local to the most "global" health centers, relies upon the stability of many other kinds of categories, including diagnostic ones. Standards for clinical diagnosis of dengue have recently been reexamined, with a view to making this kind of travel more seamless.

45. Brosius (1999) identifies the interplay of the technical and the emotional as the centerpiece of political ecologies. The emotional tends to be crowded out by the technical, especially in environmental debates.

46. McKay (2012) and Wendland (2010).

47. Mitchell (2002: 43).

48. Barad (2006), Ingold (2000), and Raffles (2002).

49. Broad and Orlove (2007).

50. Lakoff (2010).

51. Bender (2002) and Ingold (2000).

CONCLUSION

1. Mitman, Murphy, and Sellers (2004: 186).

2. Ingold (2000: 68).

3. Lakoff (2008).

4. For more on apolitical ecology, see Robbins (2007: 4), from which I draw the framework of rationality, culture, and sovereignty here.

5. Here, I am following Margaret Lock herself (see Lock 2013).

6. Helmreich (2009).

7. Ali and Keil (2008), King (2002, 2004), and Lakoff and Collier (2008).

8. Lock and Nguyen (2010).

9. Bateson (1979).

10. Geertz (1973).

11. Harding (2008: 25).

12. Harding (2008: 26).

13. Jasanoff (2004: 25–26).

14. Haraway (1989).

BIBLIOGRAPHY

Ackerman, Frank, and Sumreen Mirza. 2001. "Waste in the Inner City: Asset or Assault?" *Local Environment* 6 (2): 113–20.

Adams, Ben, and Durrell Kapan. 2009. "Man Bites Mosquito: Understanding the Contribution of Human Movement to Vector-Borne Disease Dynamics." *PLoS One* 4 (8): e6763.

Adams, Vincanne. 2010. "Against Global Health: Arbitrating Science, Non-science, and Nonsense through Health." In *Against Health: How Health Became the New Morality*. Jonathan Metzl and Anna Kirkland, eds. Pp. 40–60. New York: NYU Press.

Adams, Vincanne, Michelle Murphy, and Adele Clarke. 2009. "Anticipation: Technoscience, Life, Affect, Temporality." *Subjectivity* 28 (1): 246–65.

Agamben, Giorgio. 1998. *Homo sacer: Sovereign Power and Bare Life*. Palo Alto, CA: Stanford University Press.

Agrawal, Arun. 2001. "Common Property Institutions and Sustainable Governance of Resources." *World Development* 29: 1649–72.

Agrawal, Arun. 2005. "Environmentality: Community, Intimate Government, and the Making of Subjects in Kumaon, India." *Current Anthropology* 46 (2): 161–90.

Ali, S. Harris, and Roger Keil, eds. 2008. *Networked Disease: Emerging Disease in the Global City*. Malden, MA: Wiley-Blackwell.

Alley, Christopher. 2010. "Trash Becomes Them: Cross-Sectoral Dengue Fever Prevention and the Legitimization of Waste Pickers in Brazil's Informal Economy." Paper presented at the American Anthropological Association Annual Meeting, New Orleans, LA, November 17.

Allison, Maria. 2002. "Balancing Responsibility for Sanitation." *Social Science and Medicine* 55 (9): 1539–51.

Anand, Nikhil. 2011. "Pressure: The Politechnics of Water Supply in Mumbai." *Cultural Anthropology* 26 (4): 542–64.

Andaya, Elise. 2009. "The Gift of Health: Socialist Medical Practice and Shifting Material and Moral Economies in Post-socialist Cuba." *Medical Anthropology Quarterly* 23 (4): 357–74.

Anderson, Warwick. 1995. "Excremental Colonialism: Public Health and the Poetics of Pollution." *Critical Inquiry* 21 (3): 640–69.

Anderson, Warwick. 2004. "Natural Histories of Infectious Diseases: Ecological Vision in Twentieth-Century Biomedical Science." *Osiris* 19: 39–61.

Anderson, Warwick. 2006. *Colonial Pathologies: American Tropical Medicine, Race, and Hygiene in the Philippines*. Durham, NC: Duke University Press.

Appadurai, Arjun, ed. 1988. *The Social Life of Things: Commodities in Cultural Perspective*. Cambridge: Cambridge University Press.

Appel, Hannah C. 2012. "Walls and White Elephants: Oil Extraction, Responsibility, and Infrastructural Violence in Equatorial Guinea." *Ethnography* 13 (4): 439–65.

Arguello, D. Fermin. 2009. "Dengue Virus on the Move." Paper presented at the American Society for Microbiology Annual Meeting, Philadelphia, PA, May 21.

Ashencaen-Crabtree, Sara, Christina Wong, and Faiza Mas'ud. 2001. "Community Participatory Approaches to Dengue in Sarawak, Malaysia." *Human Organization* 60 (3): 201–8.

Babb, Florence. 2001. *After Revolution: Mapping Gender and Cultural Politics in Neoliberal Nicaragua*. Austin: University of Texas Press.

Babb, Florence. 2004. "Recycled Sandalistas: From Revolution to Resorts in the New Nicaragua." *American Anthropologist* 106 (3): 541–55.

Barad, Karen. 2003. "Posthumanist Performativity: Toward an Understanding of How Matter Comes to Matter." *Signs: Journal of Women in Culture and Society* 28 (3): 801–31.

Barad, Karen. 2007. *Meeting the Universe Halfway: Physics and the Entanglement of Matter and Meaning*. Durham, NC: Duke University Press.

Barreto, Pablo Emilio. 2001. *Ciudad Sandino: 31 Años*. Managua: IMISA, Alcaldía de Ciudad Sandino, Movimientos Comunales de Nicaragua.

Basso, Keith. 1996. *Wisdom Sits in Places: Landscape and Language among the Western Apache*. Albequerque: University of New Mexico Press.

Bateson, Gregory. 1979. *Mind and Nature: A Necessary Unity*. New York: E. P. Dutton.

Bateson, Gregory. 2000 [1972]. *Steps to an Ecology of Mind*. Chicago: University of Chicago Press.

Beck, Ulrich. 1992. *Risk Society: Towards A New Modernity*. London: Sage.

Beisel, Uli. 2010. "Jumping Hurdles with Mosquitoes." *Environment and Planning D* 28 (1): 46–49.

Belli, Gioconda. 2002. *The Country under My Skin: A Memoir of Love and War*. New York: Anchor Books.

Bender, Barbara. 2002. "Time and Landscape." *Current Anthropology* 43 (suppl. 4): S103–12.

Berlant, Lauren. 2002. "Intimacy: A Special Issue." *Critical Inquiry* 24 (2): 281–88.

Besky, Sarah. 2013. *The Darjeeling Distinction: Labor and Justice on Fair-Trade Tea Plantations in India*. Berkeley: University of California Press.

Biehl, Joao. 2005. *Vita: Life in a Zone of Social Abandonment*. Berkeley: University of California Press.

Biehler, Dawn. 2007. *In the Crevices of the City: Public Health, Urban Housing, and the Creatures We Call Pests, 1900–2000.* Ph.D. dissertation, Department of Geography, University of Wisconsin–Madison.

Birn, Anne-Emanuelle, Sarah Zimmerman, and Richard Garfield. 2000. "To Decentralize or Not to Decentralize, Is That the Question? Nicaraguan Health Policy under Structural Adjustment in the 1990s." *International Journal of Health Services* 30 (1): 111–28.

Biruk, Crystal. 2012. "Seeing Like a Research Project: Producing 'High-Quality Data' in AIDS Research in Malawi." *Medical Anthropology* 31 (4): 347–66.

Bourdieu, Pierre. 1977. *Outline of a Theory of Practice.* Cambridge: Cambridge University Press.

Bourdieu, Pierre. 1986. "The Forms of Capital," trans. Richard Nice. In *Handbook of Theory of Research for the Sociology of Education.* John Richardson, ed. Pp. 241–58. New York: Greenwood Press.

Bourgois, Philippe. 2002. *In Search of Respect: Selling Crack in El Barrio.* Cambridge: Cambridge University Press.

Bowker, Geoffrey, and Susan Leigh Star. 1999. *Sorting Things Out: Classification and Its Consequences.* Cambridge, MA: MIT Press.

Brada, Betsey. 2011. " 'Not Here': Making the Spaces and Subjects of Global Health in Botswana." *Culture, Medicine and Psychiatry* 35 (2): 285–312.

Briggs, Charles. 2003. *Stories in the Time of Cholera: Racial Profiling during a Medical Nightmare.* With Clara Mantini-Briggs. Berkeley: University of California Press.

Broad, Kenneth, and Benjamin Orlove. 2007. "Channeling Globality: The 1997–98 El Niño Climate Event in Peru." *American Ethnologist* 34 (2): 285–302.

Brosius, J. Peter. 1999. "Green Dots, Pink Hearts: Displacing Politics from the Malaysian Rainforest." *American Anthropologist* 101 (1): 36–57.

Brotherton, P. Sean. 2012. *Revolutionary Medicine: Health and the Body in Post-Soviet Cuba.* Durham, NC: Duke University Press.

Brown, Peter. 1997. "Culture and the Global Resurgence of Malaria." In *The Anthropology of Infectious Disease: International Health Perspectives.* Marcia Inhorn and Peter Brown, eds. Pp. 119–40. New York: Routledge.

Brunkard, Joan Marie, Jose Luis Robles Lopez, Josue Ramirez, Enrique Cifuentes, Stephen Rothenberg, Elizabeth Hunsperger, Chester Moore, Regina Brussolo, Norma Villareal, and Brent Haddad. 2007. "Dengue Fever Seroprevalence and Risk Factors, Texas-Mexico Border." *Emerging Infectious Diseases* 13 (10): 1477–83.

Buhs, Joshua. 2002. "The Fire Ant Wars: Nature and Science in the Pesticide Controversies of the Late Twentieth Century." *Isis* 93 (3): 377–400.

Caldeira, Theresa. 2001. *City of Walls: Crime, Segregation and Citizenship in São Paolo.* Berkeley: University of California Press.

Campos, Luisa Amanda, Veronica Chammorro, Emperatriz Lugo, Byron Acevedo, and Alejandro Uriza. 2003. *Estrategia de Comunicacion Social para Cambios de Conducta sobre Dengue: Nicaragua.* Managua: Pan American Health Organization.

Candea, Matei. 2010. "'I Fell in Love with Carlos the Meerkat': Engagement and Detachment in Human-Animal Relations." *American Ethnologist* 37 (2): 241–58.

Carse, Ashley. 2012. "Nature as Infrastructure: Making and Managing the Panama Canal Watershed." *Social Studies of Science* 42 (4): 539–63.

Carson, Rachel. 1962. *Silent Spring.* New York: Houghton Mifflin.

Carter, Eric. 2007. "Development Narratives and the Uses of Ecology: Malaria Control in Northwest Argentina: 1890–1940." *Journal of Historical Geography* 33 (3): 619–50.

Carter, Eric. 2008. "State Visions, Landscape, and Disease: Discovering Malaria in Argentina, 1890–1920." *Geoforum* 39 (1): 278–93.

Carter, Eric. 2012. *Enemy in the Blood: Malaria, Environment, and Development in Argentina.* Tuscaloosa: University of Alabama Press.

Carter, Eric. 2014. "Malaria Control in the Tennessee Valley Authority: Health, Ecology, and Metanarratives of Development." *Journal of Historical Geography* 4: 111–27.

Castree, Noel, and Bruce Braun. 2001. *Social Nature: Theory, Practice, and Politics.* Malden, MA: Wiley-Blackwell.

Castro, Arrachu, Yasmin Khawja, and James Johnston. 2010. "Social Inequalities and Dengue Transmission in Latin America." In *Plagues and Epidemics: Infected Spaces Past and Present.* Ann Herring and Alan Swedlund, eds. Pp. 231–49. New York: Berg.

Centers for Disease Control and Prevention (CDC). 2014. "Our Story." www.cdc.gov/about/history/ourstory.htm. Accessed April 9, 2014.

Choy, Timothy, Lieba Faier, Michael Hathaway, Miyako Inoue, Shiho Satsuka, and Anna Tsing. 2009. "A New Form of Collaboration in Cultural Anthropology: Matsutake Worlds." *American Ethnologist* 36 (2): 380–403.

Chwatt, Leonard. 1977. "Ronald Ross, William Gorgas, and Malaria Eradication." *American Journal of Tropical Medicine and Hygiene* 26 (2): 1071–79.

Community Information and Epidemiological Technologies International (CIET). 2006. "The SEPA Model: CIET's Approach to Communication. Executive Report 2006." www.ciet.org/_documents/SEPA%20Exec%200306.pdf. Accessed December 15, 2013.

Confalonieri, U., B. Menne, R. Akhtar, K. L. Ebi, M. Hauengue, R. S. Kovats, B. Revich, and A. Woodward, 2007. "Human Health." In *Climate Change 2007: Impacts, Adaptation and Vulnerability. Contribution of Working Group II to the Fourth Assessment Report of the Intergovernmental Panel on Climate Change.* M. L. Parry, O. F. Canziani, J. P. Palutikof, P. J. van der Linden, and C. E. Hanson, eds. Pp. 391–431. Cambridge: Cambridge University Press.

Crane, Johanna. 2013. *Scrambling for Africa: AIDS, Expertise, and the Rise of American Global Health Science.* Ithaca, NY: Cornell University Press.

Cronon, William. 1990. *Nature's Metropolis: Chicago and the Great West.* New York: W. W. Norton.

Cueto, Marcos. 2007. *The Value of Health: A History of the Pan American Health Organization.* Rochester, NY: University of Rochester Press.

Davis, Mike. 2006. *Planet of Slums*. London: Verso.

Deleuze, Gilles, and Felix Guattari. 1987. *A Thousand Plateaus: Capitalism and Schizophrenia*. Minneapolis: University of Minnesota Press.

Dick, Olivia, José San Martin, Romeo Montoya, Jorge del Diego, Betzana Zambrano, and Gustavo Dayan. 2012. "Review: The History of Dengue Outbreaks in the Americas." *American Journal of Tropical Medicine and Hygiene* 87 (4): 584–93.

Donahue, John. 1986. *The Nicaraguan Revolution in Health: From Somoza to the Sandinistas*. South Hadley, MA: Bergin and Garvey.

Dore, Elizabeth. 2006. *Myths of Modernity: Peonage and Patriarchy in Nicaragua*. Durham, NC: Duke University Press.

Douglas, Mary. 2002 [1966]. *Purity and Danger: An Analysis of Concepts of Pollution and Taboo*. London: Routledge.

Elder, Peter, and Linda Lloyd. 2006. "Achieving Behaviour Change for Dengue Control: Methods, Scaling Up and Sustainability." Working paper for the Scientific Working Group on Dengue Research, convened by the Special Programme for Research and Training in Tropical Diseases, Geneva, October 1–5.

Endy, Timothy, Scott Weaver, and Kathryn Hanley. 2010. "Dengue Virus: Past, Present and Future." In *Frontiers in Dengue Virus Research*. Kathryn Hanley and Scott Weaver, eds. Pp. 3–12. Norfolk, UK: Caister Academic Press.

Escobar, Arturo. 1995. *Encountering Development: The Making and Unmaking of the Third World*. Princeton, NJ: Princeton University Press.

Escobar, Arturo. 1999. "After Nature: Steps to an Anti-essentialist Political Ecology." *Current Anthropology* 40 (1): 1–30.

Escobar, Arturo. 2008. *Territories of Difference: Place, Movements, Life*, Redes. Durham, NC: Duke University Press.

Escobar, Cristina. 2002. "Clientelism and Citizenship: The Limits of Democratic Reform in Sucre, Colombia." *Latin American Perspectives* 29 (5): 20–47.

Ewig, Christina. 1999. "The Strengths and Limits of the NGO Women's Movement Model: Shaping Nicaragua's Democratic Institutions." *Latin American Research Review* 34 (3): 75–102.

Farmer, Paul. 1992. *AIDS and Accusation: Haiti and the Geography of Blame*. Berkeley: University of California Press.

Farmer, Paul. 1999. *Infections and Inequalities: The Modern Plagues*. Berkeley: University of California Press.

Fassin, Didier. 2004. "Public Health as Culture: The Social Construction of the Childhood Lead Poisoning Epidemic in France." *British Medical Bulletin* 69 (1): 167–77.

Fassin, Didier. 2005. "Compassion and Repression: The Moral Economy of Immigration Policies in France." *Cultural Anthropology* 20 (3): 362–87.

Fassin, Didier. 2009. "Another Politics of Life Is Possible." *Theory, Culture and Society* 26 (5): 44–60.

Feeny, David, Fikret Berkes, Bonnie McCay, and James Acheson. 1990. "The Tragedy of the Commons: Twenty-Two Years Later." *Human Ecology* 18 (1): 1–19.

Feld, Stephen, and Keith Basso, eds. 1996. *Senses of Place*. Santa Fe, NM: School for Advanced Research Press.

Ferguson, Harry. 2008. "Liquid Social Work: Welfare Interventions as Mobile Practices." *British Journal of Social Work* 38 (3): 561–79.

Ferguson, James. 1994. *The Anti-politics Machine: Development, Depoliticiztion, and Bureaucratic Power in Lesotho*. Minneapolis: University of Minnesota Press.

Fisher, Joshua. 2013. "Fair or Balanced? The Other Side of Fair Trade in a Nicaraguan Sewing Cooperative." *Anthropological Quarterly* 86 (2): 527–57.

Forsyth, Timothy. 2003. *Critical Political Ecology: the Politics of Environmental Science*. New York: Routledge.

Foucault, Michel. 1984. *The Foucault Reader*. Paul Rabinow, ed. New York: Pantheon.

Foucault, Michel. 1990. *The History of Sexuality: An Introduction*. New York: Vintage.

Foucault, Michel. 1997. *Ethics: Subjectivity and Truth*. Paul Rabinow, ed. Robert Hurley et al., trans. New York: New Press.

Foucault, Michel. 2008. *The Birth of Biopolitics: Lectures at the College de France 1978–1979*. Graham Burchell, trans. New York: Palgrave McMillan.

Foucault, Michel. 2009. *Security, Territory, Population: Lectures at the College de France*. New York: Palgrave Macmillan.

Fox, Jonathan. 1994. "The Difficult Transition from Clientelism to Citizenship: Lessons from Mexico." *World Politics* 46 (2): 151–84.

Frankenberg, Ronald. 1988. "Your Time or Mine? An Anthropological View of the Tragic Temporal Contradictions of Biomedical Practice." *International Journal of Health Services* 18 (1): 11–34.

Franklin, Sarah. 2007. *Dolly Mixtures: The Remaking of Geneaology*. Durham, NC: Duke University Press.

Freccero, Carla. 2011. "Carnivorous Virility; or, Becoming-Dog." *Social Text* 29 (1): 177–95.

Freeman, James. 2010. "From the Little Tree, Half a Block toward the Lake: Popular Geography and Symbolic Discontent in Post-Sandinista Nicaragua." *Antipode* 42 (2): 336–73.

Freire, Paolo. 2000. *Pedagogy of the Oppressed*. 30th ed. Myra Bergman Ramos, trans. New York: Continuum.

Gal, Susan. 2002. "A Semiotics of the Public/Private Distinction." *Differences* 13 (1): 77–95.

Gandy, Matthew. 2005. "Cyborg Urbanization: Complexity and Monstrosity in the Contemporary City." *International Journal of Urban and Regional Research* 29 (1): 26–49.

Gaonkar, Dilip, and Elizabeth Povinelli. 2003. "Technologies of Public Forms: Circulation, Transfiguration, Recognition." *Public Culture* 15 (3): 385–97.

Garcia, Angela. 2010. *The Pastoral Clinic: Addiction and Dispossession along the Rio Grande*. Berkeley: University of California Press.

Garfield, Richard, and Glen Williams. 1992. *Health Care in Nicaragua: Primary Care under Changing Regimes.* New York: Oxford University Press.

Geertz, Clifford. 1973. *The Interpretation of Cultures.* New York: Basic Books.

Gell, Alfred. 1992. *The Anthropology of Time: Cultural Constructions of Temporal Maps and Images.* Oxford: Berg.

Ghertner, Asher. 2010. "Calculating without Numbers: Aesthetic Governmentality in Delhi's Slums." *Economy and Society* 39 (2): 185–217.

Gladwell, Malcom. 2002. "Fred Soper and the Global Malaria Eradication Programme." *Journal of Public Health Policy* 23 (4): 479–97.

Gobat, Michael. 2005. *Confronting the American Dream: Nicaragua under U.S. Imperial Rule.* Durham, NC: Duke University Press.

Goldman, Mara, Paul Nadasdy, and Matthew Turner, eds. 2011. *Knowing Nature: Conversations at the Intersection of Political Ecology and Science Studies.* Chicago: University of Chicago Press.

Goldstein, Daniel. 2004. *The Spectacular City: Violence and Performance in Urban Bolivia.* Durham, NC: Duke University Press.

Goldstein, Donna. 2003. *Laughter Out of Place: Race, Class, Violence, and Sexuality in a Rio Shantytown.* Berkeley: University of California Press.

Good, Byron. 1994. *Medicine, Rationality, and Experience: An Anthropological Perspective.* Cambridge: Cambridge University Press.

Good, Mary-Jo DelVecchio. 2001. "The Biotechnical Embrace." *Culture, Medicine, and Psychiatry* 25 (4): 395–410.

Grosz, Elizabeth. 1995. *Space, Time and Perversion: Essays on the Politics of Bodies.* New York: Routledge.

Gubler, Duane. 1989. "*Aedes aegypti* and *Aedes aegypti*-Borne Disease Control in the 1990s: Top-Down or Bottom Up?" *American Journal of Tropical Medicine and Hygiene* 40 (6): 571–78.

Gubler, Duane. 1997. "Dengue and Dengue Hemorrhagic Fever: Its History and Resurgence as a Global Public Health Problem." In *Dengue and Dengue Hemorrhagic Fever.* Duane Gubler and Goro Kuno, eds. Pp. 1–23. New York: CAB International.

Gubler, Duane. 2002. "Epidemic Dengue/Dengue Hemorrhagic Fever as a Public Health, Social and Economic Problem in the 21st Century." *Trends in Microbiology* 10 (2): 100–103.

Gubler, Duane, and Gary Clark. 1996. "Community Involvement in the Control of *Aedes aegypti*." *Acta Tropica* 61 (2): 169–79.

Gubler, Duane, and Goro Kuno. 1997. *Dengue and Dengue Hemorrhagic Fever.* New York: CAB International.

Guyer, Jane. 2007. "Prophecy and the Near Future: Thoughts on Macroeconomic, Evangelical, and Punctuated Time." *American Ethnologist* 34 (3): 409–21.

Guzman, Maria. 2005. "Deciphering Dengue: The Cuban Experience." *Science* 309 (5740): 1495–97.

Guzman, Maria, Scott Halstead, Harvey Artsob, Phillipe Buchy, Jeremy Farrar, Duane Gubler, Elizabeth Hunsperger, Axel Kroeger, Harold Margolis, Eric

Martinez, Michael Nathan, Jose Luis Pellegrino, Cameron Simmons, Suttee Yoksan, and Rosanna Peeling. 2010. "Dengue: A Continuing Global Threat." *Nature Reviews Microbiology* 8 (12 suppl.): S7–16.

Hacking, Ian. 1991. "How Should We Do the History of Statistics?" In *The Foucault Effect: Studies in Governmentality*. Graham Burchell, Colin Gordon, and Peter Miller, eds. Pp. 181–97. Chicago: University of Chicago Press.

Hale, James, Corrine Knapp, Lisa Bardwell, Michael Buchenau, Julie Marshall, Fahriye Sancar, and Jill Litt. 2011. "Connecting Food Environments and Health through the Relational Nature of Aesthetics: Gaining Insight through the Community Gardening Experience." *Social Science and Medicine* 72 (11): 1853–63.

Halstead, Scott. 2003. "Neutralization and Antibody Dependent Enhancement of Dengue Viruses." *Advances in Virus Research* 60: 421–67.

Halstead, Scott, Suntharee Rojanasuphot, and Nadhirat Sangkawibha. 1983. "Original Antigenic Sin in Dengue." *American Journal of Tropical Medicine and Hygiene* 32 (1): 154–56.

Hammond, Samantha, Angel Balmaseda, Leonel Perez, Yolanda Tellez, Saira Indira Saborío, Juan Carlos Mercado, Elsa Videa, Yoryelin Rodriguez, Maria Angeles Perez, Ricardo Cuadra, Sorayon Solano, Julio Rocha, Wendy Idiaquez, Alcides Gonzales, and Eva Harris. 2005. "Differences in Dengue Severity in Infants, Children, and Adults in a 3-Year Hospital-Based Study in Nicaragua." *American Journal of Tropical Medicine and Hygiene* 73 (6): 1063–70.

Han, Clara. 2012. *Life in Debt: Times of Care and Violence in Neoliberal Chile.* Berkeley: University of California Press.

Haraway, Donna. 1988. "Situated Knowledges: The Science Question in Feminism and the Privilege of Partial Perspective." *Feminist Studies* 14 (3): 575–99.

Haraway, Donna. 1989. "The Biopolitics of Postmodern Bodies: Determinations of Self in Immune System Discourse." *Differences* 1 (1): 3–43.

Haraway, Donna. 2008. *When Species Meet.* Minneapolis: University of Minnesota Press.

Hardin, Garrett. 1968. "The Tragedy of the Commons." *Science* 162 (3859): 1243–48.

Harding, Sandra. 2008. *Sciences from Below: Feminisms, Postcolonialities, Modernities.* Durham, NC: Duke University Press.

Harries-Jones, Peter. 1995. *A Recursive Vision: Ecological Understanding and Gregory Bateson.* Toronto: University of Toronto Press.

Harris, Eva. 1998. *A Low-Cost Approach to PCR: Appropriate Transfer of Biomolecular Techniques.* New York: Oxford University Press.

Harris, Olivia. 1984. "Households as Natural Units." In *Of Marriage and the Market.* 2nd ed. Kate Young, Carol Wolkowitz, and Rosalyn McCullagh, eds. Pp. 136–55. London: Routledge.

Harvey, David. 1996. *Justice, Nature, and the Geography of Difference.* Oxford: Blackwell.

Hecht, Gabrielle. 2010. "Hopes for the Radiated Body: Uranium Miners and Transnational Technopolitics in Namibia." *Journal of African History* 51 (2): 1–22.

Heintze, Carl, M. V. Garrido, and A. Kroeger. 2007. "What Do Community-Based Dengue Control Programmes Achieve? A Systematic Review of Published Evaluations." *Transactions of the Royal Society of Tropical Medicine and Hygiene* 101 (4): 317–25.

Helmreich, Stefan. 2009. *Alien Ocean: Anthropological Voyages in Microbial Seas.* Berkeley: University of California Press.

Helmreich, Stefan, and Kath Weston. 2006. "Kath Weston's *Gender in Real Time: Power and Transience in a Visual Age.*" *Body and Society* 12 (3): 103–21.

Heynen, Nik, Maria Kaika, and Erik Swyngedouw, eds. 2006. *In the Nature of Cities: Urban Political Ecology and the Politics of Urban Metabolism.* New York: Routledge.

Higgins, Michael and Tanya Coen. 1992. *Oigame Oigame! Struggle and Social Change in a Nicaraguan Urban Community.* Boulder, CO: Westview Press.

Hinchliffe, Steve, John Allen, Stephanie Lavau, Nick Bingham, and Simon Carter. 2013. "Biosecurity and the Topologies of Infected Life: From Borderlines to Borderlands." *Transactions of the Institute of British Geographers* 38 (4): 531–43.

Hinchliffe, Steve, and Sarah Whatmore. 2006. "Living Cities: Toward a Politics of Conviviality." *Science as Culture* 15 (2): 123–38.

Hodges, Matt. 2008. "Rethinking Time's Arrow: Bergson, Deleuze, and the Anthropology of Time." *Anthropological Theor* 8 (4): 399–429.

Holston, James. 2008. *Insurgent Citizenship: Disjunctions of Democracy and Modernity in Brazil.* Princeton, NJ: Princeton University Press.

Howe, Cymene. 2013. *Intimate Activism: The Struggle for Sexual Rights in Postrevolutionary Nicaragua.* Durham, NC: Duke University Press.

Hunt, Kate, and Carole Emslie. 2001. "Commentary: The Prevention Paradox in Lay Epidemiology–Rose Revisited." *International Journal of Epidemiology* 30 (3): 442.

Hutchinson, Sharon. 1996. *Nuer Dilemmas: Coping with Money, War, and the State.* Berkeley: University of California Press.

Ingold, Tim. 2000. *The Perception of the Environment: Essays in Livelihood, Dwelling, and Skill.* New York: Routledge.

Ingold, Tim. 2007. *Lines: A Brief History.* New York: Routledge.

Ingold, Tim. 2008. "Bindings against Boundaries: Entanglements of Life in an Open World." *Environment and Planning A* 40 (8): 1796–810.

Ingold, Tim. 2011. *Being Alive: Essays on Movement, Knowledge, and Description.* New York: Routledge.

James, Erica. 2004. "The Political Economy of 'Trauma' in Haiti in the Democratic Era of Insecurity." *Culture, Medicine, and Psychiatry* 28 (2): 127–49.

Jasanoff, Sheila. 2004. "Ordering Knowledge, Ordering Society." In *States of Knowledge: The Co-production of Science and Social Order.* Sheila Jasanoff, ed. Pp. 13–45. New York: Routledge.

Keck, Frédéric. 2008. "From Mad Cow Disease to Bird Flu: Transformations of Food Safety in France." In *Biosecurity Interventions: Global Health and Security in Question.* Andrew Lakoff and Stephen Collier, eds. Pp. 195–226. New York: Columbia University Press.

Kelly, Ann. 2012. "The Experimental Hut: Hosting Vectors." *Journal of the Royal Anthropological Institute* 18 (suppl. 1): S145–60.

Kelly, Ann, and Uli Beisel. 2011. "Neglected Malarias: The Front Lines and Back Alleys of Global Health." *BioSocieties* 6 (1): 71–87.

Kendall, Carl. 1998. "The Role of Formal Qualitative Research in Negotiating Community Acceptance: The Case of Dengue Control in El Progreso, Honduras." *Human Organization* 57 (2): 217–21.

Kendall, Carl, Patricia Hudelson, Elli Leontsini, Peter Winch, Linda Lloyd, and Fernando Cruz. 1991. "Urbanization, Dengue and the Health Transition: Anthropological Contributions to International Health." *Medical Anthropology Quarterly* 5 (3): 257–68.

King, Nicholas. 2002. "Security, Disease, Commerce: Ideologies of Post-colonial Global Health." *Social Studies of Science* 32 (5–6): 763–89.

King, Nicholas. 2004. "The Scale Politics of Emerging Diseases." *Osiris* 19: 62–76.

Kinkela, David. 2011. *DDT and the American Century: Global Health, Environmental Politics, and the Pesticide that Changed the World.* Chapel Hill, NC: University of North Carolina Press.

Kirksey, Eben, and Stefan Helmreich. 2010. "The Emergence of Multispecies Ethnography." *Cultural Anthropology* 25 (4): 545–76.

Kleinman, Arthur. 1988. *The Illness Narratives: Suffering, Healing, and the Human Condition.* New York: Basic Books.

Kleinman, Arthur, Veena Das, and Margaret Lock, eds. 1997. *Social Suffering.* Berkeley: University of California Press.

Koch, Erin. 2011. "Local Microbiologies of Tuberculosis: Insights from the Republic of Georgia." *Medical Anthropology* 30 (1): 81–101.

Koch, Erin. 2013. "Tuberculosis Is a Threshold: The Making of a Social Disease in Post-Soviet Georgia." *Medical Anthropology* 32 (4): 309–24.

Kohn, Eduardo. 2007. "How Dogs Dream: Amazonian Natures and the Politics of Transspecies Engagement." *American Ethnologist* 34 (1): 3–24.

Krieger, Nancy, ed. 2005. *Embodying Inequality: Epidemiologic Perspectives.* Amityville, MA: Baywood.

Krieger, Nancy, and George Davey-Smith. 2004. "'Bodies Count' and Body Counts: Social Epidemiology and Embodying Inequality." *Epidemiologic Reviews* 26 (1): 92–103.

Kuan, Guillermina, Aubree Gordon, William Aviles, Oscar Ortega, Samantha Hammond, Douglas Elizondo, Andrea Nunez, Josefina Coloma, Angel Balmaseda, and Eva Harris. 2009. "The Nicaraguan Pediatric Dengue Cohort Study: Study Design, Methods, Use of Information Technology, and Extension to Other Infectious Diseases." *American Journal of Epidemiology* 170 (1): 120–29.

Kuno, Goro, Duane Gubler, and Antony Oliver. 1993. "Use of 'Original Antigenic Sin' Theory to Determine the Serotypes of Previous Dengue Infections." *Transactions of the Royal Society of Tropical Medicine and Hygiene* 87 (1): 103–5.

Kyle, Jennifer, and Eva Harris. 2008. "Global Spread and Persistence of Dengue." *Annual Review of Microbiology* 62: 71–92.

Lakoff, Andrew. 2008. "The Generic Biothreat, or, How We Became Unprepared." *Cultural Anthropology* 23 (3): 399–428.

Lakoff, Andrew. 2010. "Two Regimes of Global Health." *Humanity* 1 (1): 59–79.

Lakoff, Andrew, and Stephen Collier. 2008. "The Problem of Securing Health." In *Biosecurity Interventions: Global Health and Security in Question.* Andrew Lakoff and Stephen Collier, eds. Pp. 7–33. New York: Columbia University Press.

Lancaster, Roger. 1988. *Thanks to God and the Revolution: Popular Religion and Class Consciousness in the New Nicaragua.* New York: Columbia University Press.

Lancaster, Roger. 1992. *Life Is Hard: Machismo, Danger, and the Intimacy of Power in Nicaragua.* Berkeley: University of California Press.

LaRamée, Pierre, and Erica Polakoff. 1997. "The Evolution of the Popular Organizations in Nicaragua." In *The Undermining of the Sandinista Revolution.* Gary Prevost and Harry Vanden, eds. Pp. 141–206. New York: St. Martin's Press.

Latour, Bruno. 2005. *Reassembling the Social: An Introduction to Actor-Network Theory.* New York: Oxford University Press.

Levins, Richard, and Richard Lewontin. 1985. *The Dialectical Biologist.* Cambridge: Harvard University Press.

Li, Tania. 2007. *The Will to Improve: Governmentality, Development, and the Practice of Politics.* Durham, NC: Duke University Press.

Lien, Marianne, and John Law. 2011. "'Emergent Aliens': On Salmon, Nature, and Their Enactment." *Ethnos* 76 (1): 65–87.

Lindenbaum, Shirley, and Margaret Lock. 1993. *Knowledge, Power, and Practice: The Anthropology of Medicine and Everyday Life.* Berkeley: University of California Press.

Litt, Jill, Mah-J Soobader, Mark Turbin, James Hale, Michael Buchenau, and Julie Marshall. 2011. "The Influence of Social Involvement, Neighborhood Aesthetics, and Community Garden Participation on Fruit and Vegetable Consumption." *American Journal of Public Health* 101 (8): 1466–73.

Livingston, Julie. 2005. *Debility and the Moral Imagination in Botswana.* Durham, NC: Duke University Press.

Lock, Margaret. 1993. *Encounters with Aging: Mythologies of Menopause in Japan and North America.* Berkeley: University of California Press.

Lock, Margaret. 2001. "The Tempering of Medical Anthropology: Troubling Natural Categories." *Medical Anthropology Quarterly* 15 (4): 478–92.

Lock, Margaret. 2013. "The Lure of the Epigenome." *The Lancet* 381 (9881): 1896–97.

Lock, Margaret, and Vinh-Kim Nguyen. 2010. *An Anthropology of Biomedicine.* Malden, MA: Wiley-Blackwell.

Lockwood, Jeffrey. 1999. "Agriculture and Biodiversity: Finding Our Place within This World." *Agriculture and Human Values* 16 (4): 365–79.

Lockwood, Jeffrey. 2002. *Grasshopper Dreaming: Reflections on Killing and Loving.* Boston: Skinner House.

Low, Setha. 1996. "Spatializing Culture: The Social Production and Social Construction of Public Space in Costa Rica." *American Ethnologist* 23 (4): 861–79.

Low, Setha. 2000. *On the Plaza: The Politics of Public Space and Culture.* Austin: University of Texas Press.

Lowe, Celia. 2006. *Wild Profusion: Biodiversity Conservation in an Indonesian Archipelago.* Princeton, NJ: Princeton University Press.

Lowe, Celia. 2010. "Viral Clouds: Becoming H5N1 in Indonesia." *Cultural Anthropology* 25 (4): 625–49.

Lowy, Ilana. 1997. "Epidemiology, Immunology, and Yellow Fever: The Rockefeller Foundation in Brazil, 1923–1939." *Journal of the History of Biology* 30 (3): 397–417.

Lugo, Emperatriz, Gilberto Moreno, Marcus Zacchariah, Maria Lopez, Josepha Lopez, Marco Delgado, Sonia Valle, Perla Espinosa, Mario Salgado, Roselo Perez, Samantha Hammond, and Eva Harris. 2005. "Identification of *Aedes albopictus* in Urban Nicaragua." *Journal of the American Mosquito Control Association* 21 (3): 325–27.

Mansfield, Becky. 2008. "Health as a Nature-Society Question." *Environment and Planning A* 40 (5): 1015–19.

Marcus, George. 1998. *Ethnography through Thick and Thin.* Princeton, NJ: Princeton University Press.

Marston, Sallie, J. P. Jones, and Keith Woodward. 2005. "Human Geography without Scale." *Transactions of the Institute of British Geographers* 30 (4): 416–32.

Martin, Emily. 1994. *Flexible Bodies: Immunity from the Days of Polio to the Age of AIDS.* Boston: Beacon Press.

Marx, Karl. 1976 [1867]. *Capital.* Vol. 1. New York: Penguin Books.

Matthews, Robert G. 2008. "Metals Meltdown Burns Scrap Dealers." *The Wall Street Journal* 10, sec. Business. http://online.wsj.com/article/SB122480823113965077 .html. Accessed November 4, 2008.

McKay, Ramah. 2012. "Documentary Disorders: Managing Medical Multiplicity in Maputo, Mozambique." *American Ethnologist* 39 (3): 545–61.

McNeill, John. 2010. *Mosquito Empires: Ecology and War in the Greater Caribbean, 1640–1914.* New York: Cambridge University Press.

Meade, Teresa. 1986. " 'Civilizing Rio de Janeiro': The Public Health Campaign and the Riot of 1904." *Journal of Social History* 20 (2): 301–22.

Medina, Martin. 2007. *The World's Scavengers: Salvaging for Sustainable Consumption and Production.* Lanham, MD: AltaMira.

Medina, Martin. 2008. "The Informal Recycling Sector in Developing Countries: Organizing Waste Pickers to Enhance Their Impact." *Gridlines: Sharing Knowledge, Experiences, and Innovation in Public-Private Partnerships in Infrastructure* 44: 1–4.

Mendez, Jennifer. 2005. *From the Revolution to the Maquiladoras: Gender, Labor, and Globalization in Nicaragua.* Durham, NC: Duke University Press.

Midgley, Claire, Martha Bajwa-Joseph, Sirijitt Vasanawathana, Bridget Wills, Aleksandra Flanagan, Emily Waiyaiya, Hac Bac Tran, Alison Cowper, Pojchong Chotiyarnwon, Jonathan Grimes, Sutee Yoksan, Prida Malasit, Cameron Simmons, Juthathip Mongkolsapaya, and Gavin Screaton. 2011. "An In-Depth

Analysis of Original Antigenic Sin in Dengue Virus Infection." *Journal of Virology* 85 (1): 410–21.

Milchman, Alan, and Alan Rosenberg. 2007. "The Aesthetic and Ascetic Dimensions of an Ethics of Self-Fashioning: Nietzsche and Foucault." *Parrhesia* 2: 44–65.

Mintz, Sidney. 1960. *Worker in the Cane: A Puerto Rican Life History*. New Haven, CT: Yale University Press.

Mitchell, Timothy. 2002. *Rule of Experts: Egypt, Techno-politics, Modernity*. Berkeley: University of California Press.

Mitman, Gregg, Michelle Murphy, and Christopher Sellers. 2004. "Introduction: A Cloud over History." *Osiris* 19: 1–17.

Miyazaki, Hirokazu. 2003. "The Temporalities of the Market." *American Anthropologist* 105 (2): 255–65.

Mol, Annemarie. 2002. *The Body Multiple: Ontology in Medical Practice*. Durham, NC: Duke University Press.

Montoya, Rosario. 2003. "House, Street, Collective. Revolutionary Geographies and Gender Transformation in Nicaragua, 1979–99." *Latin American Research Review* 38 (2): 61–93.

Moore, Henrietta. 1994. *A Passion for Difference: Essays in Anthropology and Gender*. Cambridge: Polity Press.

Moore, Sarah. 2008. "The Politics of Garbage in Oaxaca, Mexico." *Society and Natural Resources* 21 (7): 597–610.

Morris, Kenneth. 2010. *Unfinished Revolution: Daniel Ortega and Nicaragua's Struggle for Liberation*. Chicago: Chicago Review Press.

Munn, Nancy. 1992. "The Cultural Anthropology of Time: A Critical Essay." *Annual Review of Anthropology* 21: 93–123.

Murphy, Edward. 2004. "Developing Sustainable Peripheries: The Limits of Citizenship in Guatemala City." *Latin American Perspectives* 31 (6): 48–68.

Murphy, Michelle. 2006. *Sick Building Syndrome and the Problem of Uncertainty: Environmental Politics, Technoscience, and Women Workers*. Durham, NC: Duke University Press.

Murray, Douglas. 1994. *Cultivating Crisis: The Human Cost of Pesticides in Latin America*. Boulder, CO: Westview Press.

Nadasdy, Paul. 2003. *Hunters and Bureaucrats: Power, Knowledge, and Aboriginal-State Relations in the Southwest Yukon*. Vancouver: University of British Columbia Press.

Nadasdy, Paul. 2007. "The Gift in the Animal: The Ontology of Hunting and Human-Animal Sociality." *American Ethnologist* 34 (1): 25–43.

Nading, Alex. 2011. "Foundry Values: Artisanal Aluminum Recyclers, Economic Involution, and Skill in Periurban Managua." *Urban Anthropology* 40 (3–4): 319–60.

Nading, Alex. 2012. "'Dengue Mosquitoes Are Single Mothers': Biopolitics Meets Ecological Aesthetics in Nicaraguan Community Health Work." *Cultural Anthropology* 27 (4): 572–96.

Nading, Alex. 2013a. "Humans, Animals, and Health: From Ecology to Entanglement." *Environment and Society: Advances in Research* 4: 60–78.

Nading, Alex. 2013b. "'Love Isn't There in Your Stomach': A Moral Economy of Medical Citizenship among Nicaraguan Community Health Workers." *Medical Anthropology Quarterly* 27 (1): 84–102.

Napier, David. 2012. "Nonself Help: How Immunology Might Reframe the Enlightenment." *Cultural Anthropology* 27 (1): 122–37.

Nash, Linda. *Inescapable Ecologies: A History of Environment, Disease, and Knowledge.* Berkeley: University of California Press.

Neves, Katja. 2005. "Chasing Whales with Bateson and Daniel." *Australian Humanities Review* 35. www.australianhumanitiesreview.org/archive/Issue-June -2005/katja.html. Accessed December 14, 2013.

Neves, Katja. 2009. "Urban Botanical Gardens and the Aesthetics of Ecological Learning: A Theoretical Discussion and Preliminary Insights from Montreal's Botanical Garden." *Anthropologica* 51 (1): 145–57.

Nguyen, Vinh-Kim. 2010. *The Republic of Therapy: Triage and Sovereignty in West Africa's Time of AIDS.* Durham, NC: Duke University Press.

Nichter, Mark. 2008. *Global Health: Why Cultural Representations, Social Relations, and Biopolitics Matter.* Tucson: University of Arizona Press.

Normile, Dennis. 2013. "First New Dengue Virus Type in 50 Years." *AAAS Science Insider* [blog], October 21. http://news.sciencemag.org/health/2013/10/first-new -dengue-virus-type-50-years#disqus_thread.

O'Neill, Kate. 2010. "A Vital Fluid: Risk, Controversy, and the Politics of Blood Donation in the Era of 'Mad Cow Disease.'" *Public Understanding of Science* 12 (4): 359–80.

O'Neill, Kevin. 2010. *City of God: Christian Citizenship in Postwar Guatemala.* Berkeley: University of California Press.

Ogden, Laura. 2011. *Swamplife: People, Gators, and Mangroves Entangled in the Everglades.* Minneapolis: University of Minnesota Press.

Oliver-Smith, Anthony. 1996. "Anthropological Research on Hazards and Disasters." *Annual Review of Anthropology* 25: 303–28.

Packard, Randall. 1997. "Malaria Dreams: Postwar Visions of Health and Development." *Medical Anthropology* 17 (3): 279–96.

Packard, Randall. 2007. *The Making of a Tropical Disease: A Short History of Malaria.* Baltimore: Johns Hopkins University Press.

Paley, Julia. 2001. *Marketing Democracy: Power and Social Movements in Post-dictatorship Chile.* Berkeley: University of California Press.

Parks, Will, and Linda Lloyd. 2004. *Planning Social Mobilization for Dengue Fever Control and Prevention: A Step-by-Step Guide.* Geneva: World Health Organization.

Patz, Jonathan, Diarmid Campbell-Lindrum, Tracey Holloway, and Jonathan Foley. 2005. "Impact of Regional Climate Change on Human Health." *Nature* 438: 310–17.

Paxson, Heather. 2008. "Post-Pasteurian Cultures: The Microbiopolitics of Raw-Milk Cheese in the United States." *Cultural Anthropology* 23 (1): 15–47.

Perez, Denis, Pierre Lefevre, Lizet Sanchez, and Patrick Van der Stuyft. 2007. "Comment on: What Do Community-Based Dengue Control Programmes Achieve? A Systematic Review of Published Evaluations." *Transactions of the Royal Society of Tropical Medicine and Hygiene* 101 (6): 630–31.

Perez, Maria Angeles, Aubree Gordon, Felix Sanchez, Federico Narvaez, Gamaliel Gutierrez, Oscar Ortega, Andrea Nuñez, Eva Harris, and Angel Balmaseda. 2010. "Severe Coinfections of Dengue and Pandemic Influenza A H1N1 Viruses." *Pediatric Infectious Disease Journal* 29 (11): 1052–55.

Peterson, Alan, and Deborah Lupton. 1996. *The New Public Health: Health and Self in the Age of Risk.* London: Sage.

Petryna, Adriana. 2004. "Biological Citizenships: The Science and Politics of Chernobyl-Exposed Populations." *Osiris* 19: 250–65.

Pfol, Stephen. 2005. "New Global Technologies of Power: Cybernetic Capitalism and Social Inequality." In *The Blackwell Companion to Social Inequalities.* Mary Romero and Eric Margolis, eds. Pp. 546–92. Cambridge, MA: Blackwell.

Pichardo, Luvy. 1993. *Historia del OPEN III.* Managua: Alcaldía de Managua, Dirección General de Cultura y Turismo Municipal.

Pink, Sarah. 2008. "An Urban Tour: The Sensory Sociality of Ethnographic Place-Making." *Ethnography* 9 (2): 175–96.

Porter, Natalie. 2012. "Risky Zoographies: The Limits of Place in Avian Influenza Management." *Environmental Humanities* 1 (1): 103–21.

Porter, Natalie. 2013. "Bird Flu Biopower: Strategies for Multispecies Coexistence in Viet Nam." *American Ethnologist* 40 (1): 132–48.

Prevost, Gary, and Harry Vanden, eds. 1997. *The Undermining of the Sandinista Revolution.* New York: St. Martin's Press.

Purcell, Mark. 2002. "Excavating Lefebvre: The Right to the City and Its Urban Politics of the Inhabitant." *GeoJournal* 58 (2–3): 99–108.

Quesada, James. 1998. "Suffering Child: An Embodiment of War and Its Aftermath in Nicaragua." *Medical Anthropology Quarterly* 12 (1): 51–73.

Rabinow, Paul. 2002. *French DNA: Trouble in Purgatory.* Chicago: University of Chicago Press.

Rabinow, Paul, and Nikolas Rose. 2006. "Biopower Today." *Biosocieties* 1 (2): 195–217.

Raffles, Hugh. 2002. *In Amazonia: A Natural History.* Princeton, NJ: Princeton University Press.

Raffles, Hugh. 2010. *Insectopedia.* New York: Vintage.

Ramos, Mary, Fermin Arguello, Christine Luxemburger, Luz Quiñones, Jorge Muñoz, Mark Beatty, Jean Lang, and Kay Tomashek. 2008. "Epidemiological and Clinical Observations on Patients with Dengue in Puerto Rico: Results from the First Year of Enhanced Surveillance—June 2005–May 2006." *American Journal of Tropical Medicine and Hygiene* 79 (1): 123–27.

Rappaport, Roy. 1984 [1968]. *Pigs for the Ancestors: Ritual in the Ecology of a New Guinea People*. New Haven, CT: Yale University Press.

Redfield, Peter. 2013. *Life in Crisis: The Ethical Journey of Doctors without Borders*. Berkeley: University of California Press.

Reichman, Daniel. 2011. *The Broken Village: Coffee, Migration, and Globalization in Honduras*. Ithaca, NY: Cornell University Press.

Reiter, Paul and Greg Murphy. 2007. "Interview: Paul Reiter, Ph.D. Global Warming Won't Spread Malaria." *EIR Science and Environment*. April 6: 52–56.

Remmer, Karen. 1991. "The Political Impact of Economic Crisis in the 1980s." *American Political Science Review* 85 (3): 777–800.

Rifkin, Susan. 1996. "Paradigms Lost: Toward a New Understanding of Participation in Public Health Programmes." *Acta Tropica* 61 (2): 79–92.

Rigau-Perez, Jose. 1998. "The Early Use of Breakbone Fever (*Quebranta Huesos, 1771*) and *Dengue* (1801) in Spanish." *American Journal of Tropical Medicine and Hygiene* 59 (2): 272–74.

Robbins, Paul. 2000. "The Practical Politics of Knowing: State Environmental Knowledge and Local Political Economy." *Economic Geography* 76 (2): 126–44.

Robbins, Paul. 2007. *Lawn People: How Grasses, Weeds, and Chemicals Make Us Who We Are*. Philadelphia: Temple University Press.

Robbins, Paul. 2012. *Political Ecology: A Critical Introduction*. 2nd ed. New York: Blackwell.

Roberts, Elizabeth. 2012. *God's Laboratory: Assisted Reproduction in the Andes*. Berkeley: University of California Press.

Rocheleau, Diane, Barbara Thomas-Slayter, and Esther Wangari, eds. 1996. *Feminist Political Ecology: Global Issues and Local Experiences*. New York: Routledge.

Rodgers, Dennis. 2004. "'Disembedding' the City: Crime, Insecurity, and Spatial Organization in Managua, Nicaragua." *Environment and Urbanization* 16 (2): 113–24.

Rodgers, Dennis. 2008. "A Symptom Called Managua." *New Left Review* 49: 103–20.

Rose, Carol. 1986. "The Comedy of the Commons: Custom, Commerce, and Inherently Public Property." *University of Chicago Law Review* 53 (3): 711–81.

Rose, Nikolas. 2007. *The Politics of Life Itself: Biomedicine, Power, and Subjectivity in the Twenty-First Century*. Princeton, NJ: Princeton University Press.

Rose, Nikolas, and Carlos Novas. 2005. "Biological Citizenship." In *Global Assemblages*. Aihwa Ong and Stephen Collier, eds. Pp. 439–63. New York: Blackwell.

Rush, Benjamin. 1789. *Medical Inquiries and Observations*. Vol. 1. Philadelphia: Pritchard and Hall.

Said, Edward. 1979. *Orientalism*. New York: Vintage.

Sanchez, Lizet, Veerle Vanlerberghe, Lázara Alfonso, Maria del Carmen Marquetti, Maria Guzman, Juan Bisset, and Patrick van der Stuyft. 2006. "Aedes Aegypti Larval Indices and Risk for Dengue Epidemics." *Emerging Infectious Diseases* 12 (5): 800–806.

Sawyer, Suzana, and Arun Agrawal. 2000. "Environmental Orientalisms." *Cultural Critique* 45: 71–108.

Scheper-Hughes, Nancy. 1992. *Death without Weeping: The Violence of Everyday Life in Brazil*. Berkeley: University of California Press.

Scheper-Hughes, Nancy, and Margaret Lock. 1987. "The Mindful Body: A Prolegomenon to Future Work in Medical Anthropology." *Medical Anthropology Quarterly* 1 (1): 6–41.

Schlager, Edella, and Elinor Ostrom. 1992. "Property-rights Regimes and Natural Resources: A Conceptual Analysis." *Land Economics* 68 (3): 249–62.

Schleissmann, Donald. 1967. "Initiation of the *Aedes aegypti* Eradication Programme of the United States." *Bulletin of the World Health Organization* 36 (4): 604–9.

Scott, James. 1976. *The Moral Economy of the Peasant: Rebellion and Subsistence in Southeast Asia*. New Haven, CT: Yale University Press.

Seabrook, John. 2008. "American Scrap: An Old-School Industry Globalizes." *New Yorker*. January 14: 46–59.

Sen, Amartya. 1990. "Gender and Co-operative Conflicts." In *Persistent Inequalities: Women and World Development*. Irene Tinker, ed. Pp. 123–49. New York: Oxford University Press.

Serres, Michel. 2007 [1982]. *The Parasite*. Lawrence R. Schehr, trans. Minneapolis: University of Minnesota Press.

Shaw, Ian, Paul Robbins, and John Paul Jones. 2010. "A Bug's Life: Spatial Ontologies of Mosquito Management." *Annals of the Association of American Geographers* 100 (2): 373–92.

Shillington, Laura. 2008. "Being(s) in Relation at Home: Socio-natures of Patio 'Gardens' in Managua, Nicaragua." *Social and Cultural Geography* 9 (7): 755–76.

Shillington, Laura. 2013. "Right to Food, Right to the City: Household Urban Agriculture, and Socionatural Metabolism in Managua, Nicaragua." *Geoforum* 44 (1): 103–11.

Shukin, Nicole. 2009. *Animal Capital: Rendering Life in Biopolitical Times*. Minneapolis: University of Minnesota Press.

Singer, Merrill. 2009. *Introduction to Syndemics: A Critical Systems Approach to Public and Community Health*. San Francisco, CA: Jossey-Bass.

Slosek, Jean. 1986. "*Aedes Aegypti* in the Americas: A Review of Their Interaction with the Human Population." *Social Science and Medicine* 23 (3): 249–57.

Standish, Katherine, Guillermina Kuan, William Avilés, Angel Balmaseda, and Eva Harris. 2010. "High Dengue Case Capture Rate in Four Years of a Cohort Study in Nicaragua Compared to National Surveillance Data." *PLoS Neglected Tropical Diseases* 4 (3): e633.

Stapleton, Darwin. 2004. "Lessons of History? Anti-malaria Strategies of the International Health Board and the Rockefeller Foundation from the 1920s to the Era of DDT." *Public Health Reports* 119 (2): 206–15.

Star, Susan Leigh. 1991. "Power, Technology, and the Phenomenology of Conventions: On Being Allergic to Onions." In *A Sociology of Monsters: Essays on Power, Technology, and Domination*. John Law, ed. Pp. 26–56. New York: Routledge.

Strathern, Marilyn. 1992. *Reproducing the Future: Anthropology, Kinship, and the New Reproductive Technologies.* Manchester, UK: Manchester University Press.

Suarez, Roberto, Maria Fernanda Olarte, M. F. A. Ana, and U. Catalina Gonzalez. 2005. "Is What I Have Just a Cold or Is It Dengue? Addressing the Gap between the Politics of Dengue Control and Daily Life in Villavicencio-Colombia." *Social Science and Medicine* 61 (2): 495–502.

Sutter, Paul. 2007. "Nature's Agents or Agents of Empire? Entomological Workers and Environmental Change during the Construction of the Panama Canal." *Isis* 98 (4): 724–54.

Swyngedouw, Erik. 2004. *Social Power and the Urbanization of Water: Flows of Power.* Oxford: Oxford University Press.

Taubes, Gary. 1997. "Resurgent Mosquitoes: Dengue in Cuba." *Science* 277 (5323): 174.

Taussig, Michael. 1980. "Reification and the Consciousness of the Patient." *Social Science and Medicine* 14: 3–13.

Tesler, Laura. 2006. " 'Now There Is No Treatment for Anyone': Health Care Seeking in Neoliberal Nicaragua." Ph.D. dissertation, Department of Anthropology, University of Arizona.

Thompson, E. P. 1971. "The Moral Economy of the English Crowd in the Eighteenth Century." *Past and Present* 50: 76–136.

Tobias, Saul. 2005. "Foucault on Freedom and Capabilities." *Theory Culture and Society* 22 (4): 65–85.

Toledo-Romani, Maria, Veerle Vanlerberghe, Dennis Perez, Pierre Lefevre, Enrique Ceballos, Digna Bandera, Alberto Baly Gil, and Patrick van der Stuyft. 2007. "Achieving Sustainability of Community-Based Dengue Control in Santiago de Cuba." *Social Science and Medicine* 64 (4): 976–88.

Tsing, Anna. 2005. *Friction: An Ethnography of Global Connection.* Princeton, NJ: Princeton University Press.

Tsing, Anna. 2012. "Unruly Edges: Mushrooms as Companion Species" *Environmental Humanities* 1 (1): 141–54.

Turner, Victor. 1966. *The Ritual Process: Structure and Anti-structure.* Chicago: Aldine.

Turner, Victor, and Edward Bruner, eds. 1986. *The Anthropology of Experience.* Champaign: University of Illinois Press.

USDHEW (U.S. Department of Health, Education, and Welfare). 1965a. Ae. aegypti *Handbook Series: Source Reduction Reference Handbook.* Atlanta, GA: U.S. Department of Health, Education and Welfare, Public Health Service, Division of Disease Prevention and Environmental Control, National Communicable Disease Center, *Aedes aegypti* Eradication Program.

USDHEW (U.S. Department of Health, Education, and Welfare). 1965b. *CDC* Aedes aegypti *Handbook.* Series no 1. Atlanta, GA: U.S. Department of Health, Education and Welfare, Public Health Service, Division of Disease Prevention and Environmental Control, National Communicable Disease Center, *Aedes aegypti* Eradication Program.

Walker, Thomas, ed. 1991. *Revolution and Counterrevolution in Nicaragua.* Boulder, CO: Westview.

Walker, Thomas, ed. 1997. *Nicaragua without Illusions: Regime Transition and Structural Adjustment in the 1990s.* Wilmington, DE: Scholarly Resources.

Weir, Lorna, and Eric Mykhalovskiy. 2010. *Global Public Health Vigilance: Creating a World on Alert.* New York: Routledge.

Wendland, Claire. 2010. *A Heart for the Work: Journeys through an African Medical School.* Chicago: University of Chicago Press.

Wendland, Claire. 2012. "Moral Maps and Medical Imaginaries: Clinical Tourism at Malawi's College of Medicine." *American Anthropologist* 114 (1): 108–22.

Werner, David. 1992. "Foreword." In *Health Care in Nicaragua: Primary Care under Changing Regimes.* Richard Garfield and Gary Williams, eds. Pp. v–xi. New York: Oxford University Press.

West, Paige. 2006. *Conservation Is Our Government Now: The Politics of Ecology in Papua New Guinea.* Durham, NC: Duke University Press.

Whiteford, Linda. 1997. "The Ethnoecology of Dengue Fever." *Medical Anthropology Quarterly* 11 (2): 202–23.

Whiteford, Linda. 2000. "Local Identity, Globalization and Health in Cuba and the Dominican Republic." In *Global Health Policy, Local Realities: The Fallacy of the Level Playing Field.* Linda Whiteford and Lenore Manderson, eds. Pp. 57–78. Boulder, CO: Lynne Reinner.

Whiteford, Linda, and Lenore Manderson, eds. 2000. *Global Health Policy, Local Realities: The Fallacy of the Level Playing Field.* Boulder, CO: Lynne Reinner.

Wickham-Crowley, Timothy. 1992. *Guerillas and Revolution in Latin America: A Comparative Study of Insurgents and Regimes since 1956.* Princeton, NJ: Princeton University Press.

Wilcox, Bruce, and Rita Colwell. 2005. "Emerging and Reemerging Infectious Diseases: Biocomplexity as an Interdisciplinary Paradigm." *EcoHealth* 2 (4): 244–57.

Williams, Raymond. 1977. *Marxism and Literature.* Oxford: Oxford University Press.

Wilson, Bradley. 2010. "Indebted to Fair Trade: Coffee and Crisis in Nicaragua." *Geoforum* 41 (1): 84–92.

WHO (World Health Organization). 2009. *Dengue: Guidelines for Diagnosis, Treatment, Prevention, and Control.* Geneva: WHO.

WHO (World Health Organization). 2012. *Communication for Behavioral Impact (COMBI): A Toolkit for Behavioral and Social Communication in Outbreak Response.* Geneva: WHO.

Zeiderman, Austin. 2012. "On Shaky Ground: The Making of Risk in Bogotá." *Environment and Planning A* 44 (7): 1570–88.

Zhan, Mei. 2005. "Civet Cats, Fried Grasshoppers, and David Beckham's Pajamas: Unruly Bodies after SARS." *American Anthropologist* 107 (1): 31–42.

Zompi, Simona, and Eva Harris. 2013. "Original Antigenic Sin in Dengue Revisited." *Proceedings of the National Academy of Sciences of the USA* 110 (22): 8761–62.

Zompi, Simona, Magelda Montoya, Marie Pohl, Angel Balmaseda, and Eva Harris. 2012. "Dominant Cross-Reactive B Cell Response during Secondary Acute Dengue Virus Infection in Humans." *PLOS Neglected Tropical Diseases* 6 (3): e1568.

INDEX

Bolaños, Enrique, 51, 58
Brazil, 229n25, 230n30
brigadistas: compensation, 111, 150, 167, 182,
    206, 219n52; demographics of, 8, 15, 43,
    151; ecological aesthetic, 15–16, 118–19,
    132; enjoyment of job, 115–16, 118, 127;
    equipment, 119, 120*fig;* as evangelical
    ecologists, 94, 95–96, 99, 113; grassroots
    activism, 43, 44, 45–46; killing of
    mosquitoes, 132, 138; perspectives on
    individualism, 55–58; post-revolution
    roles, 51, 219nn52,54; relationship to
    MINSA, 43–44, 51, 146, 219n54; sense
    of place, 91; SEPA visits, 149–54, 153*fig,*
    157; tensions embodied by, 146, 147–48,
    153, 154, 206, 234n11; understanding of
    entanglement, 116–17, 132–33, 140;
    women as, 15, 135–36, 138. *See also*
    house-to-house mosquito inspections
Briggs, Charles, 65, 161, 221n5
Brotherton, Sean, 161

Cabo Gracias a Dios, 30
Cachorros, Los, 42–49
Calles Para el Pueblo (Streets for the
    People), 33
Camino Verde, 150
Candea, Matei, 233n93
carretoneros (private, informal collectors),
    226n29
Carter, Eric, 122, 212n16, 229n26
casa bases, 170
casas de seguridad, 41
Casey, Edward, 19
catastrophes: making meaning from,
    178–79; in Nicaragua, 29–32, 39–40,
    41, 49
cauces (sewer ditches), 38, 59
CDC (Centers for Disease Control and
    Prevention), 123–25, 124*fig,* 229n28
CDS (Committees for the Defense of
    Sandinismo), 47, 50, 195, 218n39
Cecilia, 135–36
celestes, 115
Centers for Disease Control and Preven-
    tion (CDC), 123–25, 124*fig,* 229n28
Central American Free Trade Agreement,
    58

Chamorro, Violeta Barrios de, 47, 51
chatarra (recyclable materials), 62, 67, 75
chatarreros (buyer of recyclables): business
    practices, 71; daily tasks, 62–64, 63*fig;*
    multiple identities of, 76, 84; ownership
    questions, 69–70; patron–client
    relations, 69; Plan Chatarra and, 75–78,
    82, 83–84
children, in dengue prevention campaigns,
    140, 151
chora, 227n40
Christianity, evangelical, 92–94, 99, 112,
    219n52
churequeros. See scavengers
CIET (Community Information and
    Epidemiological Technologies
    International), 149–50
"Citizen Power," 51, 219n54
Ciudad Sandino: catastrophes, 29–32, 49;
    cauces, 38–40; cotton industry, 34–37,
    59; dengue as unifying factor in, 14;
    electricity, 49–50; exclusionary spaces,
    100, 100*f,* 226n28; garbage collection
    and recycling, 61–62, 62*fig,* 63*fig,*
    226n29; geographical complexity, 16–17;
    history, 13–14; as independent munici-
    pality, 53; infrastructure construction,
    31, 39, 40, 216n7; map, xvii*map;* naming
    of, 42, 91, 93; OPEN settlements, 30,
    37–39, 41, 42; political uprising, 41–42;
    post-hurricane reconstruction, 53–54,
    144; public health approaches, 31, 32,
    42–49, 51–58, 60; religious demograph-
    ics, 219n52; residential landscape, 1–2,
    103, 209n1; slum characteristics, 216n7;
    Somoza stones, 32–34; water supplies,
    38–39; *zonas francas,* 58–60. *See also*
    dump conflict
Clarke, Maura, 2
clients: in *chatarra* business, 68, 69, 75, 78,
    80, 84; in distribution of wealth and
    power, 68; patron–client relations, 68,
    85, 222n17, 224n28
climate change, 64, 65, 179, 221n3
CNDR (National Diagnostic and
    Reference Center [Nicaragua]), 176, 192
coinfections, 175–76, 185–86, 238n39
collective citizenship, 38, 55–58, 59–60

collective property, 223n18
colonialism, 228nn19,22
Columbus, Christopher, 30
COMBI (Communication for Behavioral Impact), 154–57, 158, 159
common property resources, 223n18, 223n20
Communicable Disease Center (CDC), 123–25, 124*fig*, 229n28
community, as entanglement, 25–26, 211n14
Community Information and Epidemiological Technologies International (CIET), 149–50
consumerism, 69
contact zone, 137
contra insurgency, 21, 47
cotton industry, 34–37, 59
CPC (Councils of Citizen Power), 143–44, 146, 153, 165–66
critical medical anthropology, 10, 13, 100, 202
Cronon, William, 209n1
Cruz, Oswaldo, 122, 229n25
Cuba, 159–60, 235n31
Cuesta del Plomo (Lead Ridge), 41–42
cultura, 52–53, 209n3

data collection, *vs.* narratives, 159–62
date-events, 237n29
DDT: banning of, 128, 231n43; in eradication efforts, 46, 122–23, 128, 229n28, 230n31
declarations, emergency, 190, 193–94
dengue: antigenic sin fable, 95–96; Ciudad Sandino united by, 14; climate change and, 221n3; diagnostic difficulties, 170–71, 174, 176; ecology of, 202–4; exposure rates, 5; factors influencing spread of, 46, 130–32; H1N1 coinfection, 175–76, 185–86, 237n29, 238n39; history of, 130–31, 232n58; during Ortega's second presidency, 46, 51–52, 217n36; pediatric cohort study, 148–49; political entanglements, 146–48, 159; rates of infection, 8, 12; reemergence of, 128, 138, 231n42; seasonal epidemics, 16, 173, 177–80, 185; second infections, 7, 11–12, 94–95, 174, 212n21; as set of

attachments, 10–11, 26, 112–14, 180, 211n12; similarities to H1N1, 185–86; symptoms, 1, 4, 7–8; temporal entanglements, 11–12, 171–76, 177–80; term etymology, 209n4; tracking difficulties, 12; transmission of, 130, 231n53; viral serotypes, 7, 94–95, 131
dengue hemorrhagic fever (DHF), 7, 132, 174, 210n7
dengue prevention campaigns: biopolitics of, 212n17; under CDS (Committees for the Defense of Sandinismo), 46–47, 129; challenges, 144–45, 152; under Chamorro government, 47–49; connection to hygiene and sanitation, 121–22; control *vs.* eradication, 118–19, 160, 167; historical background, 121–22, 229n28, 230n33; local adjustments to, 9, 97, 160, 161; during Ortega's second presidency, 46, 51–52, 57, 58*fig,* 146, 217n36; participatory, 129–30, 140, 145–47, 168, 218n46, 231n49; Rockefeller programs, 48, 122, 218n48, 230nn30,31; social development agendas and, 122, 229n28; under Somoza regime, 46, 123; women's roles in, 9, 15, 135, 138. *See also under* MINSA
DengueWatch, 191–92, 194
denuncias, 163–64, 186–88, 192, 196, 198
detachment, 233n93
DHF (dengue hemorrhagic fever), 7, 132, 174, 210n7
Dionisio, *chatarrero,* 69
diseases, emergent, 22, 215n47
diseases, emerging infectious, 198, 204–5
diseases, "global," 204
doctor/doctora usage, 238n34
Domingos Rojinegros, 46–47, 129
Donahue, John, 44
don/doña usage, 238n34
Dora, *brigadista,* 55–57
dump conflict, 67–68, 70, 71–73, 77, 78

earthquake, Managua (1972), 30, 41
ecological aesthetics, 15–16, 118–19, 132, 139–40
effective geography, 179–80

egomorphism, 135

Egypt, 197

electricity, 49–50

emergencies: *brigadistas'* livelihoods as, 182; declaration of, 183–84, 188–92, 193–96; politics of, 178, 192–93, 194–96, 238n41, 239n44; seasonality of, 177–80, 185; technical *vs.* emotional aspects, 196, 239n45

emergent diseases, 22, 215n47

emerging infectious diseases (EIDs), 198, 204–5

endemic channels, 189–91, 190*fig*, 194, 198

enhanced surveillance, 149–51

entanglements: of bodies, 15–16, 91–92, 213n30; bodies and environment, 10, 64, 118; *brigadistas'* understanding of, 116–17, 132–33, 140; community interaction as, 25–26, 211n14; defined, 11, 202; disease-related, 13, 197, 202, 204–5, 212n26; as enacted condition, 203; as framework for understanding dengue, 10–11; of houses, 98, 226n30; human–nonhuman, 11, 132, 197, 206–7; knowledge as factor in, 16; *oikos/polis* dichotomy and, 226n37; patterns of attachment and, 112–14; in play, 137, 140; politics and, 13, 15, 98, 146–48, 159, 213n30; routines of, 226n30; sanitation-related, 69; scientific and political practices, 159–62; seasonal, 177–80; temporal dimension of, 11–12. *See also* temporal incongruities

environment: caring for, 118–19; connection to bodies, 10, 64, 118; individual responsibility for, 48, 64–65, 78, 162, 218n46

environmental sanitation approach, 122, 229n26

epidemic threshold, 189

EPTISA, 54

Esteban, 170–71, 172, 173–74, 187

Eugenia, MINSA psychologist, 22, 23, 195–96

European Union (EU), 53–54

evangelical Christianity, 92–94, 99, 112, 219n52

evangelical ecology, 95–96, 99, 113

"fallacy of the level playing field," 235n35

Farmer, Paul, 22, 224n27

Fassin, Didier, 147, 237n31

Fatima, dengue patient, 1–5, 7–8, 17, 20

Feliciana, MINSA nurse, 3–4, 5, 20, 38, 41

Felipe, Ciudad Sandino resident, 49–50

Fenosa, 49–50

Ferguson, Harry, 108

Fillermina, *brigadista,* 115

floods, Managua (1970), 29–30

Flor, scavenger, 62–64

focos (breeding spots): finding and documenting, 84, 101, 115, 117–18, 126–27; perceptions about, 158; streets as, 6

Foucault, Michel, 139, 213n30, 227n5, 232n59

Francisco, *celeste,* 119, 123, 126, 128, 138

Freire, Paolo, 44

FSLN (Sandinista National Liberation Front): base communities, 43, 44; branches of government, 51, 219n54; CDS (Committees for the Defense of Sandinismo), 47, 50, 195, 218n39; effect of contra insurgency on, 47; infrastructure campaigns, 32–33, 144; movements contributing to, 216n12; during Ortega's second presidency, 51–52, 144, 146; overthrow of Somoza dynasty, 21; social innovations, 44

garbage. *See* waste

garbage, ownership of, 69–70, 222n12, 223n18

garbage collectors: *carretoneros,* 226n29; daily tasks, 61–62, 62*fig*; in dump conflicts, 67–68, 70, 71–72, 73–74, 77, 78. *See also* scavengers

Geertz, Clifford, 98–99, 205

gender issues: cultivation of bodies and, 103; dengue exposure narratives, 91; evangelical ecology, 96, 99, 113; local biologies, 210n11; metaphors for mosquitoes and dengue, 113, 134–35; mosquito control efforts, 138; in post-revolutionary Nicaragua, 137, 211n12. *See also* women

Génesis, *brigadista,* 127

private property, 223n18

private/public life dichotomy, 33, 78–79, 101, 113, 114, 226n37

PROMAPER (Integrated Project for Peripheral Managua), 43–44

property types, 222n12, 223n18

public health: Alma Ata approach, 44–45; Chamorro government approach, 47–48; community engagement with, 6, 9; individual responsibility for, 7, 65, 145, 162–63; as moral and ethical responsibility, 98; vs. openness, 9; Ortega government approach, 51, 186–87, 192; seasonal entanglements affecting, 179–80; temporal models of, 199; as underresourced, 171; women's roles in, 137

public/private life dichotomy, 33, 78–79, 101, 113, 114, 226n37

Raffles, Hugh, 161, 179–80, 212n17, 227n2, 235n39

Ramos, Miguel, 40

Reagan, Ronald, 21

recolectores. See garbage collectors

recyclables, ownership of, 69–70, 222n12, 223n18

recycling industry: effect of financial crisis on, 81–82; market growth, 67–68, 70, 78, 222n12. See also chatarreros

Reed, Walter, 121

refrains (routines of entanglement), 226n30

Reiter, Paul, 221n3

religion: evangelical Christianity, 92–94, 99, 112, 219n52; liberation theology, 24, 215n49, 219n52; Roman Catholicism, 92

research methods, 17–20

revolutionary praxis, 154

rhizomes, as trope, 212n23

Rigau-Perez, Jose, 209n4

Robbins, Paul, 12, 112, 194

Rockefeller Colony, 130

Rockefeller Foundation, 48, 122, 218n48, 230nn30,31

Roman Catholic Church, 92

Rose, Nikolas, 225n14

Ross, Ronald, 121

Rush, Benjamin, 209n4

Sanchez, Morena: attitude toward cristianos, 94; brigadista work, 20, 89, 126, 135–36; household space, 97; leadership among brigadistas, 181–82

Sandinista movement, 24, 33, 41, 215n49. See also FSLN

Sandinistas, vs. Ortegistas, 167

Sandino, Augusto César, 36

sanitary citizenship, 65, 221n5

sanitation, 66–67, 69, 121–22

scavengers: barriers to housekeeping, 106–7; business practices, 70–71; as citizens, 74–75; client–patron relationships, 68, 78, 84–85; as community of resource users, 223n18; daily tasks, 62, 63fig; economic contribution of, 222n12; effect of Plan Chatarra on, 75–76, 82, 83–84; labor organization, 71–72, 74, 223n24; as perceived harborers of disease, 3–4, 84; protests by, 67–68, 71–72, 77, 78, 222n15; as stewards of environmental health, 6, 222n12, 223n24; as supporters of family members, 5, 70, 222n12

Schilz, Ulrich, 73–74

science, politics and, 206

self-fashioning, aesthetics of, 139

Sellers, Christopher, 201

SEPA (Socializing Evidence for Participatory Action): emphasis on data, 153–54, 156, 159; house visits, 151–53; program expansion, 150, 234n22; relationship to CPCs, 153; relationship to MINSA, 153–54; strategy, 149–52, 154, 155, 157

Serres, Michel, 224n28

Shaw, Ian, 112

Shillington, Laura, 209n1

SILAIS (Integrated Health Attention System), 47, 48–49, 218n43

Singer, Merrill, 237n31

sin metaphors, 95–96, 112, 113

socialism, 44, 47, 77, 112. See also FSLN

social norms, 108–9, 113

social relationships: as healthy entanglement, 25–26, 211n14; in house-to-house mosquito inspections, 120, 125–26, 128, 138, 153; objective facts as, 174